ENDOMETRIOSIS

Endometriosis

Current Understanding and Management

EDITED BY

ROBERT W. SHAW

MD, FRCOG, FRCS(Ed.), MFFP
Department of Obstetrics and Gynaecology
University of Wales College of Medicine
Heath Park, Cardiff, UK

Blackwell
Science

Editorial Offices:
Osney Mead, Oxford OX2 0EL
25 John Street, London WC1N 2BL
23 Ainslie Place, Edinburgh EH3 6AJ
238 Main Street, Cambridge
Massachusetts 02142, USA
54 University Street, Carlton
Victoria 3053, Australia

Other Editorial Offices:
Arnette Blackwell SA
1, rue de Lille, 75007 Paris
France

Blackwell Wissenschafts-Verlag GmbH
Kurfürstendamm 57
10707 Berlin, Germany

Zehetnergasse 6, A-1140 Wien
Austria

First published 1995
Reprinted 1996

Set by DP Photosetting, Aylesbury, Bucks
Printed and bound in Great Britain
by Bell & Bain Ltd, Glasgow

DISTRIBUTORS

Marston Book Services Ltd
PO Box 87
Oxford OX2 0DT
(*Orders:* Tel: 01865 791155
Fax: 01865 791927
Telex: 837515)

North America
Blackwell Science, Inc.
238 Main Street
Cambridge, MA 02142
(*Orders:* Tel: 800 215-1000
617 876-7000
Fax: 617 492-5263)

Australia
Blackwell Science Pty Ltd
54 University Street
Carlton, Victoria 3053
(*Orders:* Tel: 03 9347 0300
Fax: 03 9349 3016)

A catalogue record for this title
is available from the British Library

ISBN 0–86542–821–2

Library of Congress
Cataloging-in-Publication Data

Endometriosis: current understanding
and management/edited by
Robert W. Shaw.
p. cm.
ISBN 0–86542–821–2
1. Endometriosis. I. Shaw,
Robert W. (Robert Wayne)
[DNLM: 1. Endometriosis—
physiopathology.
2. Endometriosis—therapy.
WP 390 E565 1994]
RG483.E53E555 1994
618.1—dc20 94-36488
CIP

Contents

List of Contributors, vii

Preface, xi

Part 1: Cellular Pathophysiology

1 Pathogenesis and Aetiology: Questions, Questions, Questions, 3
J.L.H. Evers

2 Morphology, Ultrastructure and Receptors in Untreated and Treated Endometriotic Implants, 16
H. Ochs and K.-W. Schweppe

3 Morphology of the Implant: Two- and Three-dimensional Evaluation, 38
J. Donnez, M. Nisolle and F. Casanas-Roux

4 Peritoneal Environment in Endometriosis, 47
G.A.J. Dunselman

5 Immune System, 75
D.H. Barlow and S. Fernández-Shaw

Part 2: Clinical Features

6 Ovarian Endometriosis, 97
I.A. Brosens

7 Pelvic Pain and Endometriosis, 112
C.M. MacLaverty and R.W. Shaw

8 Infertility and Endometriosis, 147
S. Ingamells and E.J. Thomas

9 Classification of Endometriosis, 168
M.J. Canis, F.H. Loh, A. Wattiez, J.L. Pouly, E. Glowaczover and J. Raiga

Part 3: Medical Treatments

10 Medical and Endocrine Modulatory Treatments, 187
P.C. Lindsay

11 Evaluation of Treatment with Gonadotrophin-releasing Hormone Analogues, 206
R.W. Shaw

Part 4: Surgical Treatments

12 Conservative Laparoscopic Treatment of Ovarian Endometriosis, 237
M. Nisolle and J. Donnez

13 Techniques for Ablation and Excision of Endometriosis, 248
M.J. Canis, S. Boughizane, F.H. Loh, J.L. Pouly, A. Wattiez, H. Manhes, G. Mage and M.-A. Bruhat

14 Surgical Treatment of Deeply Infiltrating Endometriosis, 264
P.R. Koninckx and D. Martin

15 Role of Assisted Reproduction in Endometriosis, 282
N.N. Amso

Index, 297

List of Contributors

NAZAR N. AMSO MB, ChB, MRCOG, *Consultant Obstetrician and Gynaecologist, Department of Obstetrics and Gynaecology, Queen Elizabeth Hospital, Gateshead, Tyne and Wear, NE9 6SX, UK*

DAVID H. BARLOW MA, BSc, MD, FRCOG, *Nuffield Professor of Obstetrics and Gynaecology, University of Oxford, Women's Centre, The John Radcliffe Hospital, Headington, Oxford, OX3 9DU, UK*

S. BOUGHIZANE MD, *Service de Gynécologie Obstétrique Reproduction Humaine, Polyclinique de l'Hôtel Dieu, Université Clermont-Ferrand I, 13 Boulevard Charles-De-Gaulle, F-63000 Clermont-Ferrand Cedex 1, France*

IVO A. BROSENS MD, PhD, *Professor of Obstetrics & Gynaecology, University Hospital Gasthuisberg, Herestraat 49, B-3000 Leuven, Belgium*

MAURICE-ANTOINE BRUHAT MD, *Professor and Head of Department of Gynecology, Polyclinique de l'Hôtel Dieu, Université Clermont-Ferrand I, 13 Boulevard Charles-De-Gaulle, F-63000 Clermont-Ferrand Cedex 1, France*

MICHAEL J. CANIS MD, *Service de Gynécologie Obstétrique Reproduction Humaine, Polyclinique de l'Hôtel Dieu, Université Clermont-Ferrand I, 13 Boulevard Charles-De-Gaulle, F-63000 Clermont-Ferrand Cedex I, France*

FRANÇOISE CASANAS-ROUX *Infertility Research Unit, Department of Gynecology, Catholic University of Louvain, Cliniques Universitaires Saint-Luc, Avenue Hippocrate 10, B-1200 Bruxelles, Belgium*

JACQUES DONNEZ MD, PhD, *Chairman and Head, Department of Gynecology, Catholic University of Louvain, Cliniques Universitaires Saint-Luc, Avenue Hippocrate 10, B-1200 Bruxelles, Belgium*

GERARD A.J. DUNSELMAN MD, *Associate Professor, Department of Obstetrics & Gynaecology, Academic Hospital Maastricht, PO Box 5800, NL 6202 AZ Maastricht, The Netherlands*

JOHANNES L.H. EVERS MD, *Professor of Obstetrics and Gynaecology, Department of Obstetrics & Gynaecology, Academic Hospital Maastricht, PO Box 5800, NL 6202 AZ Maastricht, The Netherlands*

SYLVIA FERNÁNDEZ-SHAW MD, DPhil, *Clinical Research Fellow, Nuffield Department of Obstetrics and Gynaecology, University of Oxford, The John Radcliffe Hospital, Headington, Oxford, OX3 9DU, UK*

ERIC GLOWACZOVER MD, *Service de Gynécologie Obstétrique Reproduction Humaine, Polyclinique de l'Hôtel Dieu, Université Clermont-Ferrand I, 13 Boulevard Charles-De-Gaulle, F-63000 Clermont-Ferrand Cedex I, France*

SUSAN INGAMELLS BM, PhD, *Wellcome Trust Research Fellow, University of Southampton, Princess Anne Hospital, Coxford Road, Southampton, SO9 4HA, UK*

PHILIPPE R. KONINCKX MD, PhD, *Professor, Department of Obstetrics and Gynecology, and Head, Division of Endoscopic Surgery, University Hospital Gasthuisberg, Catholic University Leuven, Herestraat 49, B-3000 Leuven, Belgium*

PETER C. LINDSAY MA, MRCOG, *Lecturer and Senior Registrar, Department of Obstetrics and Gynaecology, Llandough Hospital, Penlan Road, Llandough, Penarth, South Glamorgan, CF64 2XX, UK*

F.H. LOH MB, BS, MRCOG, MMed (Obst. & Gynae.), *Lecturer, Department of Obstetrics and Gynaecology, National University Hospital, National University of Singapore, Lower Kent Ridge Road, Singapore 0511*

CAOILIN M. MACLAVERTY MB, ChB, *Clinical Research Fellow, Department of Obstetrics and Gynaecology, University of Wales College of Medicine, Heath Park, Cardiff, CF4 4XN, UK*

H. MANHES MD, *Service de Gynécologie Obstétrique Reproduction Humaine, Polyclinique de l'Hôtel Dieu, Université Clermont-Ferrand I, 13 Boulevard Charles-De-Gaulle, F-63000 Clermont-Ferrand Cedex 1, France*

GÉRARD MAGE MD, *Service de Gynécologie Obstétrique Reproduction Humaine, Polyclinique de l'Hôtel Dieu, Université Clermont-Ferrand I, 13 Boulevard Charles-De-Gaulle, F-63000 Clermont-Ferrand Cedex 1, France*

D. MARTIN *Baptist Memorial Hospital, University of Tennessee, Memphis, Tennessee, USA*

MICHELLE NISOLLE *Infertility Research Unit, Department of Gynecology, Catholic University of Louvain, Cliniques Universitaires Saint-Luc, Avenue Hippocrate 10, B-1200 Bruxelles, Belgium*

H. OCHS *Department of Obstetrics and Gynaecology, University of Münster, Scholossplatz 2, D-4400 Münster, Germany*

JEAN LUC POULY MD, *Professor and Director of the Infertility Unit, Departement de Gynécologie Obstétrique et Reproduction Humaine, Centre Hospitalier Universitaire, BP 69, F-63033 Clermont-Ferrand Cedex 1, France*

J. RAIGA MD, *Service de Gynécologie Obstétrique Reproduction Humaine, Polyclinique de l'Hôtel Dieu, Université Clermont-Ferrand I, 13 Boulevard Charles-De-Gaulle, F-63000 Clermont-Ferrand Cedex 1, France*

KARL-WERNER SCHWEPPE (Prof. Dr Medicine), *Chairman, Department of Obstetrics and Gynecology, KKH Ammerland Academic Teaching Hospital of the University of Gottingen, Lange Strasse 38, D-26655 Westerstede, Germany*

ROBERT W. SHAW MD, FRCOG, FRCS (Ed.), MFFP, *Professor and Head, Department of Obstetrics and Gynaecology, University of Wales College of Medicine, Heath Park, Cardiff, CF4 4XN, UK*

ERIC J. THOMAS MB, BS, MD, MRCOG, *Professor of Obstetrics and Gynaecology, University of Southampton, Princess Anne Hospital, Coxford Road, Southampton, SO9 4HA, UK*

A. WATTIEZ MD, *Service de Gynécologie Obstétrique Reproduction Humaine, Polyclinique de l'Hôtel Dieu, Université Clermont-Ferrand I, 13 Boulevard Charles-De-Gaulle, F-63000 Clermont-Ferrand Cedex 1, France*

Preface

Endometriosis remains a challenging condition for clinicians, research scientists and patients alike. The difficulties include problems of explanation of aetiology, pathophysiology and progression; problems of its recognition, both symptomatically and at endoscopy; and problems of determining who, when, how and for how long to treat individuals once its presence has been confirmed.

Our understanding of the pathological features in what has become a spectrum of disease, including the interplay of the immune mechanisms and the role of cellular growth factors and cytokines, has added significantly to our knowledge of the disorder in recent years. However, despite this insight into an increasingly recognized condition, it is still unclear how best to treat the disease.

The contributors to this book are established international clinical researchers in the field of endometriosis and have reviewed and summarized the current understanding of the various components of the disease. In addition, they have, where possible, indicated selection and treatment options in management.

I trust that the book will prove of equal interest to clinicians and researchers, and provide pointers to future advances in what is a long-standing and distressing disorder for many women.

R.W. Shaw
September 1994

Part 1
Cellular Pathophysiology

Chapter 1
Pathogenesis and Aetiology: Questions, Questions, Questions

J.L.H. EVERS

Introduction

Why do we never get an answer
when we're knocking on the door
with a thousand million questions . . .
The Moody Blues
A Question of Balance, 1970

Why do women menstruate? Why do hardly any other mammals menstruate? Why has the endometrium to be shed at the end of the menstrual cycle? How does one viable tissue (the functional layer of the endometrium) detach from another viable tissue (the basal layer)? Does normal endometrium reach the normal abdominal cavity during a normal menstruation in a normal woman? Is regurgitated endometrium removed from the normal abdominal cavity by the normal peritoneal defence system? Under which conditions does regurgitated endometrium attach to the peritoneum? Why does regurgitated endometrium attach to the peritoneum in some women, and not in others? How does regurgitated endometrium attach to the peritoneum? Is endometriosis always visible to the naked eye? Is endometriosis a progressive disease or is it self-limiting? Does endometriosis cause infertility, or is it an epiphenomenon? Why is endometriosis found more frequently nowadays? Or isn't it? Is painful endometriosis a separate disease? Is deep endometriosis of the rectovaginal septum similar to adenomyosis externa? Why does ovarian endometriosis form cysts, whereas these are not found at other locations? Do there exist more differences between peritoneal and ovarian endometriosis? Questions, questions, questions.

The clinical case of the woman with severe pelvic pain and only minimal endometriosis is about as common as the woman without any complaint who is accidentally found to have severe endometriosis at an infertility laparoscopy. Do we really know anything about this mysterious disease? In this chapter I want to explore the facts that exist in evidence of the aetiology and pathogenesis of endometriosis. I will limit myself to six of the deluge of questions.

How does viable endometrium detach from its basal layer?

Apart from some subhuman primates, some bats and the elephant shrew, the human female is the only menstruating mammal [1]. In normal, cycling endometrium, glandular epithelium undergoes rapid growth and remodelling during the follicular phase of the cycle. Growth ceases during the luteal phase and, in the absence of the continued progesterone-dominated environment of pregnancy, the arteries supplying the superficial layer of the endometrium constrict during the late luteal phase of the menstrual cycle, in response to the failing progesterone drive. Glandular activity decreases and loss of interstitial fluid occurs. Eventually the feeding arteries close down, making the superficial zone ischaemic. After some time the constricted arteries open up again, the walls of the damaged surface vessels burst to release blood into the stroma, and ultimately patches of tissue separate from the basal layer of the endometrium [2]. Metalloproteinases of the stromelysin family, collagenase and the extracellular matrix-degrading enzyme matrilysin are expressed in endometrium and probably play a role in endometrial growth, remodelling, breakdown and possibly in the establishment of ectopic endometriotic tissue and in determining its invasive properties [3].

Why do women menstruate?

The process of menstruation has fascinated, frightened and troubled people of all cultures and societies throughout history. Religious and worldly authorities have felt obliged to devise rules and regulations for women during the time of their menstrual period. Contact with the menstrual effluent would spoil the crops, tarnish the fruits and make the wine go sour. Attendance of women at religious functions during their periods usually was not allowed and amenorrhoea, on the other hand, was a reason for divorce. Ever since Hippocrates, menstruation has been considered a detoxification process of the female body, and it was not until Aristotle that it was recognized that a relationship existed between menstruation and conception. Contrary to endometriosis research, most research of menstruation has been aimed at the 'how' rather than the 'why'. By trying to elucidate the mechanisms involved, doctors have tried to offer appropriate and rational therapies for menstrual abnormalities. Still we are faced with the problem of the 'why'.

Few people, even few medical doctors, recognize that menstruation is a rare event in the animal kingdom. Apart from humans, only a few subhuman primates and two non-primate species, see above, have been found to menstruate. Little is known about their cyclic endometrial development. Finn [1] in a beautifully written monograph, recently reviewed our knowledge of the phenomenon of menstruation and concluded that the decidual cell reaction in the uterine stroma is a human-species-specific adaption of the endometrial inflammatory response that allows the implanting blastocyst to develop safely inside the uterine tissues, where usually this inflammatory response would have been directed at removal and destruction of the invading foreign object. The premenstrual condition in women whereby the uterus is prepared in advance so as to be able to withstand the invasion of the blastocyst is considered by Finn [1] to represent the latest stage in the evolution of implantation, with menstruation being the price to pay for the fact that during the menstrual cycle the human endometrium goes a stage further in the preparation of the stroma for implantation than does the uterus of non-menstruating species. The decidual reaction of the endometrial stroma cells represents a stage of differentiation which does not allow them to return to their former undifferentiated state again. If cells cannot be maintained, they must be discarded. As a result, in order for our species to survive, monthly menstruation troubles its female members.

How does shed endometrium reach the abdominal cavity?

Sampson [4], in 1927, was the first to note blood escaping from the fimbrial end of the Fallopian tubes when surgery was performed during the menstrual period. Whether the refluxed endometrium implants on the peritoneal lining of the pelvic organs (metastasis theory) or whether it induces a local metaplastic response in the peritoneum, leading to the neogenesis of endometrial tissue by mesothelial metaplasia at the ectopic site (metaplasia theory [5]), is still an unsolved problem and a matter of arduous debate among distinguished 'endometriologists' [6, 7]. Most students of endometriosis, however, favour the implantation theory nowadays as the most important explanation for the pathogenesis of endometriosis [8], although not all aspects of the disease may be explained by this theory. Endometrial metaplasia of the peritoneal serosa may constitute an additional (and not an opposing) explanation: endometrial cells or cell products may stimulate metaplasia after they have been transported to a susceptible site in the abdominal cavity. Merrill [9] implanted millipore filters containing vital endometrium tissue in the abdominal cavity of rabbits. Although these filters will not allow cells to pass, endometrium-like glandular tissue, but not stroma, was found at subsequent histologic examination of the connective tissue adjacent to the filters. The same occurred when only devitalized endometrium was enclosed in the filters. Although the type of tissue induced, because of the lack of stroma, did not fulfil all criteria for a diagnosis of endometriosis to be established, this study offers suggestive evidence that subcellular substances from (even decaying) endometrium are apparently capable of inducing endometrial metaplasia in mesothelium.

The reflux implantation theory of Sampson [4] is supported by the distribution of lesions in the abdominal cavity [10], the demonstration of the viability of shed menstrual endometrium in tissue culture [11], the immunohistochemical characteristics of retrogradely shed endometrium and its similarities to *in situ* endometrium, antegradely shed endometrium and endometriosis lesions in the peritoneal cavity [12], the capacity of adhesion and proliferation of peritoneal cells obtained from the peritoneal fluid during the early follicular phase of the cycle [13], the high prevalence of endometriosis in girls with congenital menstrual outflow tract obstruction [14] and animal experiments in which endometriosis was induced by the creation of uteropelvic fistulas [15]. The reflux implantation theory is based on the assumption that retrograde menstruation takes place, and that viable endometrial cells reach the abdominal cavity, attach to the peritoneal lining and implant. Goodall [16] observed spill of blood in about 50% of laparotomies performed during menstruation. Blumenkrantz and coworkers [17] reported that nine of 11 women undergoing peritoneal dialysis had blood in the dialysate during their periods. Halme and coworkers [18] found red discoloration of the peritoneal fluid (PF) in 90% of patients with patent tubes, laparoscoped during their menstrual periods. Blood was found by Liu and Hitchcock [19] in 76%. van der Linden and coworkers [12] found endometrial cells in the PF during the early follicular phase of the cycle in all of the 16 patients in their study. Kruitwagen and coworkers [13] were able to demonstrate the presence of endometrial cells in 79% of their early follicular phase PF samples and showed these cells to be viable in culture.

We may conclude from these studies that viable endometrial cells reach the abdominal cavity via the Fallopian tubes during the menstrual period in most, if not all, women with patent tubes. The volume of regurgitated menstrual debris may be determined by anatomic-mechanical predispositions. Ayers and Friedenstab [20] showed uterotubal junction hypotonia in endometriosis patients as compared with (infertile) controls. Their findings seem to be corroborated by Bartosik and coworkers [21], who found more endometrial cells to reach the abdominal cavity during flushing of the tubes in endometriosis patients. Whether the sheer volume or also the tissue properties of the regurgitated menstrual debris determines that endometriosis will develop in some patients and not in others and whether differences in their peritoneal defence system contribute to the problem still remain to be elucidated.

Why is regurgitated endometrium not always disposed of by the peritoneal defence system?

In women with endometriosis a local, sterile inflammation occurs in the peritoneal cavity [22–24]. On theoretical grounds this inflammation may be a response to menstrual debris, either regurgitated through the Fallopian tubes or shed locally by the endometriotic implants [12]. Haney and coworkers [25] have shown the latter mechanism to be the less likely one. Elicitation of a reactive inflammatory response may be considered the body's first line of defence against the development of endometriosis. If the defence mechanism fails or if the aggression is too voluminous or too strong, viable endometrial cells will implant and develop into clinical endometriosis. The association between the sterile inflammation of the PF and infertility remains to be elucidated [25–28].

The peritoneal response to the invasion of regurgitated menstrual debris is directed at incapacitation, destruction and removal of these cells. This should prevent the adhesion of viable endometrial cells to the peritoneal lining, and their subsequent development into endometriotic lesions. An inadequate response of this defence mechanism has been suggested as a facilitating factor for the development of endometriosis. Immunologic factors have been the subject of many studies in this respect, although it should be stressed that no increased occurrence of immunologic disorders has been found in endometriosis patients [29–35].

Drake and coworkers [22] have reported increased volumes of PF in women with endometriosis, and have interpreted this as a sign of inflammation.

Macrophages are involved in phagocytosis and, through their secretory products, in inflammatory reactions. They constitute the dominant cell type in the PF cell population [36]. Macrophages are involved in the initiation of the inflammatory response as antigen-presenting cells and, in the active phase, as tumoricidal and microbicidal cells. Upon stimulation, resident peritoneal macrophages produce factors that stimulate proliferation of monocytes in the bone marrow. These monocytes travel to the site of violation of homoeostasis (i.e. the peritoneal cavity) to take part, as activated macrophages, in the inflammatory response and defence reaction. In this respect they may be considered the garbage collection and disposal system of the peritoneal cavity. Halme and coworkers [24] found increased activation of peritoneal macrophages in infertile women with mild endometriosis. Proteolytic enzymes, lysozyme, γ-interferon, interleukins 1 and 2 (IL-1 and IL-2), tumour necrosis factor (TNF) and growth factors are amongst the secretory products of activated macrophages [37–40].

Also the other major cell types of the immune system, T lymphocytes, B lymphocytes and natural killer (NK) cells, have been studied in PF of endometriosis patients. All cells have the capacity to produce cytokines, and cytokines in turn activate T cells, B cells, NK cells and macrophages. Of particular interest in this regard is the finding by Dunselman and coworkers [36] that, although activated macrophages show increased *in vitro* phagocytosis of sheep red blood cells, their capability to show chemiluminescence after ingestion of zymosan is decreased. This suggests that, in endometriosis patients, macrophages may lack, even when activated in other respects, sufficient capacity to clear the pelvic cavity of regurgitated menstrual debris, i.e. of viable endometrial cells. This is in accordance with an immunologic basis for the development of endometriosis, as suggested by Steele and coworkers [41], who found reduced cell-mediated cytotoxicity toward autologous endometrial cells. More recently, Oosterlynck and coworkers [42] reported defective NK cell activity in endometriosis patients, also resulting in decreased cellular immunity.

From the isolated reports on defence mechanisms in the peritoneal cavity published so far, one may conclude that a highly reactive peritoneal inflammatory response exists in endometriosis patients, which may lower cycle fecundity through interference with intra-abdominal and intratubal reproductive processes. On the other hand, indications exist that isolated defects in these activated immunocompetent cells may explain why endometrial cells may implant and develop into endometriotic lesions. Furthermore, the adhesion of viable endometrial cells may even be facilitated by secretory products of the activated macrophages, e.g. fibronectin [43], and their outgrowth stimulated by inflammatory-cell-derived growth factors, e.g. epidermal growth factor (EGF), transforming growth factor α (TGF-α), TGF-β and IGF-1 [44–46]. Human breast cancer research has revealed that reduction of E-cadherin expression may play an important role in invasion and metastasis of neoplasms [47]. E-cadherin is usually strongly expressed on cell–cell boundaries of normal, non-neoplastic tissue. Oka and coworkers [47] showed that the expression of EGF-receptor tended to be positive in E-cadherin positive breast cancers. Zhang and coworkers [48] tested macrophage-conditioned media on an endometrial cancer cell line, ECC-1. They found that the media of six stage III/IV endometriosis patients demonstrated a mitogenic effect, which was blocked by an antibody to EGF. Most macrophage-conditioned media from stage I/II endometriosis patients lacked this effect. When purified cytokines were tested in the tritium-thymidine uptake assay, only EGF and TGF-α were mitogenic on ECC-1, whereas TNF, IL-1 and platelet-derived growth factor (PDGF) had no effect [48].

Does endometrium attach to the peritoneal lining?

Malignant tumour research has shown that, after separation of individual or groups of tumour cells from the primary tumour, the three crucial steps of invasion are: adherence of the tumour cells to the host tissue cells, local proteolysis associated with breakdown of the extracelluar matrix and migration into the colonized tissue [49]. Regurgitated endometrial cells possess the capacity to attach to the peritoneal lining, as shown by van der Linden and coworkers [12]. These authors concluded from their work that the expression pattern of cell adhesion molecules indicates that the loss of cell adhesion properties may play a role in the shedding of endometrial tissue during menstruation and that integrins, and perhaps cadherins, may also be operative in attachment of endometrial tissue fragments to the peritoneum. The demonstration of the expression of cell adhesion molecules by cells in menstrual effluent, endometrium and PF, as well as in endometriosis lesions, is no strict evidence that endometriosis originates from endometrium by retrograde shedding of viable tissue fragments. However, all cells potentially involved in the pathogenesis of endometriosis possess the property to express integrin and cadherin cell adhesion molecules during the menstrual phase of the cycle. Although the exact mechanism by which endometrial cells might attach to the peritoneal serosa is still not clear, and although the first endometrial cell making contact with the first serosal cell still has to be sighted, it has been established [50] that early endometriosis invades the peritoneal extracelluar matrix: products of local proteolysis, e.g. the aminoterminal propeptide of type III collagen, accumulate in the PF of patients with endometriosis, especially those with early, active lesions. van der Linden and coworkers [12] showed E-cadherin to be expressed in *in situ* endometrial epithelial cells of 16 of 16 women, however, it was expressed in only one of 16 endometrial cells retrieved from their PF during the menstrual period. Similarity with the loss of E-cadherin expression in invasive breast cancer would suggest a potential role for cadherins in invasive endometriosis. After cell division has resumed, the new endometrial implant will soon reach a critical tissue volume. From then onwards, it will have to rely on new vessel ingrowth for support of its further outgrowth and development. In an elegant series of experiments, Oosterlynck and coworkers [51] investigated the presence of angiogenic factors in PF from 24 endometriosis patients and compared the results with those in 24 controls. Angiogenesis was assayed by placing glass fibre filters impregnated with PF on the exposed chorioallantoic membrane of chicken embryos. The PF of endometriosis patients appeared to contain more angiogenic activity than the PF of controls. The reaction remained after charcoal treatment of the PF. TGF-α, TGF-β, TNF-α and EGF all have angiogenic properties. These factors can be produced by activated macrophages. They may, however, also be secreted by endometrial cells, or by immunocompetent cells amidst them. Haining and coworkers [52], in an immunocytochemical study, have shown one of the angiogenic growth factors, EGF, to be produced in eutopic and ectopic endometrium. EGF receptors are present in endometrium as well as in endometriosis [53, 54].

Is endometriosis a progressive disease?

In 1987, David Redwine [55] drew our attention to the age-related evolution in colour appearance of endometriosis. He found the mean age of endometriosis patients to increase from 21.5 years, for those with clear papules only, via 26.3 years, for those with red lesions, and 29.5 years, for those with white lesions, to 31.9 years, for those with black lesions. The age range of patients with clear papules only was 17–26 years, the age range of patients with black plus any other lesions was 17–43, and of patients with black lesions only, 20–52 years. No patient over the age of 31 was found to present clear lesions any more. These findings suggest that endometriosis in many patients is a self-limiting disease. The early, non-pigmented papules (with invasive activity into the extracelluar matrix of the host tissue) evolve into well-vascularized, hyperaemic, red lesions, and finally are subdued by the peritoneal defence system and develop into the familiar black and blue powderburn lesions, poorly vascularized, quiescent and surrounded by white fibrotic tissue. One wonders what the age range was of those (rare) patients that have been described in the literature [56–58] who showed invisible, i.e. microscopic, lesions only.

The concept of spontaneous resolution of endometriosis is corroborated by the composition of the patient groups usually described in treatment studies. Typically, patients with American Fertility Society (AFS) stage I and II disease constitute the majority of cases, whereas the group of patients belonging to stage III and IV is usually much smaller, irrespective of whether only surgical or also medical treatment studies are considered.

Although several studies have suggested that medical treatment of endometriosis is effective in inhibiting progression of endometriosis, other investigations have cast doubt upon this conclusion. If a second-look laparoscopy is performed during medical suppression of endometriosis and the findings are compared with the findings at first-look laparoscopy (when the pelvic environment was moist, active, with productive endometriotic foci and their inherent hyperaemia, haemorrhage, secretion and inflammatory reaction), one may erroneously conclude that the less active, and therefore less visible, foci in the dry, inactive pelvis reflect regression or even resolution of endometriosis. After suppression has been discontinued, however, the foci will become reactivated again and the disease will return to its original path of development [59]. The final answer to the question of whether endometriosis is a progressive disease will have to come from long-term prospective investigations studying spontaneous evolution of peritoneal lesions without therapeutic interference. This will require performing a second-look laparoscopy in a patient who has not received any treatment in the interval since her first laparoscopy. It is obvious that such groups will be difficult to collect. We may already learn something, however, from the evolution of disease as detailed in the no-treatment or placebo groups of the few randomized controlled studies published so far. Thomas and Cooke [60] showed, in 17 placebo-treated patients who underwent a laparoscopy before and after 6 months of placebo treatment, unchanged or even diminished endometriosis in 53%, but an increment in 47%. Similar figures were obtained by other investigators [61, 62]. Mahmood and Templeton [62] noted improvement among 27% of untreated patients, an increment in 64% and an unchanged situation in 9%. Many other studies give indirect evidence that endometriosis is progressive [63–67]. D'Hooghe and coworkers [68] studied the spontaneous evolution of endometriosis in baboons and reported a significant increase in the number of lesions at relaparoscopy at 10 months. The new lesions were mainly subtle, atypical (67%) and localized on the uterine peritoneum. Progression of endometriosis did not, however, go beyond revised American Fertility Society (RAFS) stage I. Repeat laparoscopies in 10 baboons with an initially normal pelvis showed endometriosis to be present in seven after 10–12 months. They conclude endometriosis to be moderately progressive in the baboon, but never beyond the borders of RAFS stage I. Remodelling of endometriosis lesions within stage I took place within a period of several months.

Answers, answers, answers, please!

From all published evidence we may conclude that endometriosis appears to be a dynamic disease, especially in the early phase, with subtle, atypical lesions emerging and vanishing again. In the end, however, the peritoneal defence system will prevail and the disease will be contained in the majority of patients. When doing repeat laparoscopies in young patients, one should be prepared to encounter more advanced histological types of lesions, which do not necessarily have to indicate more advanced stages of the disease: the classical, blue and black powderburn spots and blueberry lesions reflect the extinguishing phase of the dynamic endometriotic process, and herald its inactivated histological end-stage. The dynamic phase of the disease may involve a varying interval of each patient's life, and medical suppression of the activity of the implants during this interval may lead one to conclude erroneously that treatment has been effective. If subsequently (after the end of medical suppression of the activity of the lesions) ovarian activity resumes and the lesions are stimulated again by ovarian steroids, their productive activity returns. Recurrence of disease may be diagnosed if at that stage a laparoscopy is performed, whereas in reality only reactivation of temporarily obscured lesions has occurred. The suppressed, dormant (but never absent) lesions produce mucus again, desquamation occurs and there is reaction by the surrounding tissue. The inflammatory response, the local hyperaemia and the neogenesis of vessels accentuate the presence of previously invisible endometriotic lesions and make them visible again. Endometriosis resumes its temporarily halted natural course of development, tissue remodelling occurs again, the battle between the aggressor and the defence resumes and waxing and waning of the several types of lesions, red, white and black, can be found again. Brosens has likened this situation to mushrooms (I.A. Brosens, personal communication): there exists a hidden, invisible network of mycelia which gives rise to the emergence of mushrooms that develop, stabilize and disappear again. Until the soil on which they grow is exhausted, the mushrooms will come and go.

Conclusion

In order to fully understand this mysterious disease we will have to learn where the spores come from, what makes them sometimes form mycelia, what determines the (limited) period of turnover of mushrooms and why the fungus eventually disappears again. It is only after these processes have been understood that we might try to comprehend why in the occasional patient the disease is not self-limiting, and why in this patient the aggressor wins. Identification of specific characteristics of these patients will help us to distinguish between those patients who will not benefit from extended diagnostic and therapeutic procedures and those who will need permanent medical attention in order to prevent the disease from deteriorating into the severe forms that we every so often encounter in our clinics.

References

1 Finn CA. Why do women and some other primates menstruate? *Perspect Biol Med* 1987 **30**: 566–574.

2 Edwards RG. *Conception in the Human Female*, 1980, pp. 463–464. London, Academic Press.

3 Rodgers WH, Osteen KG, Matrisian LM, Navre M, Giudice LG, Gorstein F. Expression and localization of matrilysin, a matrix metalloproteinase, in human endometrium during the reproductive cycle. *Am J Obstet Gynecol* 1993 **168**: 253–260.

4 Sampson JA. Peritoneal endometriosis due to menstrual dissemination of endometrial tissue into the peritoneal cavity. *Am J Obstet Gynecol* 1927 **14**: 422–469.

5 Meyer R. Ueber den Stand der Frage der Adenomyositis und Adenomyome in Algemeinen und Insbesondere ueber Adenomyositis seroepithelialis und Adenomyometritis sarcomatosa. *Zbl f Gynaekol* 1919 **43**: 745–750.

6 Kruitwagen RFPM. Retrograde menstruation. In: Brosens IA, Donnez J (eds). *The Current Status of Endometriosis Research and Management*, 1992, pp. 3–19. Carnforth, Parthenon Publishing Group.

7 Fujii S. Metaplasia: secondary Muellerian system and endometriosis. In: Brosens IA, Donnez

J (eds). *The Current Status of Endometriosis Research and Management*, 1992, pp. 19–34. Carnforth, Parthenon Publishing Group.
8 Dunselman GAJ. *Endometriosis, Clinical and Experimental Aspects* (Thesis), 1988. Maastricht, Fertility Foundation Publishing Group.
9 Merrill JA. Endometrial induction of endometriosis across millipore filters. *Am J Obstet Gynecol* 1966 **94**: 780–789
10 Jenkins S, Olive DL, Haney AF. Endometriosis: pathogenetic implications of the anatomic distribution. *Obstet Gynecol* 1986 **67**: 335–338.
11 Keettel WC, Stein RJ. The viability of cast-off menstrual endometrium. *Am J Obstet Gynecol* 1951 **61**: 440–442.
12 van der Linden PJQ, de Goeij AFPM, Denselman GAJ *et al.* Expression of integrins and E-cadherin in cells from menstrual effluent, endometrium, peritoneal fluid, peritoneum, and endometriosis. *Fertil Steril* 1994 **61**: 85–90.
13 Kruitwagen RF, Poels LG, Willemsen WN, de Ronde IJ, Jap PH, Rolland R. Endometrial epithelial cells in peritoneal fluid during the early follicular phase. *Fertil Steril* 1991 **55**: 297–303.
14 Sanfilippo JS, Wakim NG, Schikler KN, Yussman MA. Endometriosis in association with uterine anomaly. *Am J Obstet Gynecol* 1986 **154**: 39–43.
15 Te Linde RW, Scott RB. Experimental endometriosis. *Am J Obstet Gynecol* 1950 **60**: 1147–1173.
16 Goodall JR. *A Study of Endometriosis, Endosalpingosis, Endocervicosis, and Peritoneo-ovarian Sclerosis: a Clinical and Pathologic Study*, 1943. Philadelphia, J.B. Lippincot.
17 Blumenkrantz MJ, Gallagher N, Bashore RA, Tenckhoff H. Retrograde menstruation in women undergoing chronic peritoneal dialysis. *Obstet Gynecol* 1981 **57**: 667–670.
18 Halme J, Hammond MG, Hulka JF, Raj SG, Talbert LM. Retrograde menstruation in healthy women and in patients with endometriosis. *Obstet Gynecol* 1984 **64**: 151–154.
19 Liu DT, Hitchcock A. Endometriosis: its association with retrograde menstruation, dysmenorrhoea and tubal pathology. *Br J Obstet Gynaecol* 1986 **93**: 859–862.
20 Ayers JWT, Friedenstab AP. Utero-tubal hypotonia associated with pelvic endometriosis. *Fertil Steril* 1985 Ann Meeting: 131.
21 Bartosik D, Jacobs SL, Kelly LJ. Endometrial tissue in peritoneal fluid. *Fertil Steril* 1986 **46**: 796–800.
22 Drake TS, Metz SA, Grunert GM, O'Brien WF. Peritoneal fluid volume in endometriosis. *Fertil Steril* 1980 **34**: 27–31.
23 Haney AF, Muscato JJ, Weinberg JB. Peritoneal fluid cell populations in infertility patients. *Fertil Steril* 1981 **35**: 696–698.
24 Halme J, Becker S, Hammond MG, Raj MH, Raj S. Increased activation of pelvic macrophages in infertile women with mild endometriosis. *Am J Obstet Gynecol* 1983 **145**: 333–337.
25 Haney AF, Jenkins S, Weinberg JB. The stimulus responsible for the peritoneal fluid inflammation observed in infertile women with endometriosis. *Fertil Steril* 1991 **56**: 408–413.
26 Halme J. Role of peritoneal inflammation in endometriosis-associated infertility. *Ann N Y Acad Sci* 1991 **622**: 266–274.
27 Boutten A, Dehoux M, Edelman P *et al.* IL6 and acute phase plasma proteins in peritoneal fluid of women with endometriosis. *Clin Chim Acta* 1992 **210**: 187–195.
28 Cirkel U, Ochs H, Mues B, Zwadlo G, Sorg C, Schneider HP. Inflammatory reaction in endometriotic tissue: an immunohistochemical study. *Eur J Obstet Gynecol Reprod Biol* 1993 **48**: 43–50.
29 Fernandez Shaw S, Hicks BR, Yudkin PL, Kennedy S, Barlow DH, Starkey PM.

Anti-endometrial and anti-endothelial auto-antibodies in women with endometriosis. *Hum Reprod* 1993 **8**: 310–315.

30 Cunningham DS, Hansen KA, Coddington CC. Changes in T-cell regulation of responses to self antigens in women with pelvic endometriosis. *Fertil Steril* 1992 **58**: 114–119.

31 Gorai I, Ishikawa M, Onose R, Hirahara F, Minaguchi H. Antiendometrial autoantibodies are generated in patients with endometriosis. *Am J Reprod Immunol* 1993 **29**: 116–123.

32 D'Cruz OJ, Wild RA. Evaluation of endometrial tissue specific complement activation in women with endometriosis. *Fertil Steril* 1992 **57**: 787–795.

33 Rajkumar K, Malliah V, Simpson CW. Identifying the presence of antibodies against endometrial antigens. A preliminary study. *J Reprod Med* 1992 37: 552–556.

34 Wild RA, Shivers CA, Medders D. Detection of antiendometrial antibodies in patients with endometriosis: methodological issues. *Fertil Steril* 1992 **58**: 518–521.

35 Kilpatrick DC, Haining RE, Smith SS. Are cardiolipin antibody levels elevated in endometriosis? *Fertil Steril* 1991 **55**: 436–437.

36 Dunselman GA, Hendrix MG, Bouckaert PX, Evers JL. Functional aspects of peritoneal macrophages in endometriosis of women. *J Reprod Fertil* 1988 **82**: 707–710.

37 Fakih H, Baggett B, Holtz G, Tsang KY, Lee JC, Williamson HO. Interleukin-1: a possible role in the infertility associated with endometriosis. *Fertil Steril* 1987 **47**: 213–217.

38 Fukumatsu Y, Katabuchi H, Miyamura S *et al.* Activated macrophages in the peritoneal fluid of women with endometriosis: examination of the intracytoplasmic localization of endogenous peroxidase and interleukin-1. *Nippon Sanka Fujinka Gakkai Zasshi* 1992 **44**: 529–536.

39 Mori H, Sawairi M, Nakagawa M *et al.* Peritoneal fluid interleukin-1 beta and tumor necrosis factor in patients with benign gynecologic disease. *Am J Reprod Immunol* 1991 **26**: 62–67.

40 Braun DP, Gebel H, Rotman C, Rana N, Dmowski WP. The development of cytotoxicity in peritoneal macrophages from women with endometriosis. *Fertil Steril* 1992 **57**: 1203–1210.

41 Steele RW, Dmowski WP, Marmer DJ. Immunologic aspects of human endometriosis. *Am J Reprod Immunol* 1984 **6**: 33–36.

42 Oosterlynck DJ, Meuleman C, Waer M, Vandeputte M, Koninckx PR. The natural killer activity of peritoneal fluid lymphocytes is decreased in women with endometriosis. *Fertil Steril* 1992 **58**: 290–295.

43 Kauma S, Clark MR, White C, Halme J. Production of fibronectin by peritoneal macrophages and concentration of fibronectin in peritoneal fluid from patients with or without endometriosis. *Obstet Gynecol* 1988 **72**: 13–18.

44 Simms JS, Chegini N, Williams RS, Rossi AM, Dunn WAJ. Identification of epidermal growth factor, transforming growth factor-alpha, and epidermal growth factor receptor in surgically induced endometriosis in rats. *Obstet Gynecol* 1991 **78**: 850–857.

45 Hammond MG, Oh ST, Anners J, Surrey ES, Halme J. The effect of growth factors on the proliferation of human endometrial stromal cells in culture. *Am J Obstet Gynecol* 1993 **168**: 1131–1136.

46 Ferriani RA, Charnock Jones DS, Prentice A, Thomas EJ, Smith SK. Immunohistochemical localization of acidic and basic fibroblast growth factors in normal human endometrium and endometriosis and the detection of their mRNA by polymerase chain reaction. *Hum Reprod* 1993 **8**: 11–16.

47 Oka H, Shiozaki H, Kobayashi K *et al.* Expression of E-cadherin cell adhesion molecules in human breast cancer tissues and its relationship to metastasis. *Cancer Res* 1993 **53**: 1696–1701.

48 Zhang RJ, Wild RA, Medders D, Gunupudi SR. Effects of peritoneal macrophages from patients with endometriosis on the proliferation of endometrial carcinoma cell line ECC-1. *Am J Obstet Gynecol* 1991 **165**: 1842–1846.

49 Liotta LA. Cancer cell invasion and metastasis. *Sci Am* 1992 **266**: 54–59, 62–63.
50 Spuijbroek MD, Dunselman GA, Menheere PP, Evers JL. Early endometriosis invades the extracelluar matrix. *Fertil Steril* 1992 **58**: 929–933.
51 Oosterlynck DJ, Meuleman C, Sobis H, Vandeputte M, Koninckx PR. Angiogenic activity of peritoneal fluid from women with endometriosis. *Fertil Steril* 1993 **59**: 778–782.
52 Haining RE, Cameron IT, van Papendorp C *et al.* Epidermal growth factor in human endometrium: proliferative effects in culture and immunocytochemical localization in normal and endometriotic tissues. *Hum Reprod* 1991 **6**: 1200–1205.
53 Henzen Logmans SC, van der Burg ME, Foekens JA *et al.* Occurrence of epidermal growth factor receptors in benign and malignant ovarian tumors and normal ovarian tissues: an immunohistochemical study. *J Cancer Res Clin Oncol* 1992 **118**: 303–307.
54 Prentice A, Thomas EJ, Weddell A *et al.* Epidermal growth factor receptor expression in normal endometrium and endometriosis: an immunohistochemical study. *Br J Obstet Gynaecol* 1992 **99**: 395–398.
55 Redwine DB. Age-related evolution in color appearance of endometriosis. *Fertil Steril* 1987 **48**: 1062–1063.
56 Nisolle M, Paindaveine B, Bourdon A *et al.* Histologic study of peritoneal endometriosis in infertile women. *Fertil Steril* 1990 **53**: 984–988.
57 Vasquez G, Cornillie F, Brosens IA. Peritoneal endometriosis: scanning electron microscopy and histology of minimal pelvic endometriotic lesions. *Fertil Steril* 1984 **42**: 696–703.
58 Murphy AA, Green WR, Bobbie D, dela Cruz ZC, Rock JA. Unsuspected endometriosis documented by scanning electron microscopy in visually normal peritoneum. *Fertil Steril* 1986 **46**: 522–524.
59 Evers JL. The second-look laparoscopy for evaluation of the result of medical treatment of endometriosis should not be performed during ovarian suppression. *Fertil Steril* 1987 **47**: 502–504.
60 Thomas EJ, Cooke ID. Impact of gestrinone on the course of asymptomatic endometriosis. *Br Med J Clin Res Ed* 1987 **294**: 272–274.
61 Telimaa S. Danazol and medroxyprogesterone acetate inefficacious in the treatment of infertility in endometriosis. *Fertil Steril* 1988 **50**: 872–875.
62 Mahmood TA, Templeton A. The impact of treatment on the natural history of endometriosis. *Hum Reprod* 1990 **5**: 965–970.
63 Brosens IA. Evolution of endometriotic lesions: is endometriosis a progressive disease? *Prog Clin Biol Res* 1990 **323**: 151–156.
64 Koninckx PR, Meuleman C, Demeyere S, Lesaffre E, Cornillie FJ. Suggestive evidence that pelvic endometriosis is a progressive disease, whereas deeply infiltrating endometriosis is associated with pelvic pain. *Fertil Steril* 1991 **55**: 759–765.
65 Lanzone A, Marana R, Muscatello R *et al.* Serum CA-125 levels in the diagnosis and management of endometriosis. *J Reprod Med* 1991 **36**: 603–607.
66 Stovall DW, Halme J. Endometriosis and associated pathology. *Curr Opin Obstet Gynecol* 1991 **3**: 853–858.
67 DeCherney AH. Endometriosis: recurrence and retreatment. *Chin Ther* 1992 **14**: 766–772.
68 D'Hooge TM, Bambra CS, Isahakia M, Koninckx PR. Evolution of spontaneous endometriosis in the baboon (*Papio anubis, Papio cynocephalus*) over a 12-month period. *Fertil Steril* 1992 **58**: 409–412.

Chapter 2
Morphology, Ultrastructure and Receptors in Untreated and Treated Endometriotic Implants

H. OCHS AND K.-W. SCHWEPPE

Introduction

The diagnosis of endometriosis still presents us with several problems resulting from similarities in clinical symptoms to other benign or non-benign gynaecological diseases. Gynaecological symptoms may give a diagnostic help to the suspicion of endometriosis. Although there are the well-known complaints of dysmenorrhoea (present in 78% of patients), pelvic pain (39%) and deep dyspareunia (32%), none of the investigations until now have found a clear-cut relation to either localization or stage of the disease [1,2]. Nevertheless these symptoms have been characterized in more detail. The endometriosis-associated dysmenorrhoea extends to the pre- and post-menstrual phase and is typically secondary (acquired) and progressive rather than primarily existent. Pelvic pain and tenderness, however, vary in quality and quantity seemingly irrespective of the localization of the lesion, although the studies of Konninckx *et al.* [3] and Cornillie *et al.* [4] indicate the symptom 'pelvic pain' to be related to the depth of the lesion in the peritoneal layer. Dyspareunia is typically experienced on deep penetration in the presence of lesions on the uterosacral ligaments or in the rectovaginal septum.

Atypical bleeding patterns are the leading symptom of a variety of gynaecological diseases, but may also characterize endometriosis patients. Premenstrual spotting and meno- or metrorrhagia are frequently noted [5]. On the other hand cyclical rectal bleeding or haematuria are pathognomonic for the disease. Although rarely observed (< 2%), this symptom gives strong evidence for bowel or bladder involvement. Painful micturition or defecation at the time of menstruation may be the first signs of the progressing disease.

Macroscopic aspect

Gynaecological examination may visualize endometriotic lesions as clear, red or bluish cysts or nodules in the vagina or on the cervix. Macroscopic diagnosis is often misleading and cannot substitute histological confirmation, even if bleeding from these lesions at the time of menstruation is rare, but impressive. Palpation detects induration of the uterosacral ligaments or nodules in the pouch of Douglas or the rectovaginal septum. Endometriosis in the ovaries can lead to large cysts even beyond the pelvis, which can be palpated. Fixation of the uterus in retroversion and immobilization of the ovaries, by adhesion formation, may additionally add to the suspicion of the diagnosis of endometriosis. In the case of bladder or bowel involvement, cystoscopy or rectosigmoidoscopy will be necessary. Ultrasound examination of the pelvis gives some more information about clinical findings, although haemorrhagic functional cysts of the ovary may give the same picture sonographically. Even though a specificity of 90% by ultrasound examination has been published [6], we feel that operative intervention is still needed to further ascertain the diagnosis.

For visualization of endometriotic implants in the abdominal cavity, diagnostic laparoscopy is the method of choice. The lesions have quite a characteristic, even though variable, appearance. Besides the classical 'black powderburn' foci, which are usually associated with endometriosis, the disease includes red, yellow, white, blue and brown implants. In addition, there was the investigation of Jansen and Russell [7], who described non-pigmented endometriosis, i.e. non-haemorrhagic lesions, as an addition to the variety of other appearances. Different types of growth and progression in relation to the peritoneal surface are described by polyp-like or papular implants in contrast to scarred lesions or even deeply infiltrating growth. Relationship to the activity of the implant has been suggested [8] as well as a correlation to the age of the patient [9].

These varieties in appearance give the possibility of missing the correct diagnosis because other lesions of the pelvic organs may look identical at laparoscopy. Haemorrhagic ovarian cysts of functional origin, haemangioma and dilated vessels and scarred residuals from preceding operations may give the same macroscopic impression. Additional confirmation is needed. One such method was the 'thermocolour test' inaugurated by Semm [10]. Turning red and brownish lesions into black colour, this test allows the chance of including therapy (thermocoagulation) and diagnosis in one step. On the other hand, it demands a haemorrhagic component of the implant and gives rise to false positive diagnoses with blood residuals of other origin than that of endometriosis. Trying to get close to the reliability of histological information without the need for traumatizing biopsies was suggested by Bühler *et al* [11] by using a cytological smear from suspicious areas. In their recently published study a sensitivity of the method of 79% was reported [11]. Despite all the above-mentioned approaches, including patient's history, clinical and laparoscopic examination with macroscopic means, a histological confirmation of the diagnosis endometriosis is still necessary. Only the microscopic proof of endometrial glands and stroma can verify the diagnosis and is preferred before invasive treatment – either surgical or medical – is started. In addition, histology enables us to study the implant itself to get more information about pathogenesis, susceptibility to hormonal treatment or importance for infertility causation. The following pages will try to elucidate data on the microscopic and ultrastructural appearance of the lesion. Morphological effects of modulating factors such as endogenous and/or exogenous steroids will be reviewed and illustrated to draw possible conclusions in order to come closer to the still unknown histogenesis and pathogenesis of endometriosis.

Histogenesis

Endometriosis is defined as the presence of endometrial glands and stroma outside the uterine cavity. Independent of the accepted aetiology and histogenesis of this pathological condition, all authors agree in the observation that the ectopic tissue resembles more or less eutopic endometrium. To date there are two main theories of development of endometriosis, for either of which clinical evidence and theoretical arguments can be given.

Metastatic theory

As early as 1940 Sampson [12] proposed his metastatic theory postulating that a retrograde menstrual flow transports desquamated endometrial fragments through the Fallopian tubes into the peritoneal cavity, and once there the still viable cells subsequently implant and grow. One basic requirement – the retrograde menstruation via patent tubes – has more recently been demonstrated in a study by Halme *et al.* [13], who observed bloody fluid at the time of menstruation in the pelvis. As this occurred in 90% of all women in their study, it was regarded as a physiological phenomenon. Additional support came from the observation of Kirshon and Poindexter [14], who saw a higher risk of endometriosis in patients with an increased retrograde blood flow – in their study, due to the use of intrauterine devices for contraception. On the other hand, the presence of viable glands and stromal cells in the peritoneal fluid alone does not necessarily lead to the development of endometriosis. Other factors, probably within the local peritoneal environment, must additionally be present to allow the tissue particles to implant and grow. Further support for Sampson's [12] 'metastatic theory' is the observation of endometriotic foci in laparotomy scars after Caesarean section or episiotomy scars following delivery. Additionally, lymphatic or vascular spread is postulated for the presence of endometriosis in extragenital localizations such as lung or skeletal muscle [15]. Finally, the anatomical distribution of endometriosis in relation to the uterine position adds further support to the transplantation hypothesis [16].

Metaplastic theory

On the other hand, Sampson's theory [12] cannot explain endometriosis in women with primary amenorrhoea [17], Müllerian anomalies without functional uterine endometrium (Meyer–Rokitansky–Küster syndrome) or the rare event of development of endometriosis in male patients [18]. In these cases, the induction of metaplastic changes in pluripotent coelomic cells, thus resulting in endometriotic tissue, gives a convincing explanation. The 'metaplastic theory' was first postulated by Meyer [19], who suggested repeated irritation of the coelomic epithelium to be the initiating factor of the metaplastic process. Novak [20] suggested that hormonal stimuli might be the activating factor. Additional support is given in some way by the studies of Murphy *et al.* [21] and Brosens *et al.* [22], who demonstrated microscopic implants of endometriosis beneath macroscopically normal peritoneum.

It is still unclear whether endometriotic implants are derived from *in situ* located pluripotential cells or generated by metastatic seeding, but it is known that genetic, endocrine and immunological factors allow the growth and spread within the pelvis and neighbouring organs (Fig. 2.1).

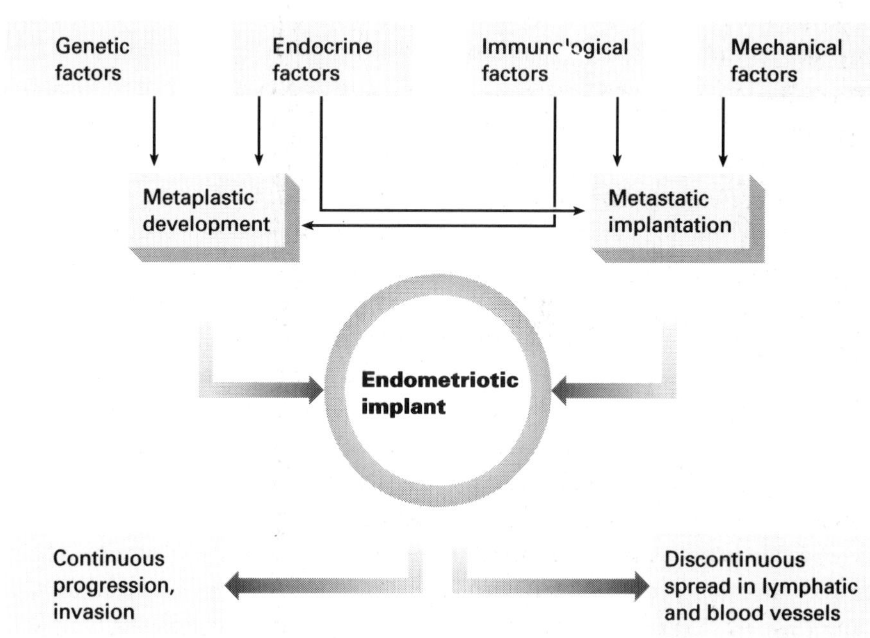

Fig. 2.1 Aetiology and histogenesis of endometriosis.

Light microscopic and ultrastructural appearances

Endometriotic tissue resembles eutopic uterine endometrium. In consequence, the two major components are present: on the one hand the epithelial component, identified as glands or as superficial epithelium, and on the other hand the mesenchymal component of stromal cells. Both cell types are pluripotential and can undergo various changes, e.g. a reaction to the influence of endogenous or exogenous hormones.

Morphological changes in the normal uterine endometrium throughout the physiological 28-day cycle have been described by numerous reports. It was the work of Noyes *et al.* [23] that first taught us how to 'date' the endometrium histologically. Even though various authors have meanwhile doubted the precision and accuracy of morphological 'dating' alone [24], this basic work still forms the 'gold standard' for studies on morphological cycle variations in eutopic and ectopic endometrium.

During the early proliferative phase the endometrium is low and shows few and narrow glands with a flat regenerating superficial epithelium. The epithelial cells are low columnar with small oval nuclei. The stromal components of the tissue are spindle-shaped and form a loose network of similar, poorly differentiated cells. In the mid-proliferative phase the effect of increasing oestrogen levels is expressed morphologically by a generalized stromal oedema and rapidly growing glands with beginning tortuosity. The epithelial cells become tall columnar and an increasing number of mitoses are seen. The late proliferative phase is characterized by a regression of the oestrogen-induced oedema and continuing growth of the glands, resulting in increasing tortuosity. The epithelial cells begin to pile up and show their nuclei at different levels, imitating a multilayer appearance. The nuclei still remain fusiform while the nuclear-cytoplasmic ratio moves toward the cytoplasm.

Although morphologic changes in the secretory phase have been described precisely day by day [25], for evaluation of cyclic changes in endometriotic foci a dating attempt in three stages of the secretory phase in accordance with the proliferative phase is possible at maximum. In the early secretory phase the glands become corkscrew-shaped while the number of mitoses decreases with the increasing influence of progesterone. The nuclear-cytoplasmic ratio is still in favour of the cytoplasm and basal vacualization pushes the nuclei towards the apical portion of the cells, where they form a uniform row. Changes in the stroma are hardly visible compared with the drastic effect seen on the epithelium. In the mid-secretory phase a dilation of the glands takes place, allowing for the secretion of glycogen into the lumen together with acid and neutral mucopolysaccharides. The nuclei again return to the base of the cells and appear round with clear or pale staining. Together with the peak of oestrogen secretion in the mid-luteal phase, another increase in stromal oedema can be observed. The late secretory phase sees the stromal oedema and glycogen secretion diminishing while spiral arteries appear, together with predecidualization of the stromal cells or their change into small granulocytes. The glandular epithelium is strongly dentated and shows residual secretion in the glandular lumen.

In the earlier comparative studies between eutopic and ectopic endometrium it was often stated that endometriosis reacts precisely in the same manner as uterine endometrium, while later findings could not support these data [26]. Only highly differentiated foci with proliferative activity demonstrate cyclic changes more or less similar to uterine endometrium (Fig. 2.2). In contrast, about one-half of implants, especially endometriotic cysts of the ovary, are poorly differentiated, demonstrating no morphological changes induced by cyclic variations of endogenous hormones (Fig 2.3). In addition, degenerative and regressive features are often found in this group (Fig 2.4). These light microscopic studies were complemented by the first electron microscopic study to compare endometriosis and simultaneously gained uterine eutopic endometrium [27]. Electron microscopic criteria for dating

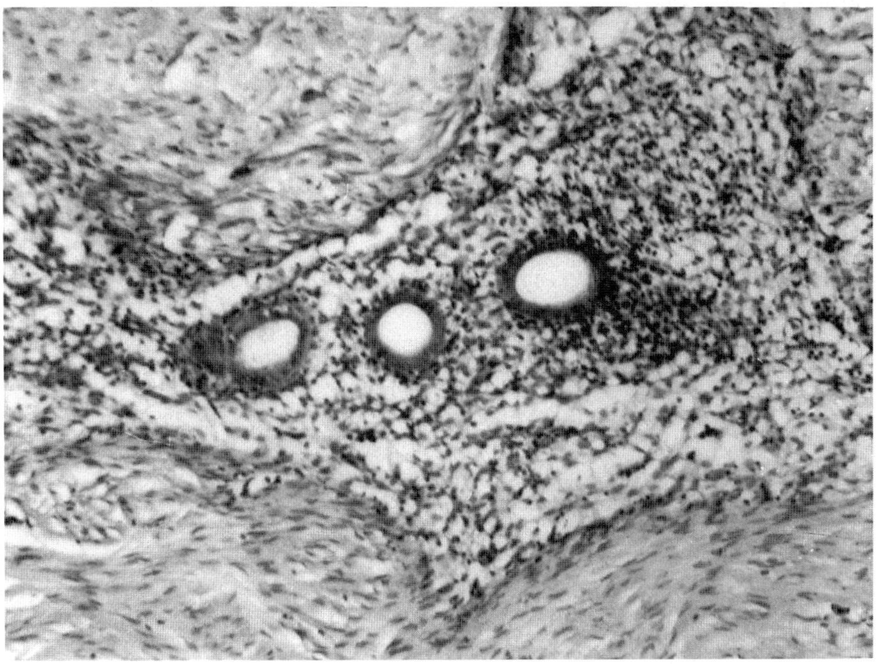

Fig. 2.2 (a) Highly differentiated endometriotic implant from the cul-de-sac showing morphological features resembling the early proliferative phase (HE staining, 65 × magnification).

Continued on p. 22

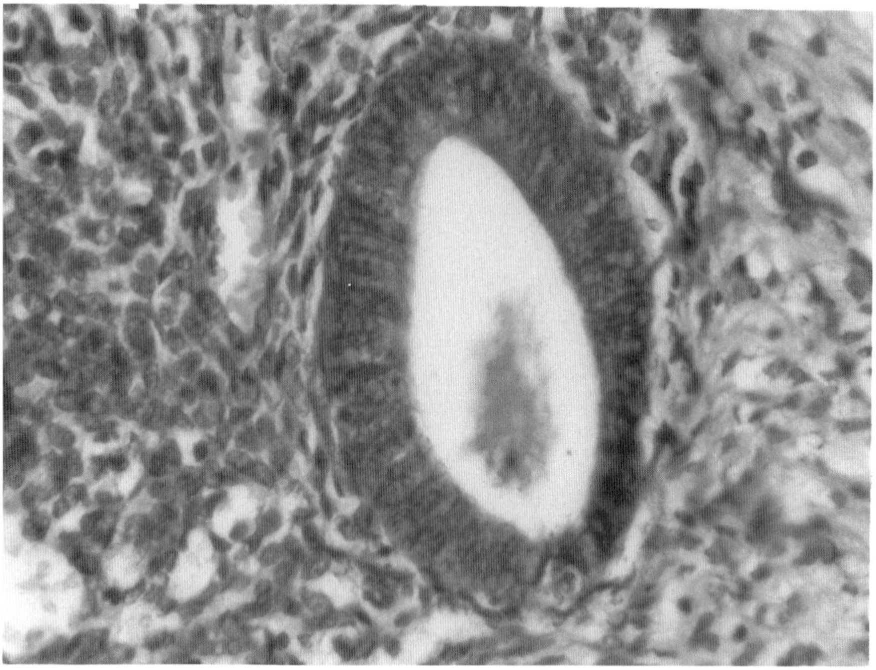

Fig. 2.2 (b) Highly differentiated endometriotic focus from the vesico-uterine pouch with characteristics of late proliferative phase of the menstrual cycle (HE staining, 120 × magnification).

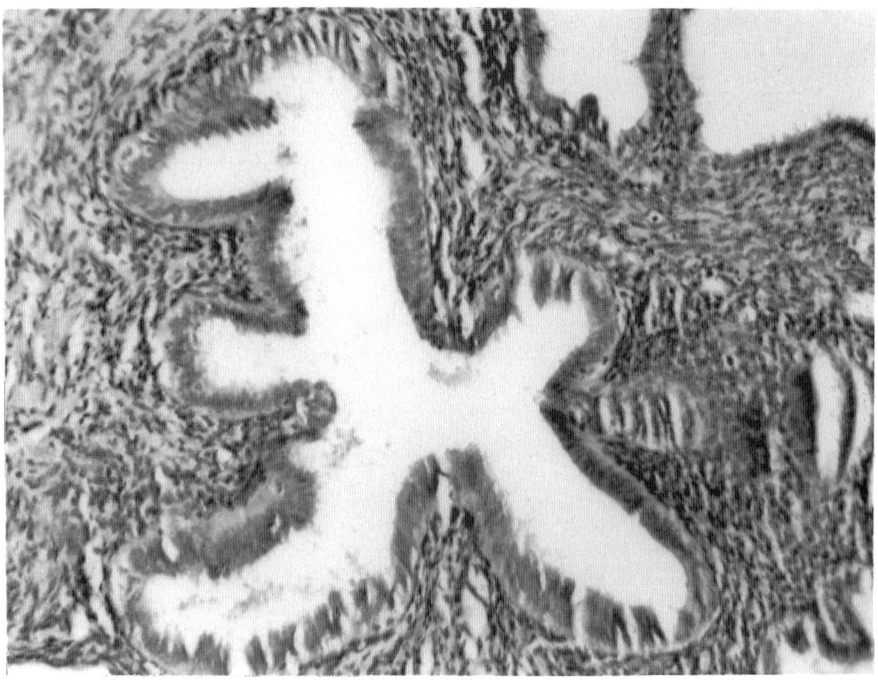

Fig. 2.2 (c) Highly differentiated, endocrine-modulated endometriotic biopsy from the surface of the right ovary with some typical secretory changes (HE staining, 110 × magnification).

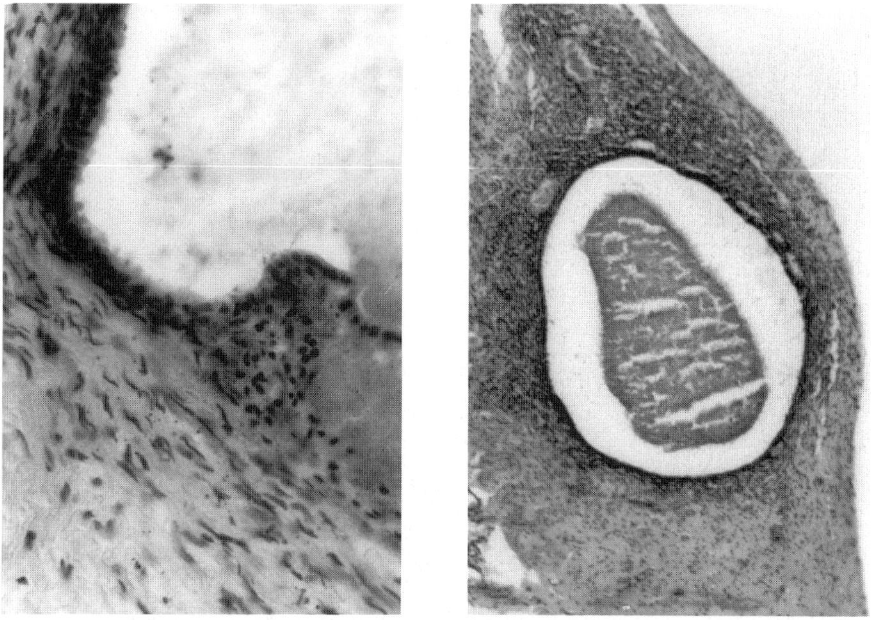

(a) (b)

Fig. 2.3 (a) Poorly differentiated endometriosis with no signs of endocrine changes; cuboidal and cylindrical epithelium partly inactive and partly with secretory changes; biopsy of the mid-proliferative phase from the lining of an ovarian cyst (HE staining, 90 × magnification). (b) No characteristics of hormonal-induced morphological features in a biopsy of the cul-de-sac taken during the mid-secretory phase of a normal cycle (HE staining, 50 × magnification).

the endometriotic foci are listed in Tables 2.1 and 2.2 (modified from [28]). The extension of the above-mentioned study [27] to 92 cases can be summarized as follows:

1 The uterine endometrium was appropriate for the stage of the cycle in all of the cases.

2 In contrast to this, endometriotic foci showed good differentiation in the proliferative phase in only 14 out of 32 implants biopsied (Fig. 2.5). One-third of the implants were clearly out of phase with the cycle and described as delayed. Another 10 endometriotic foci showed various degrees of differentiation within the same biopsy specimen; therefore dating was impossible. In eight implants only poorly differentiated glands were found, showing an autonomous proliferation without any sign of hormonal dependency. 'Ultrastructural dating' of endometriotic foci in the secretory phase of the cycle found 24 out of 60 specimens highly developed, with a reaction to hormones, all but five biopsies being delayed; 23 foci were mixed and 13 were less differentiated and without signs of endocrine modulation (Fig. 2.6).

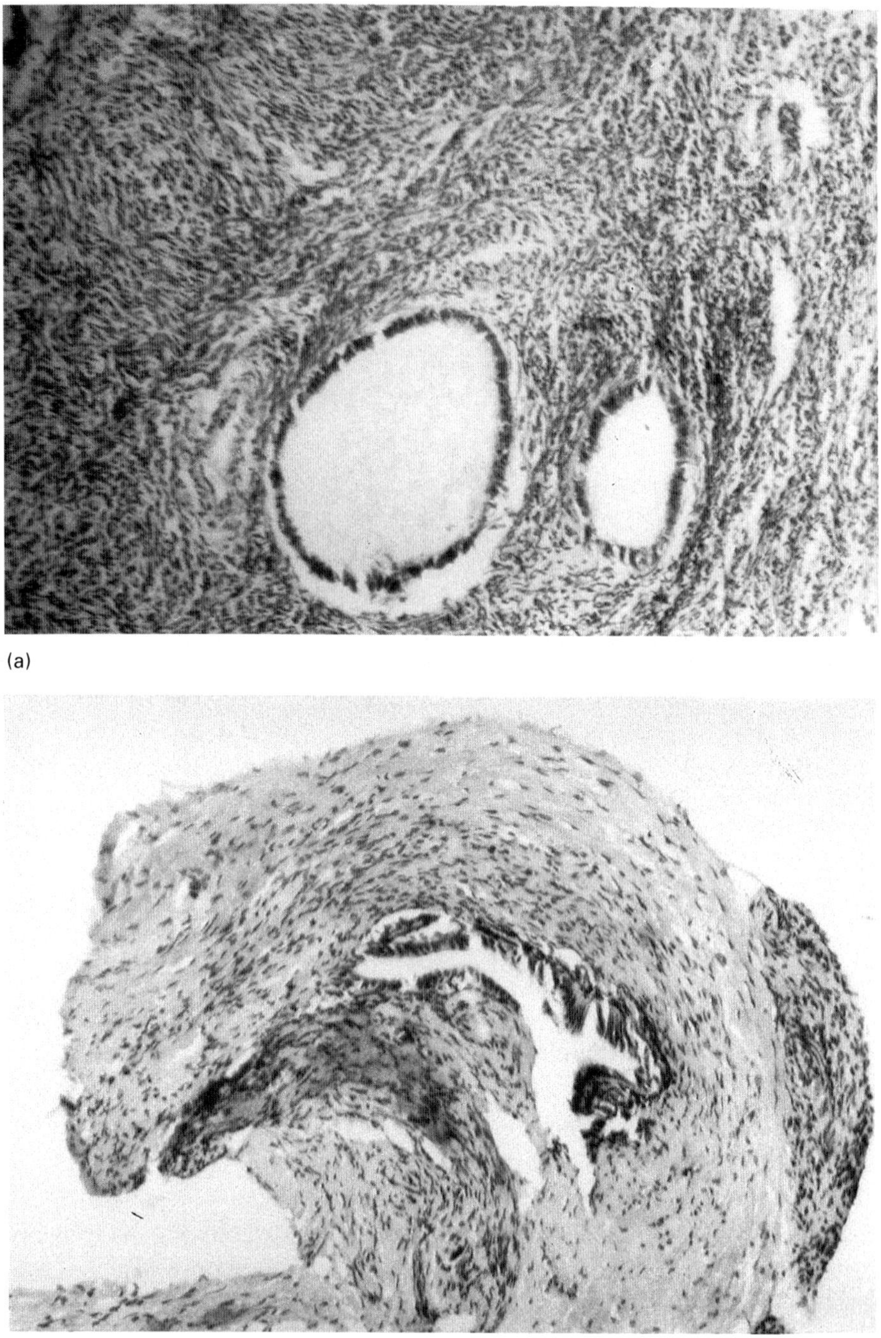

(a)

(b)

Fig. 2.4 (a) Regressive changes of the epithelial lining of endometriotic glands in a biopsy taken from the broad ligament. (HE staining, 60 × magnification). (b) Various signs of degeneration in an endometriotic focus deeply infiltrating the uterosacral ligament (HE staining, 60 × magnification).

Table 2.1 Ultrastructural characteristics of endometriosis in the proliferative phase

	Early proliferative	Mid-proliferative	Late proliferative
Membranes	Straight, uniform; microvilli up to 1.5 μm; basal lamina 300 nm	Apical projections; irregular microvilli	Large projections; irregular microvilli; basal lamina 500 nm
Nucleus	Ovoid, uniform, basal or mid-position; dark clear nucleolus	Undulating contour; basal position	Irregularly shaped; various positions
Organelles	Poorly developed	Mitochondria with more cristae; rough ER	Well-developed mitochondria; rough ER; many free ribosomes

ER, endoplasmic reticulum.

Table 2.2 Ultrastructural characteristics of endometriosis in the secretory phase

	Early secretory	Mid-secretory	Late secretory
Membranes	Irregular, large projections; stubby microvilli	Maximal projections; short microvilli	Variable projections; irregular microvilli
Nucleus	Irregular, often apical position; some invaginations	Irregular-shaped; variable position; deep invaginations	Irregular-shaped; clumping of chromatin
Organelles	Well-developed Golgi complexes, ribosomes and mitochondria	Maximal developed Golgi complexes; secretory vesicles	Variation in size; most in regression; rough ER decreased

ER, endoplasmic reticulum.

The above-described data [28] suggest an incomplete response of endometriosis to the prevalent hormonal milieu. A recent study by Metzger *et al.* [29] found evidence for the fact that this impaired responsiveness to endogenous hormones might be related to the architectural relationships between the cellular elements found in normal endometrium. The authors derived this from the observation that implants that were 'in phase' with the eutopic endometrium had more stroma surrounding the glands and the amount of fibrosis was inversely related to hormonal responsiveness.

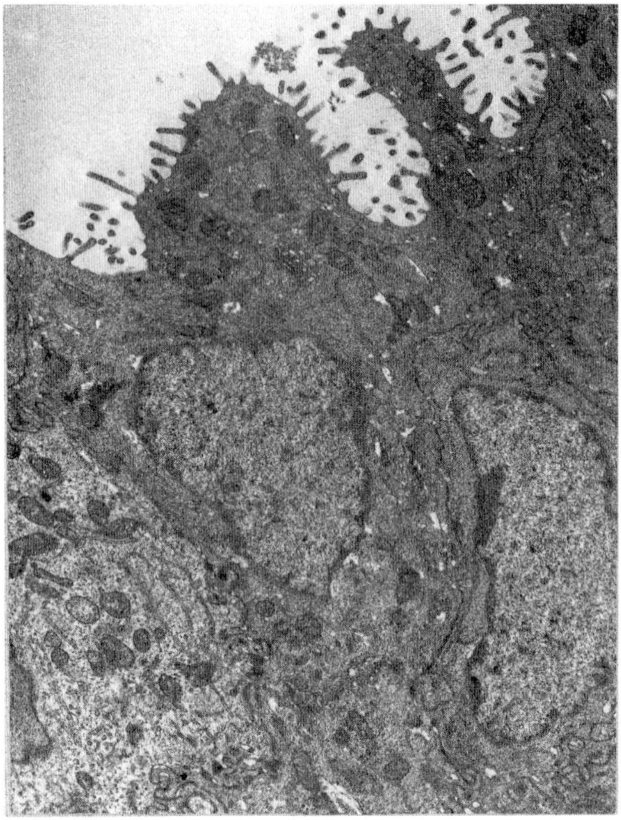

Fig. 2.5 Well-differentiated endometriotic glandular epithelium corresponding to the mid-proliferative phase of the menstrual cycle (3300 × magnification).

Histochemical characterization and proliferation markers

To further elucidate whether endometriosis and endometrium react in the same way, several histochemical factors have been investigated. In spite of the fact that, as has been suggested, the morphological response to endogenous progestins is less than to oestrogens, glycogen and acid as well as neutral polysaccharides do not differ in the two tissues. This indicates that the endometriotic tissue is able to respond to both the oestrogenic and the gestogenic stimulus [30]. The metabolism of oestrone sulphate in endometriotic tissue and in uterine endometrium in the proliferative and secretory cycle phases was clearly different in the two tissues, reaching higher levels in the eutopic than in the ectopic endometrium. Cycle variations of statistical significance were observed in the uterine endometrium only [31]. These observations were in accordance with the findings of Vihko [32], who found lower 17β-hydroxysteroid dehydrogenase (17β-HSD) activity in endometriosis than in

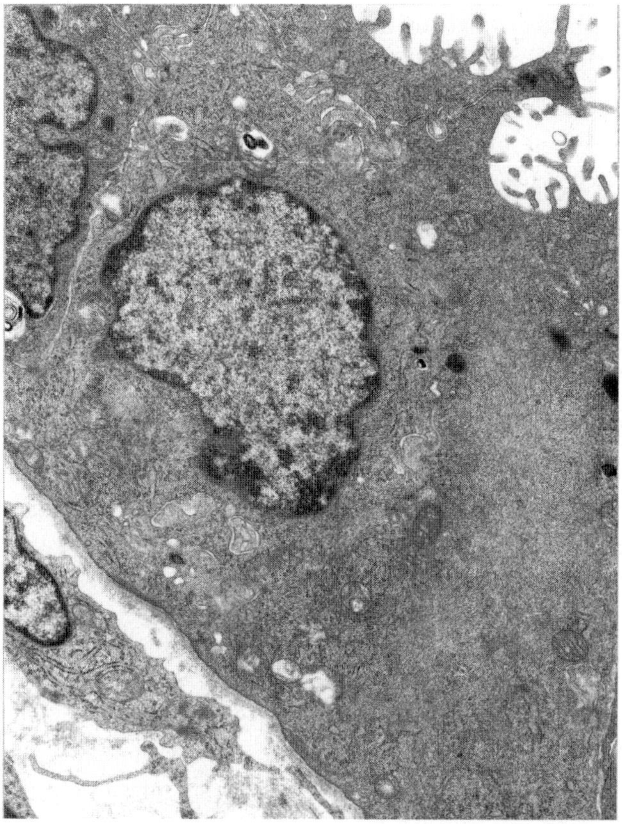

Fig. 2.6 Poorly differentiated glandular epithelium cells showing no sign of modulation by ovarian steroids (4750 × magnification).

endometrium, thus indicating an impaired steroid metabolism in the ectopic tissue.

On the other hand, morphometric studies evaluated vascularization and mitotic activity in macroscopically different peritoneal implants. Nisolle *et al.* [33] conclude that red lesions are very active and may represent the early stage of implantation, in contrast to black and brown implants, which demonstrate inactive and regressive forms. The early and proliferating lesions were further characterized by the presence of the aminoterminal propeptide of type II procollagen, indicating invasion of the extracelluar matrix [34]. Nevertheless, the basement membrane still remains continuously intact [35] and, despite this proliferation and invasion, with different degrees of dysplasia, malignancy arising within a focus of endometriosis is a rare event (far less than 1% of patients with ovarian endometriosis).

Morphological changes after medical treatment for endometriosis

Danazol

Morphological studies to evaluate the possible effects of exogenous steroids on endometriotic tissue are scarce. While as early as 1976 it was reported that danazol has a progestin-like effect on the human endometrium [36], the first systematically performed study on the morphological changes in endometriotic tissue during danazol treatment was published by Schweppe *et al.* in 1984 [37]. Sixteen patients with primary or secondary infertility were treated with 800 mg danazol daily after histological verification of the diagnosis. After 2, 4 and 6 months of hormonal therapy, tissue samples from ectopic endometrium were obtained and investigated by light microscopy and scanning electron microscopy. There were 29 glands available for evaluation. All of them were surrounded by dense inactive stroma. The epithelial layer resembled atrophic, postmenopausal endometrium, with signs of degeneration and without secretory activity (Fig. 2.7). Atypical secretory transformation as reported in earlier studies [36, 38] was not reproducible. The ultrastructural features included a decrease in amount and an increase in density of cytoplasm

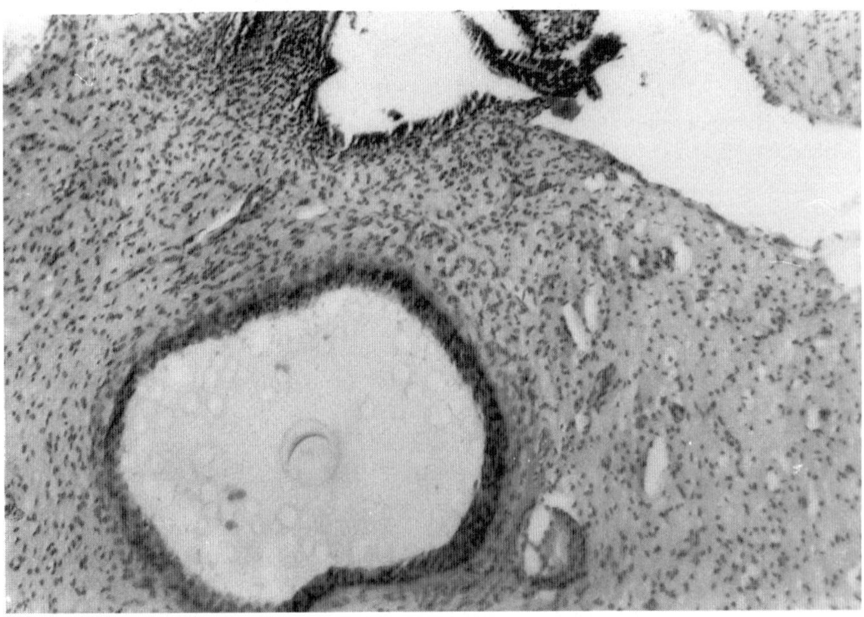

Fig. 2.7 Different degrees of degeneration and atrophic changes in the glandular structures (top) and stroma of an endometriotic focus exposed 6 months to danazol; the gland below is vital with intact epithelial layer showing the features of a proliferative arrest (HE staining, 55 × magnification).

after 2 months of treatment. The nuclei were of normal size but of irregular shape. Free ribosomes and polyribosomes were diffusely distributed in the cytoplasm but only a few parallel channels of smooth and rough endoplasmic reticulum and a few Golgi complexes were found. Only small amounts of secretion could be found in the lumen, while the cells themselves showed no secretory activity. Ciliated cells were located in small groups and generally of normal appearance. After 4 months of treatment changes in ultrastructural appearance were qualitatively the same, even though the above-mentioned criteria were more pronounced. Six months of treatment saw a less homogeneous picture in different areas of the same gland. Some cells appeared to be arrested in the early proliferative stage, with large cytoplasmic projections and normal-looking mitochondria with darkly stained cristae. In other areas, a picture of degeneration was expressed by degenerated mitochondria and a darkly stained degenerating nucleus (Fig. 2.8). Only a few cells retained a

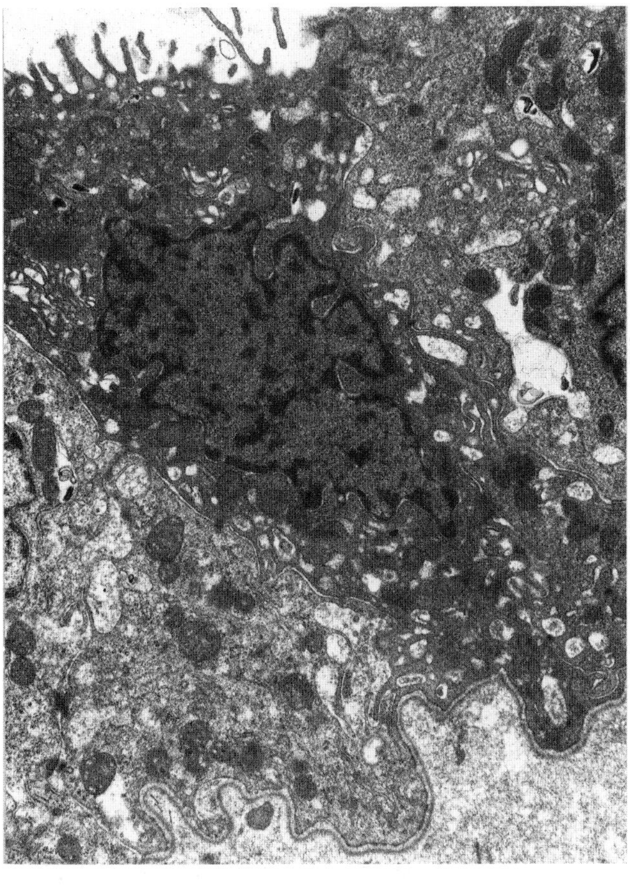

Fig. 2.8 Biopsy from an endometriotic implant after 4 months of influence of 800 mg danazol daily; the darkly stained chromatin of the nucleus and degenerative signs in the organelles of the cytoplasm are clearly seen) (2900 × magnification).

nearly homogeneously granular nucleus, without clumping of chromatin or invaginations of the nuclear envelope. The ultrastructural changes induced in endometriotic glands by danazol can be summarized:

1 Condensation of the cytoplasm, resulting mainly from loss of cellular water.

2 Irregularly curved, superficial intercellular and basal membranes, with degeneration of microvilli.

3 Poorly developed ergastoplasm, often with signs of degeneration, especially in respect to mitochondria.

4 Irregular nuclei, with clumping of chromatin.

5 Increased numbers of giant lysosomes, with homogeneously stained lipoprotein vesicles.

6 Flattening of the cell as a whole.

7 Lack of induced changes in the ciliated cells.

In conclusion, these danazol-induced changes of endometriotic foci resulted in a morphological appearance characterized as 'proliferative arrest'. This condition can be interpreted as a danazol-resistant state, and could be the explanation for no further degeneration and resumption of the disease once the medical treatment has ceased.

Gestrinone

The other steroid which has been evaluated thoroughly with respect to morphological changes is gestrinone. It has contraceptive activity when administered in a weekly dose and possesses weak progestin and marked antiprogesterone activities. Cornillie and coworkers [39] reported a marked involutionary effect on endometriotic glandular epithelium after a period of 4 months' therapy. In terms of ultrastructural features, this is expressed by lysosomal degradation, especially within the apical cytoplasm of the cells. The nucleus appeared to be indented while its chromatin was clumped and the apical microvilli were lost and cytoplasmic lysosomes were extruded. These degenerative processes resulted additionally in a concentration of damaged mitochondria within the supranuclear area. The authors stated that gestrinone-induced effects on endometriosis include a resorption of endometriotic implants by an initiation of involutionary processes similar to those occurring in the premenstrual phase of the cycle. The activation of the lysosomal system is followed by abortive apocrine secretion of cell remnants and finally, but not in all cases, the extrusion of individual epithelial cells. In another study, the effect of a short-term application (2 months) of the drug was evaluated [40]. The morphological effects in the implants had reached the same degree of degeneration and regression and the subsequent pregnancy rate was identical. Therefore the authors suggest [41] further evaluation of short-term treatment regimens in a greater number of patients.

Gonadotrophin-releasing hormone (GnRH) analogues

The effect of GnRH analogues on endometrium has been studied by Fedele and coworkers [42]. Intranasal buserelin (400 μg three times a day) resulted in morphological changes which were seen as the direct consequence of hypo-oestrogenism, resulting in a weakly proliferative or inactive epithelium. Ultrastructural analysis revealed a more marked involution of the cells, impaired cellular respiration, nuclear pyknosis and karyorrhexis. Comparable effects of the drug were seen by investigating vaginal specimens under buserelin therapy [43]. After 3 and 6 months of therapy, a marked hypotrophy with typical appearances of the menopause were observed.

In a recent study [44] we characterized residual endometriosis after a 6-month treatment with the GnRH analogue buserelin. Although in the majority of patients a marked reduction in revised American Fertility Society (RAFS) implant score was observed, in 34 of the 69 women remnants of the disease could be proved histologically. According to light microscopic criteria, regressive changes were seen in 52% of implants (Fig. 2.9), whereas 29%

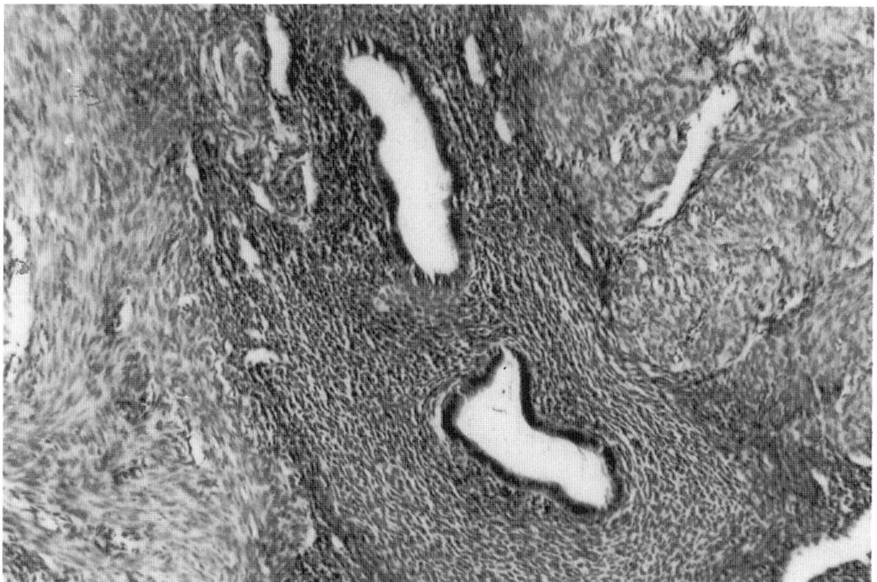

Fig. 2.9 Regressive changes of implants in the wall of an endometriotic cyst and condensed atrophic stroma after 6 months of suppression with buserelin 900 μg daily (HE staining, 55 × magnification).

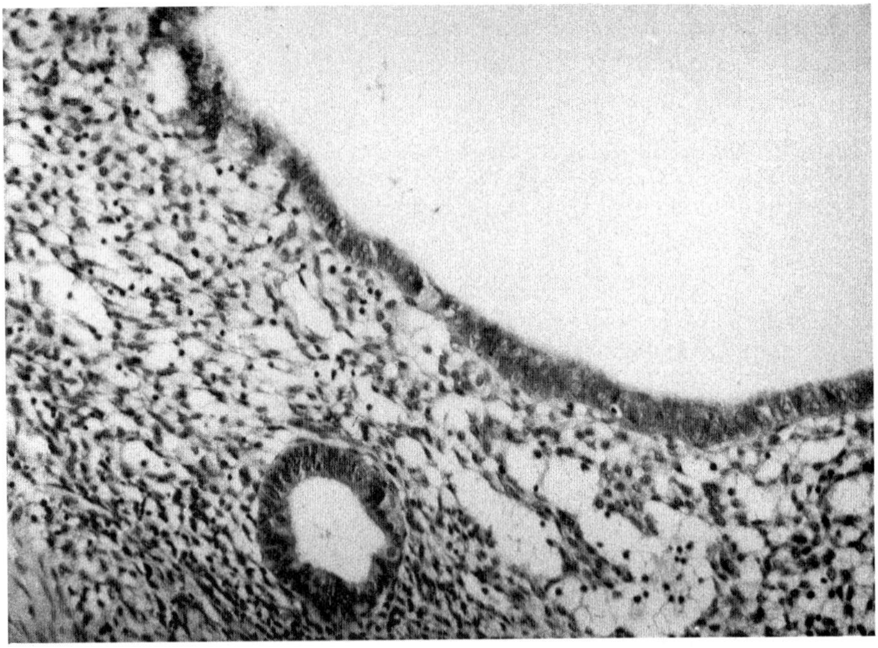

Fig. 2.10 Typical autonomously proliferative endometriotic glands in a biopsy of the peritoneum of the broad ligament after 6 months of ovarian suppression using intranasal buserelin 900 μg/day (HE staining, 65 × magnification).

presented with proliferative elements (Fig. 2.10) of the disease. In 19% proliferation and regression were seen in the same biopsy specimen. Histology did not relate to either the degree of ovarian suppression or the location of the residual endometriotic foci. The latter is in contradiction to the findings of Nisolle-Pochet *et al.* [45], who found in ovarian implants 97% of cases had residual endometriosis after GnRH therapy.

Hormone receptors in endometriotic tissue

The mechanism of action of steroid hormones on their target tissues is believed to be receptor-mediated. These receptors are cytoplasmic proteins that specifically and rapidly bind the steroid as it diffuses into the cell. In most cells of a target organ, some 10 000 of such steroid receptors exist in the cytoplasm. The concentration varies within the cycle, the hormonal pretreatment and other factors. If a steroid fails to stimulate its target organ, it is generally believed that it lacks binding sites for that specific hormone [46]. In the mechanism of action, after binding of the steroid to its cytoplasmic receptor protein the complex is then translocated into the nucleus. Here it exerts its effects on the genome by interacting with nuclear chromatin, causing the production of a specific set of messenger ribonucleic acids (RNAs) which modifies the target cell itself.

In the female genital trace the vagina, uterus, ovary and Fallopian tubes have been reported as possessing oestrogen receptors to a varying degree and with variations during the cycle. On the other hand, the synthesis of the progesterone receptor is induced by oestrogen action in hormonally responsive target cells. Androgen receptors do exist in human endometrium, but in far lower concentrations than those of the other steroid receptors. Cyclic changes of receptors within the human endometrium vary due to the effects of endogenous steroids: in the early follicular phase oestrogen receptors gradually increase to a maximum in the late proliferative phase. On the other hand, in the luteal phase of the cycle cytoplasmic oestrogen receptors gradually decrease, reaching levels even below those at the onset of the cycle. Progesterone receptor content is maximal prior to and immediately after ovulation. In the luteal phase the total concentration of progesterone receptors gradually falls, due to a sharp decrease in cytosolic receptors, while the nuclear fraction remains at high levels, corresponding to the luteal secretion of progesterone. Androgen receptor sites were far fewer and did not change noticeably during the menstrual cycle [47].

Oestrogen and progestogen receptors have been detected in endometriotic tissue by several authors. Since the first report of Tamaya *et al.* [48], who used biochemical assays, immunohistochemical detection of binding sites has been established. All authors agree that oestrogen receptors are significantly lower in endometriotic tissue than in endometriosis. In addition, hormone receptors are not found in all of the biopsies examined. Jänne and coworkers [49], as well as Bergqvist *et al.* [50], identified oestrogen receptors in no more than 30% of specimens, indicating that many endometriotic cells are not yet or are no longer capable of responding to the cyclical changes in plasma steroids.

The relation to the success of endocrine therapy has been studied extensively by Kauppila *et al.* [51]. Concentrations of cytosolic and nuclear oestrogen and progesterone receptor levels, as well as the activity of 17β-HSD, in endometrium and endometriosis were compared (Fig. 2.11). The concentrations of cytosol receptors were significantly higher in endometrium than in endometriosis. After hormonal suppressive therapy with danazol or high-dose medroxyprogesterone acetate, the activity of 17β-HSD was increased more than 10-fold, compared with that of untreated proliferative endometrium. In contrast, no increase was observed in endometriotic lesions. In addition, the concentrations of oestrogen receptors as well as progesterone receptors in uterine endometrium decreased significantly, but no differences induced by hormonal therapy were found in endometriotic tissues. The authors concluded from their studies that hormonal control of ectopic and

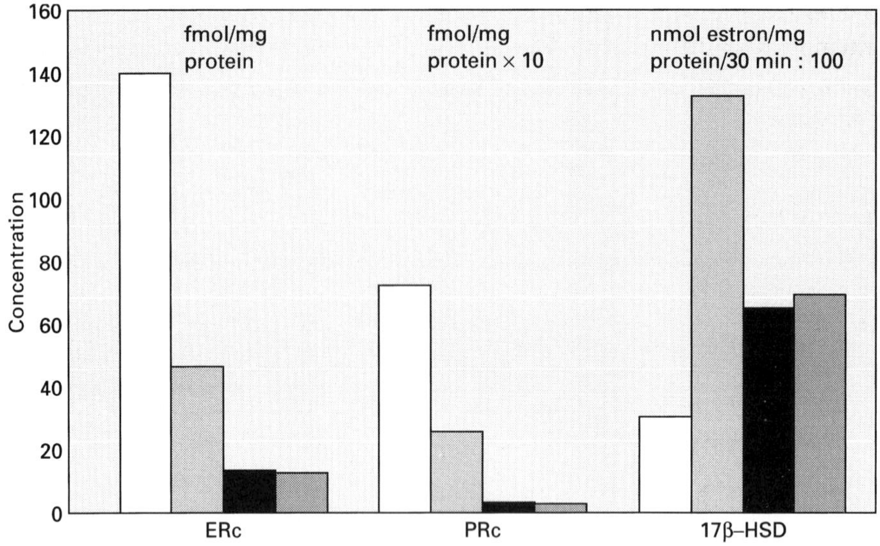

Fig. 2.11 Receptor and enzyme concentrations in uterine endometrium and endometriosis before and after therapy by ovarian suppression using danazol and/or medroxyprogesterone-acetate. White, endometrium untreated; dark grey, endometrium treated; black, endometriosis untreated; light grey, endometriosis treated. Redrawn from [51] with permission.

eutopic endometrium is different. This is in agreement with other studies mentioned in this chapter and may well add further support to the observation that clinical success of hormonal therapy is not complete and varies within patients as well as at different foci within the same patient.

In a subsequent continuation of these data, Bergqvist and Fernö [52] recently published a study to evaluate differences in oestrogen and progestogen receptor content in primary and recurrent disease. In primary endometriotic lesions, both oestrogen and progesterone receptors were significantly lower than in endometrium. In recurrent lesions, however, the progesterone receptor level was significantly higher than in ectopic tissue examined at the first diagnosis of the disease. Oestrogen receptor content revealed no difference. Whether lesions with high progesterone receptor levels tend to recur more easily, as suggested by this study, needs further investigation.

Conclusion

Derived from the above published knowledge, detailed evaluation of morphological features appears useful. Information about the relation between the two components of endometriotic tissue as well as light microscopic criteria about the degree of differentiation, the similarity to uterine endometrium and cyclic modulation may give hints whether endocrine treatment attempts may stand a chance of regressing the disease. Additional clues are given in respect to a possible explanation of pathogenetic and aetiological pathways.

References

1 Fedele L, Parazzini F, Bianchi S, Arcaini L, Candiani GB. Stage and localization of pelvic endometriosis and pain. *Fertil Steril* 1990 **53**: 155.

2 Fukaya T, Hoshiai H, Yajima A. Is pelvic endometriosis always associated with chronic pain? A retrospective study of 618 cases diagnosed by laparoscopy. *Am J Obstet Gynecol* 1993 **169**: 719.

3 Konninckx PR, Meuleman C, Demeyre S, Lesaffre E, Cornillie FJ. Suggestive evidence that pelvic endometriosis is a progressive disease whereas deeply infiltrating endometriosis is associated with pelvic pain. *Fertil Steril* 1991 **55**: 759.

4 Cornillie FJ, Oosterlynck D, Lauweryns JM, Konninckx PR. Deeply infiltrating pelvic endometriosis: histology and clinical significance. *Fertil Steril* 1990 **53**: 978.

5 Wentz AC. Premenstrual spotting: its association with endometriosis but not luteal phase inadequacy. *Fertil Steril* 1980 **39**: 656.

6 Mais V, Guerriero S, Anjossa S *et al.* The efficiency of transvaginal ultrasonography in the diagnosis of endometrioma. *Fertil Steril* 1993 **60**: 776.

7 Jansen RPS, Russell P. Non-pigmented endometriosis: clinical, laparoscopic and pathological definition. *Am J Obstet Gynecol* 1986 **115**: 1154.

8 Donnez J, Nisolle M, Casanas-Roux F. Three dimensional architectures of peritoneal endometriosis. *Fertil Steril* 1992 **57**: 980.

9 Redwine DB. Age-related evolution in color appearance of endometriosis. *Fertil Steril* 1987 **48**: 1062.

10 Semm K. *Pelviscopy and Hysteroscopy*, 1976. Stuttgart, FK Schattauer.

11 Bühler K, Thaele M, Thaele S, Schindler EM. Cytology for microscopical verification of endometriosis. In: Brosens I, Donnez J (eds). *The Current Status of Endometriosis Research and Management*, 1993 p.67. Carnforth, Parthenon Publishing Group.

12 Sampson JA. The development of the implantation theory for the origin of peritoneal endometriosis. *Am J Obstet Gynecol* 1940 **40**: 549.

13 Halme Y, Hammond MG, Hulka JF, Ray SG, Talbert LM. Retrograde menstruation in healthy women and in patients with endometriosis. *Obstet Gynecol* 1984 **64**: 151.

14 Kirshon B, Poindexter AN III. Contraception: a risk factor for endometriosis. *Obstet Gynecol* 1988 **71**: 829.

15 Javert CT. Pathogenesis of endometriosis based on endometrial homeoplasia, direct extension, exfoliation and implantation, lymphatic and hematogenous metastasis. *Cancer* 1949 **2**: 399.

16 Jenkins S, Olive DL, Haney AF. Endometriosis: pathogenic implications of the anatomic distribution. *Obstet Gynecol* 1986 **67**: 335.

17 Peress MR, Sosnowski JR, Mathur RS, Williamson HO. Pelvic endometriosis and Turner's syndrome. *Am J Obstet Gynecol* 1982 **144**: 474.

18 Martin JD Jr, Hauck AE. Endometriosis in the male. *Am Surg* 1985 **51**: 426.

19 Meyer R. Über den Stand der Adenomyositis und Adenomyome im Allgemeinen und Insbesondere über Adenomyositis serosepithelialis und Adenomyometritis sarcomatosa. *Zbl Gynäk* 1919 **43**: 745.

20 Novak E. Pelvic endometriosis. *Am J Gynecol* 1931 **22**: 826.

21 Murphy AA, Green WR, Bobby D, DelaCruz ZC, Rock JA. Unsuspected endometriosis documented by scanning electron microscopy in visually normal peritoneum. *Fertil Steril* 1986 **46**: 522.

22 Brosens I, Vasquez G, Gordts S. Scanning electron microscopy study of the pelvic peritoneum in unexplained infertility and endometriosis. (Abstract) *Fertil Steril* 1984 **41**: 215.

23 Noyes RW, Hertig AT, Rock J. Dating the endometrial biopsy. *Fertil Steril* 1950 **1**: 3.

24 Li T-C, Dockery P, Rogers AW, Cook ID. How precise is histologic dating of endometrium using the standard dating criteria? *Fertil Steril* 1989 **51**: 759.

25 Dallenbach-Hellweg G. *Histopathology of the Endometrium*, 1987. Berlin, Springer.

26 Bergqvist A, Ljungberg O, Myhre E. Human endometrium and endometriotic tissue obtained simultaneously: a comparative histologic study. *Int J Gynecol Pathol* 1984 **3**: 135.

27 Schweppe K-W, Wynn RM. Ultrastructural changes in endometriotic implants during the menstrual cycle. *Obstet Gynecol* 1981 **58**: 465.

28 Schweppe K-W, Wynn RM, Beller FK. Ultrastructural comparison of endometriotic implants and eutopic endometrium. *Am J Obstet Gynecol* 1984 **148**: 1024.

29 Metzger DA, Szpak CA, Haney AF. Histologic features associated with morphologic responsiveness of ectopic endometrium. *Fertil Steril* 1993 **59: 83.**

30 Bergqvist A, Myhre E. Glycogen and acid and neutral polysaccharides in endometriotic tissue and in uterine endometrium: a comparative histochemical study. *Int J Gynecol Pathol* 1986 **5**: 338.

31 Carlström K, Bergqvist A, Ljungberg O. Metabolism of estrone sulfate in endometriotic tissue and endometrium in proliferative and secretory cycle phases. *Fertil Steril* 1988 **49**: 229.

32 Vihko R, Isotalo H, Kauppila A, Rönnberg L, Vierikko P. Hormonal regulation of endometrium and endometriosis tissue. In: Raynaud J-P, Ojasoo T, Martini, L (eds). *Medical Management of Endometriosis*, 1984, p. 79. New York, Raven Press.

33 Nisolle M, Casanas-Roux F, Anaf V, Mine JM, Donnez J. Morphometric study of the stromal vascularization in peritoneal endometriosis. *Fertil Steril* 1993 **59**: 684.

34 Spuijbroek MDEH, Dunselman GAJ, Menheere PPCA, Evers JLH. Early endometriosis invades the extracelluar matrix. *Fertil Steril* 1992 **58**: 929.

35 Evers JLH, Willebrand D. The basement membrane in endometriosis. *Fertil Steril* 1987 **47**: 505.

36 Wentz AC, Jones GS, Sapp KC, King TM. Progestational activity of danazol in the human female subject. *Am J Obstet Gynecol* 1976 **126**: 378.

37 Schweppe K-W, Dmowski WP, Wynn RM. Ultrastructural changes in endometriotic tissue during danazol treatment. *Fertil Steril* 1984 **36**: 20.

38 Kokko E, Jänne O, Kauppila A, Rönnberg L, Vikho R. Danazol has progestin like action on the human endometrium. *Acta Obstet Gynecol Scand (Suppl)* 1981 **101**: 53.

39 Cornillie FJ, Vasquez G, Brosens I. The response of human endometriotic implants to the antiprogesterone steroid R 2323: a histological and ultrastructural study. *Path Res Pract* 1985 **180**: 647.

40 Brosens IA, Verleyen A, Cornillie F. The morphological effect of a short term medical therapy of endometriosis. *Am J Obstet Gynecol* 1987 **157**: 1215.

41 Cornillie FJ, Brosens IA, Vasquez G, Riphagen I. Histologic and ultrastructural changes in human endometriotic implants treated with the antiprogesterone steroid ethylnorgestrienone (gestrinone) during 2 months. *Int J Gynecol Pathol* 1986 **5**: 95.

42 Fedele L, Marchini M, Bianchi S *et al.* Endometrial patterns during danazol and buserelin therapy for endometriosis: comparative structural and ultrastructural study. *Obstet Gynecol* 1990 **76**: 79.

43 Fedele L, Marchini M, Bianchi S, Baglioni A, Zanotti F: Vaginal patterns during danazol

and buserelin acetate therapy for endometriosis: structural and ultrastructural study. *Fertil Steril* 1993 **59**: 1191.
44 Ochs H, Cirkel U, Schweppe K-W, Schneider HPG. Residualendometriose nach LHRH-Analogtherapie. *Geburtsh Frauenheilk* 1990 **50**: 140.
45 Nisolle-Pochet M, Casanas-Roux F, Donnez J. Histological study of ovarian endometriosis after hormonal therapy. *Fertil Steril* 1988 **49**: 423.
46 Baxter JD, Funder JW. Hormone receptors. *N Engl J Med* 1979 **301**: 1149.
47 Tamaya T, Murakami T, Okada H. Concentrations of steroid receptors in normal human endometrium in relation to the day of the menstrual cycle. *Acta Obstet Gynecol Scand* 1986 **65**: 195.
48 Tamaya T, Motoyama T, Ohono Y *et al.* Steroid receptor levels and histology of endometriosis and adenomyosis. *Fertil Steril* 1979 **31**: 396.
49 Jänne O, Kauppila A, Kokko E *et al.* Estrogen and progestin receptors in endometriosis lesions: comparison with endometrial tissue. *Am J Obstet Gynecol* 1981 **141**: 562.
50 Bergqvist A, Rannevik G, Thorell J. Estrogen and progesterone cytosol receptor concentration in endometriotic tissue and intrauterine endometrium. *Acta Obstet Gynecol Scand (Suppl)* 1981 **101**: 53.
51 Kauppila A, Vierikko P, Isotalo H, Rönnberg L, Vihko R. Cytosol estrogen and progestin receptor concentrations and 17β-hydroxysteroid dehydrogenase activities in the endometrium and endometriotic tissue. *Acta Obstet Scand Suppl* 1984 **123**: 45.
52 Bergqvist A, Fernö M: Estrogen and progesterone receptors in endometriotic tissue and endometrium: comparison according to localization and recurrence. *Fertil Steril* 1993 **60**: 63.

Chapter 3
Morphology of the Implant: Two- and Three-dimensional Evaluation

J. DONNEZ, M. NISOLLE AND F. CASANAS-ROUX

Introduction

Endometriosis most commonly affects the pelvic peritoneum close to the ovaries, including the uterosacral ligaments, the ovarian fossa peritoneum and the peritoneum of the cul-de-sac. The diagnosis of peritoneal endometriosis at the time of laparoscopy is often made by the observation of typically puckered black or bluish lesions. There are, in addition, numerous subtle appearances of peritoneal endometriosis [1–6]. These lesions, frequently non-pigmented, were diagnosed as endometriosis following confirmation by biopsy by Jansen and Russell in 1986 [7].

Morphology of typical black lesions

The typical black peritoneal endometriotic lesion results from tissue bleeding and retention of blood pigment, producing brown discoloration of tissue (Plate 3.1a, facing p. 50). Puckered black lesions are a combination of glands, stroma and intraluminal debris (Plate 3.1b, facing p. 50).

Menstrual shedding from a viable endometrial implant initiates an inflammatory reaction, which provokes a scarification process, which, in turn, encloses the implants. The presence of entrapped menstrual debris is responsible for the typical black or bluish appearance. If the inflammatory process obliterates or devascularizes the endometrial cells, eventually this discoloration disappears. A white plaque of old collagen is all that remains of the ectopic implant. Scarring of the peritoneum around endometrial implants is a typical finding. In addition to encapsulating an isolated implant, the scar may deform the surrounding peritoneum or result in the development of adhesions.

Classification and morphology of subtle appearances

The non-pigmented endometriotic peritoneal lesions include essentially the following (Table 3.1).

Table 3.1 Different appearances of peritoneal endometriosis

Black	Typical puckered black lesion
Red	Red flame-like lesions [7] Glandular excrescences [7] Petechial peritoneum [15] Areas of hypervascularization [15]
White	White opacification [7] Subovarian adhesions [7] Yellow-brown peritoneal patches [7] Circular peritoneal defects [9]

Red lesions

1 Red flame-like lesions of the peritoneum or red vesicular excrescences (Plate 3.2a, facing p. 50) more commonly affecting the broad ligament and the uterosacral ligaments. Histologically, red flame-like lesions and vesicular excrescences are due to the presence of active endometriosis surrounded by stroma (Plate 3.2b, facing p. 50).

2 Glandular excrescences on the peritoneal surface which in colour, translucency and consistency closely resemble the mucosal surface of the endometrium seen at hysteroscopy. Biopsy reveals the presence of numerous endometrial glands which are very active and mostly synchromous with eutopic endometrium.

3 Areas of petechial peritoneum or areas with hypervascularization were diagnosed as endometriosis in our recent study [8]. These lesions resemble the petechial lesions resulting from the manipulation of the peritoneum or from hypervascularization of the peritoneum. They most generally affect the bladder and the broad ligament, and, histologically, red blood cells are numerous and endometrial glands are very rare.

White lesions

1 White opacification of the peritoneum which appears as peritoneal scarring or as circumscribed patches, often thickened and sometimes raised. Histologically, white opacified peritoneum is due to the presence of an occasional retroperitoneal glandular structure and scanty stroma surrounded by fibrotic tissue or connective tissue (Plate 3.3, facing p. 50).

2 Subovarian adhesions or adherence between the ovary and the peritoneum of the ovarian fossa, which are distinct from adhesions characteristic of previous salpingitis or peritonitis. Histologically, connective tissue with sparse endometrial glands was found.

3 Yellow-brown peritoneal patches resembling *café au lait* patches. The histological characteristics are similar to those observed in white opacification, but in the yellow-brown patches the presence of the blood pigment – haemosiderin – among the stroma cells produces the *café au lait* colour.
4 Circular peritoneal defects as described by Chatman [9]. Serial section demonstrates the presence of endometrial glands in more than 50% of cases. Peritoneal endometriosis can thus be found in the visually normal peritoneum of infertile women with or without associated endometriosis.

Morphometric study of the vascularization

Vascularization

Vascularization of endometriotic implants is probably one of the most important factors of growth and invasion of endometrial glands in other tissue. A stereometric analysis was applied in order to study precisely the vascularization in peritoneal endometriotic foci. We evaluated histologically the vascularization of typical peritoneal endometriosis and its modifications according to the macroscopic appearance of peritoneal endometriosis.

A two-dimensional (2-D) image analysis program set on a Vidas computer (Kontron Bildanalyse GmbH, Eching, Germany) was completed by the interactive counting of 262 144 points.

All endometriotic lesions ($n = 220$) were analysed field by field using the objective 40 × of an Axioskop light microscope (Zeiss, Oberkochen, Germany) and a television camera (Dage – MTI, Michigan City, IN). The histological features were displayed on a television monitor and stored in the memory for processing by the measuring program. The mean of fields analysed in each case was 13.3 ± 6.7. Histologic structures of interest, such as the stroma, the glandular epithelium and lumen, capillaries and lymphocytes, were drawn moving a cursor (Plate 3.4, facing p. 50). Each different structure was discriminated and grey level images were transferred to binary images. The interactive measurements of the selected parameters (number of structures, area and perimeter of the structures per field) were appended and stored at the end of an existing data base.

Data management and evaluation was checked according to specific search criteria on the Videoplan (Kontron Bildanalyse GmbH, Eching, Germany) and displayed on the television monitor and printed.

The results concerning the capillaries are shown in Table 3.2. The number of capillaries per mm^2 of stroma, their mean surface area and the surface area ratio (capillaries/stroma) were calculated. The mitotic index was calculated in glandular epithelium and its value was 0.1‰ and 0.61‰ respectively in typical and red lesions. In white lesions, no mitosis was observed. The vascularization

Table 3.2 Morphometric study of the stromal vascularization

	Typical lesions	Subtle lesions		Treated typical lesions
	Black Group Ia *n* = 135	Red lesions Group Ib *n* = 35	White lesions Group Ic *n* = 50	Group Id *n* = 45
Number of capillaries/mm^2 stroma	243	147	206	225
Capillary mean surface (μm^2)	118 ± 84	234 ± 192*	78 ± 43†	71 ± 40†
Capillaries/stroma relative surface (%)	2.4	3.2*	1.5†	1.4†

* Significantly different from groups Ic and Id.
† Significantly different from group Ia.
From [8] with permission.

of typical peritoneal endometriosis was evaluated in 45 patients after gonadotrophin-releasing hormone agonist (GnRh-a) therapy.

Our study demonstrated significant differences between the typical (black or bluish) lesion and the 'subtle' lesion. Subtle lesions were classified as red lesions (vesicular, red flame-like and glandular excrescences) and as white lesions (white opacification, yellow-brown patches and circular peritoneal defects). When compared with typical black lesion data, the vascularization was found to be significantly higher in red lesions and significantly lower in white lesions. This change was due to an increase (red) or a decrease (white) in the volume occupied by the vessels, as proved by both the mean capillary surface area and the ratio of capillaries/stroma surface area. This change is more evident in the group of red lesions, in which the number of capillaries/mm^2 was significantly lower than in the other subgroups.

In the red lesions (Plate 3.5a, facing p. 50), the increased level of vascularization is due to a greater number of larger vessels than in the other groups. In white lesions (Plate 3.5b, facing p. 50), there was a great number of smaller vessels, and the number of capillaries was higher than in red lesions.

Moreover, the mitotic index [10] was also significantly different in the three groups. Mitotic processes permit the maintenance and the growth of peritoneal endometriosis. The absence of mitosis in white lesions proves their low 'activity' [8].

According to our data, we suggest that there are probably different types of peritoneal endometriotic lesions, in different stages of development. Red flame-like lesions and glandular excrescences are probably the first stage of early implantation of endometrial glands and stroma. The significantly higher stromal vascularization and epithelial mitotic index could be responsible for the invasion of glands and stroma into the ectopic sites.

Our results demonstrated that there was a significant decrease in the vascularization of the endometriotic foci after GnRH-a therapy. This change was not due to a reduction in the number of capillaries in the lesion but to a decrease in the area of the vessels. After GnRH-a, a predominance of smaller vessels was observed when compared with the non-treated black lesions.

This vascularization decrease, observed histologically, was in accordance with the observations made by laparoscopy after hormonal therapy. Vascular effects of the GnRH-a have also been demonstrated by Doppler on the uterine arteries [11]. The hypo-oestrogenaemia induced by GnRH-a could also have an effect on the vascular compartment of the endometriotic stroma. The reduction in the vascularization after hormonal therapy could account for the decrease in the inflammatory reaction observed around the endometriotic foci.

In conclusion, the evaluation of the stromal vascularization permitted the differentiation and classification of the different appearances of peritoneal endometriosis according to their level of vascularization. Our study proves that the 'activity' of peritoneal endometriosis is related to the vascularity.

Three-dimensional (3-D) architecture of endometriosis

A recently advanced stereographic computer technique [12–14] was applied to the investigation of the three-dimensional (3-D) architectures of peritoneal endometriosis [15], in order to elucidate further biological characteristics of peritoneal endometriotic lesions – for example, how they stereologically develop *in vivo* and how glandular epithelium and stroma are related to the surrounding tissue.

Computer-assisted reconstruction of 3-D models was developed with two main aims in mind: (i) to generate a complete multicoloured model of a complex structure which can be rotated and viewed from any angle or orientation; and (ii) to calculate the volumes and surfaces within the 3-D model automatically. The major features of the program include:

1 Input of serial section data by manual tracing, or automatic contour finding.

2 Alignment of sections.

3 Editing and reassignment of contours of individual sections.

4 Storing contour data in a file.

5 Selecting a range of sections and/or a range of elements to be used for reconstruction.

6 Reconstructing in a wire frame and/or a solid modelling mode by using parallel projection.

7 Rotating reconstruction in the *x*, *y* and *z* plane at variable magnification.
8 Viewing inside a model by cutting away part of the reconstruction using an 'electronic knife'.
9 Calculating surfaces and volumes.
10 Plotting reconstruction on a matrix or laser print.

With this program, outlines of glandular structure and endometrial stroma in the serial histological sections were traced by the digitizer, sections were aligned and contour data stored in a file. Once all the serial outlines had been digitized and stored, reconstructed (3-D) image models of these *in vivo* structures were displayed on the TV monitor. The 3-D reconstruction could generate a complete multicoloured model of the complex structure, which could be rotated and viewed from any angle or orientation.

Volumes of the reconstructed glandular and stromal structures were obtained by calculation function in the same program. Lumen volume, which is the volume attributed to the lumen, was also calculated. Ratios of lumen volume/epithelial volume/stromal volume were determined for each specimen. The χ^2 test was used for statistical analysis.

Biopsy was taken from the typical (puckered black) endometriotic implants in women with peritoneal endometriosis who had not previously received any hormonal therapy (group I) and in women who had received GnRH-a therapy for 12 weeks before biopsy (group II).

Evaluation and comments

Histologically, all the biopsy specimens showed typical epithelium and stroma of the endometrial type. The reconstructed 3-D image models of the structures in the peritoneal endometriotic lesions were displayed and a pink colour was applied for the stroma, green for the epithelium and blue for the lumen. The 3-D image models were usually indicated as a solid structure; however, models could be displayed as a transparent structure, when they were simultaneously shown with their stromal and epithelial structures.

Stereographically, two types could be easily recognized and classified:
1 The first type is composed of glands with ramifications (Plate 3.6, facing p. 50).
2 The second type is composed of cylinder-like glands without ramifications (Plate 3.7, facing p. 50).

In the first type, the lesion shows a regular distribution of the glandular epithelium in the stromal structure, which is also regular. Luminal structures are interconnected with each other. Epithelial structures appear like fingers (Plate 3.6c, facing p. 50) and seem to invade the stroma. The distribution of glandular structures in the stroma is not regular. Many glandular structures are formed inside luminal structures whose diameter varied from 22 to

Table 3.3 Stereometry of volumes of 3-D structures: percentage of the lesion attributed to the epithelium, stroma or lumen

Ratio (%)	Group I $n = 26$	Group II $n = 16$
Epithelium/lesion	19.9%	14.9%
Stroma/lesion	62.2%	51.8%
Lumen/lesion	13.2%	25.2%

Group I: Untreated patients.
Group II: After GnRH agonist (12 weeks).
From [15] with permission.

185 μm (Plate 3.6d, facing p. 50). In all groups, the 'external' stromal surface is regular (Plates 3.6a & 3.7a, facing p. 50). Like normal uterine epithelial structures, the glandular epithelium has a markedly regular luminal surface. In some cases, the lumen is dilated; in other cases, especially when the ramifications are numerous, the lumen is narrow (Plate 3.8, facing p. 50).

Volumes of epithelial, stromal and luminal structures were separately measured by computer stereometry and the results are shown in Table 3.3. The stroma/lesion ratio was respectively 62.2% and 51.8% in groups I and II. Although there was a decrease in stroma/lesion ratio in group II, when compared with group I, the difference was not significant. The epithelium/lesion ratio was respectively 19.9% and 14.9%, and the lumen/lesion ratio was respectively 13.2% and 25.2% in groups I and II. These values were significantly ($P < 0.01$) different.

Recently, computer-stereographic studies of skin tissues have been reported describing the advantages of the computer-generated 3-D models of tissue structures. The first publication on the topic of endometriosis using computer-graphic mechanical methods of reconstruction was produced by our group [15]. When compared with the 3-D models demonstrated in other studies, the present 3-D models seemed to be much better and to show more realistic appearances of structures since the structures of the reconstructed models were coloured. Furthermore, the transparent display of our 3-D models was excellent for the observation of their inside structures.

The present study demonstrates that two different types of endometrial peritoneal lesions can be differentiated: (i) a type in which glands are ramified and connected; and (ii) a type without ramification of the glands. The two different types could be correlated to the different degree of 'aggressiveness' and to the different appearances of peritoneal endometriosis.

From the present stereographic findings, one may consider that the apparently multifocal occurrence (in 2-D) of glandular epithelium in one lesion is not confirmed by the 3-D study. Indeed, in each peritoneal lesion, epithelial glands are interconnected by luminal structures. Probably, in each peritoneal lesion, epithelial structures occur in a single focus of the stroma and may then gradually develop, elongate and swell, forming luminal structures, occasionally with endometrial debris inside. During the expansion, all glands are connected and no peripheral epithelial structures become independent by loss of interconnection.

This stereometric study of volumes of 3-D structures revealed the volume distribution in peritoneal endometriosis. The ratios of epithelium, stroma and lumen/lesion observed in groups I and II indicate a stronger effect of the GnRH-a therapy on the stroma than on the epithelium. This effect could be due to the reduction in stromal vascularization induced by GnRH-a. The stromal capillary network can also be reconstructed in 3-D. In active lesions, the 3-D evaluation of the capillary network reveals the presence of a great number of larger vessels. After GnRH-a therapy (as well as in white lesions), the network is composed of smaller vessels.

The present stereographic and stereometric study has shown some new characteristics of peritoneal endometriosis. Further studies will be required to investigate the variations in the 3-D architecture of peritoneal endometriotic lesions among the different appearances of endometriosis in individual patients, among patients of different ages and among patients having different types of peritoneal endometriosis before and after hormonal therapy.

Acknowledgements

This research was partially supported by a grant from the Fonds de la Recherche Scientifique (Belgique) and a grant from Ipsen Biotech (France).

References

1 Brosens I, Vasquez G, Gordts S. Scanning electron microscopic study of the pelvic peritoneum in unexplained infertility and endometriosis. *Fertil Steril* 1984 **41**: 215.
2 Murphy AA, Green WR, Bobbie D, de la Cruz ZC, Rock JA. Unsuspected endometriosis documented by scanning electron microscopy in visually normal peritoneum. *Fertil Steril* 1986 **46**: 522.
3 Martin DC, Hubert GD, Vander Zwaag R, El-Zeky F. Laparoscopic appearances of peritoneal endometriosis. *Fertil Steril* 1989 **51**: 63.
4 Redwine DB. The distribution of endometriosis in the pelvis by age groups and fertility. *Fertil Steril* 1987 **47**: 173–175.
5 Stripling MC, Martin DC, Chatman DL, Vander Zwaag R, Poston WM. Subtle appearances of pelvic endometriosis. *Fertil Steril* 1988 **49**: 427.
6 Nisolle M, Paindaveine B, Bourdon A, Berlière M, Casanas-Roux F, Donnez J. Histologic study of peritoneal endometriosis in infertile women. *Fertil Steril* 1990 53: 984–988.

7 Jansen RPS, Russell P. Nonpigmented endometriosis: clinical laparoscopic and pathologic definition. *Am J Obstet Gynecol* 1986 **155**: 1154.

8 Nisolle M, Casanas-Roux F, Anaf V, Mine JM, Donnez J. Morphometric study of the stromal vascularization in peritoneal endometriosis. *Fertil Steril* 1993 **59**: 681.

9 Chatman DL. Pelvic peritoneal defects and endometriosis: Allen–Masters syndrome revisited. *Fertil Steril* 1981 **36**: 751.

10 Nisolle M, Casanas-Roux F, Donnez J. Histologic study of ovarian endometriosis after hormonal therapy. *Fertil Steril* 1988 **49**: 423.

11 Matta WHM, Stabille I, Shaw RW, Campbell S. Doppler assessment of uterine blood flow changes in patients with fibroids receiving the GnRH agonist Buserelin. *Fertil Steril* 1988 **49**: 1083.

12 Marchevsky AM, Gil J, Jeanty H. Computerized interactive morphometry in pathology: current instrumentation and methods. *Hum Pathol* 1987 **18**: 320–331.

13 Braverman MS, Braverman IM. Three-dimensional reconstructions of objects from serial sections using a microcomputer graphic system. *J Invest Dermatol* 1986 **86**: 290–294.

14 Ito M, Yokoyama H, Ikeda K, Sat Y. Stereographic analysis of syringomas. *Arch Dermatol Res* 1990 **282**: 17–21.

15 Donnez J, Nisolle M, Casanas-Roux F. Three-dimensional architectures of peritoneal endometriosis. *Fertil Steril* 1992 **57**: 980.

Chapter 4
Peritoneal Environment in Endometriosis

G.A.J. DUNSELMAN

Introduction

Endometriosis may be defined as a disease characterized by the presence of functional endometrial glands and stroma in ectopic locations outside the uterine cavity. The ectopic endometrial tissue responds to steroids in a way similar to eutopic endometrium. Endometriosis is linked to the reproductive years, it does not occur in premenarcheal girls and it is believed to regress in the postmenopausal years. Changes in endometriotic lesions, in the mesothelial lining of the peritoneal cavity and in the ovarian vascularization secondary to ovarian steroids and the process of retrograde menstruation alter the peritoneal environment. These functional changes are reflected in the peritoneal fluid bathing the reproductive organs in the pelvic cavity.

Since the introduction of laparoscopy the peritoneal environment has become easily accessible for research in the field of endometriosis related to the pathogenesis and to the infertility seen in this disease. In the early years of peritoneal fluid research, the main emphasis was on peritoneal fluid volume related to the time of the cycle [1–3] and peritoneal fluid steroids [1,4–7]. The peritoneal fluid constituents, cellular and biochemical, received considerable attention thereafter. After the publication of the article entitled 'How does mild endometriosis cause infertility?' [8] numerous articles were published describing changes in peritoneal fluid constituents to try to elucidate the assumed relation between mild endometriosis and subfertility (reviews in [9–13]). This cascade of articles was not restrained by that of Wheeler and Malinak [14] entitled 'Does mild endometriosis cause infertility?'

The pivotal role of the peritoneal macrophage and its products in the altered humoral and cell-mediated immunology in endometriosis patients and in the development of endometriosis was the next main issue. Easier access to monoclonal antibodies against a variety of substances and the development of commercially available cytokines have led to a new insight into the regulation and growth of eutopic and ectopic endometrial glands and stroma.

Three topics will be discussed in this chapter: the physiology of peritoneal fluid, peritoneal fluid and subfertility in endometriosis and peritoneal fluid and the development of endometriosis.

Peritoneal fluid physiology

Peritoneal fluid volume

The peritoneum is a smooth, glistening, serous membrane that lines the abdominal wall. The peritoneal cavity is normally empty except for a thin film of fluid that keeps surfaces moist. In women the peritoneal cavity is indirectly in communication with the exterior of the body by way of the Fallopian tubes [15]. Histologically the peritoneum consists of a thin layer of loose connective tissue covered by a layer of mesothelium. There is a rich supply of subperitoneal blood-vessels and lymphatics [16].

In 1922 Novak [17] reported the presence of fluid in the pouch of Douglas during clinical observations. The volume of the fluid was found to be influenced by the stage of the cycle, rising from an early proliferative mean value of 0.8 ml to a mean value of 18.7 ml after ovulation and decreasing again to a mean value of 5.4 ml in the late secretory phase [1]. These findings were corroborated in subsequent studies by other investigators [2, 3]. Women on oral contraceptives were found to harbour a small cycle-independent amount of peritoneal fluid [1].

In theory, the volume of peritoneal fluid may be influenced by secretion of fluid from the uterus and the Fallopian tubes, by exudation and reabsorption of fluid through the peritoneal lining from and to the ovarian and subperitoneal capillaries and by direct contribution from the rupturing follicle [18]. Women with a congenital absence of the uterus but with functioning ovaries appear to have an amount of peritoneal fluid comparable to that of women with a uterus [2]. The contribution of tubal secretion to the total amount of peritoneal fluid is probably low, in view of a 24-hour production of 1–2 ml [1, 19]. In addition, in patients with distally blocked tubes the volume of peritoneal fluid was not different from that in patients with patent tubes [20].

The fact that women without functioning ovarian tissue and men have a small amount of peritoneal fluid compared with ovulating women has led to the assumption that a hormonal influence on the vascular permeability exists that influences the amount of peritoneal fluid. A cycle-dependent correlation has been found between the volume of peritoneal fluid and the oestradiol levels in serum and peritoneal fluid [1]. This could be an indication of an oestrogenic effect on the permeability of vascular and peritoneal membranes. Changes in vascular permeability lead to a change of the equilibrium between inflow and outflow across the peritoneal membranes and fluid transfer after and possibly also before follicular rupture at the level of the ovarian surface [1]. Similar changes have been noted in the ovarian hyperstimulation syndrome. Vasoactive compounds like histamine and prostaglandins may play a role as well.

Contributions from the ovaries to the peritoneal fluid volume can result either from exudation from the ovarian capillaries, from transudation and exudation from the antrum of the preovulatory follicle or from release of the follicular fluid into the abdomen during ovulation. During ultrasound investigation an increase of the fluid volume in the cul-de-sac was noted after ovulation [21]. However, deposition of the follicular fluid into the abdominal cavity cannot account for the persistent high peritoneal fluid volumes throughout the luteal phase [7]. Moreover, in patients with a failure of the luteinizing follicle to rupture peritoneal fluid volumes did not differ significantly from those in ovulating women [22].

Peritoneal fluid constituents

Cellular constituents

Peritoneal fluid of women with patent tubes contains leucocytes, mesothelial cells and endometrial tissue [23, 24]. Normally peritoneal fluid contains 0.5–2.6×10^6 leucocytes/ml, of which more than 85% are macrophages [23, 25, 26]. Macrophages play an important role in maintaining homoeostasis. They are involved in phagocytosis and, through their numerous secretory products, in inflammatory and immunological reactions, in remodelling of tissues and in healing of wounds. In addition to their regulatory functions, macrophages play a central role in the cell-mediated immune response; they are involved both in the initiation of the response, as antigen-presenting cells, and in the effector phase, as inflammatory, tumoricidal and microbicidal cells.

Elements of the mononuclear phagocyte system originate in the bone marrow. Mononuclear phagocytes, after development over several days, leave the marrow and pass into the circulation as monocytes and subsequently, within hours to days, into the various tissues and compartments of the body, for instance the peritoneal cavity, where they survive for months as resident macrophages. Functional heterogeneity exists in most populations of macrophages, as a result of variable degrees of differentiation.

Once established in the tissues, macrophages can be subjected to a myriad of stimulatory and suppressive signals, particularly in instances of disturbed homoeostasis, such as inflammation. This alters their morphology, metabolism and physiology and activates them to adopt various functions [25, 27, 28]. Their responses include the secretion of some hundred different substances and their biologic activity ranges from induction of cell growth to cell death [29]. By appropriate stimulation, profound alterations can be induced in the physiology of the resident cells. Secondary to non-specific, non-immunological inflammatory stimuli, humoral and cellular, resident macrophages produce substances that cause proliferation of monocytes in the bone marrow. These monocytes, with specific functions, after reaching the peritoneal cavity are called inflammatory macrophages. Macrophages exposed to lympokines and other signals are competent to present antigen to T lymphocytes and to display microbicidal and tumoricidal activity. The mediation of macrophage activation by specifically sensitized lymphocytes is achieved by way of soluble mediators collectively referred to as lymphokines.

Important factors in regulating development and function of macrophages are the secretory products released from the macrophages themselves, which initiate many complex positive and negative feedback loops. Most functions can be down- as well as up-modulated [30].

An important concept in understanding macrophage function and regulation is the heterogeneity of macrophages within any given population. Individual capacities are not necessarily expressed uniformly by all cells [31]. The various capacities of macrophages do not all develop synchronously but rather asynchronously and even disparately [28].

Proteins

The total protein concentration in peritoneal fluid has been reported to be below that of serum [1,2]. The concentrations of total protein and of various individual proteins in the peritoneal fluid exhibited a cyclic pattern with a significant increase in the luteal phase of the cycle [2,3]. The relatively high total protein concentration of peritoneal fluid accentuates its origin as an exudation product [3].

Steroid hormones

In regularly ovulating women peritoneal fluid oestradiol and progesterone levels are comparable to serum levels in the follicular phase of the cycle [18]. After the luteinizing hormone (LH) surge and subsequent ovulation, the peritoneal fluid levels of oestradiol and progesterone rise sharply. The increase in oestradiol concentration in the postovulatory phase is more gradual than the increase in the progesterone concentration. Postovulatory levels of oestradiol in peritoneal fluid rise to 8–10 times those of serum and those of progesterone to 20–50 times [1,5,7]. The cyclic changes in peritoneal fluid concentrations of oestradiol and progesterone are directly related to ovarian activity. Women with anovulatory cycles have low values of these steroids [1]. The sources of the steroids in the peritoneal fluid are the developing follicle, the contents of the follicle and the luteinized theca interna [7]. In luteinized unruptured follicles (LUF) cycles the postovulatory peritoneal fluid levels of

(a) 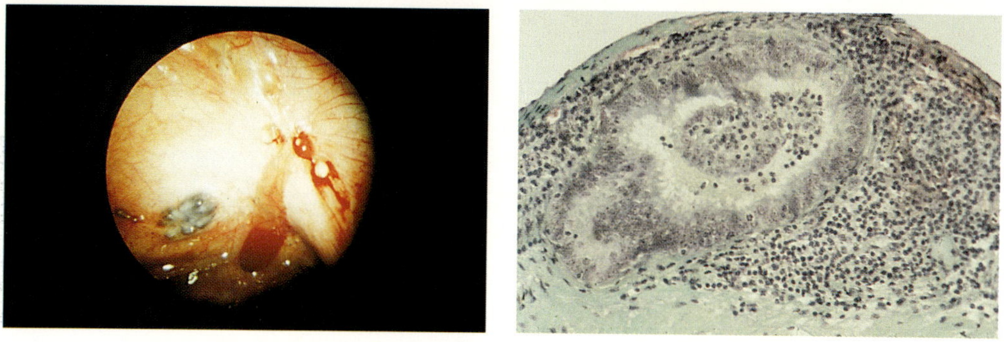 (b)

Plate 3.1 Endometriotic peritoneal lesions: typical black lesion. (a) Laparoscopic aspect; (b) histology: combination of glands, stroma and intraluminal debris.

(a) 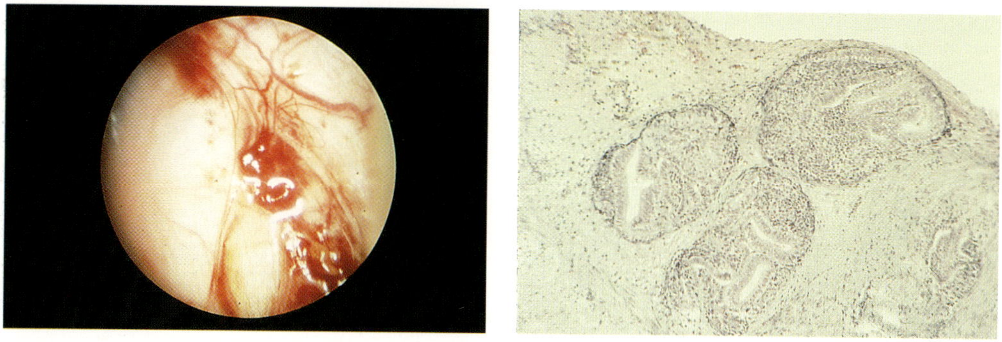 (b)

Plate 3.2 Endometrial peritoneal lesions: red flame-like lesion. (a) Laparoscopic aspect; (b) histology: active endometriotic glands surrounded by stroma.

(a) 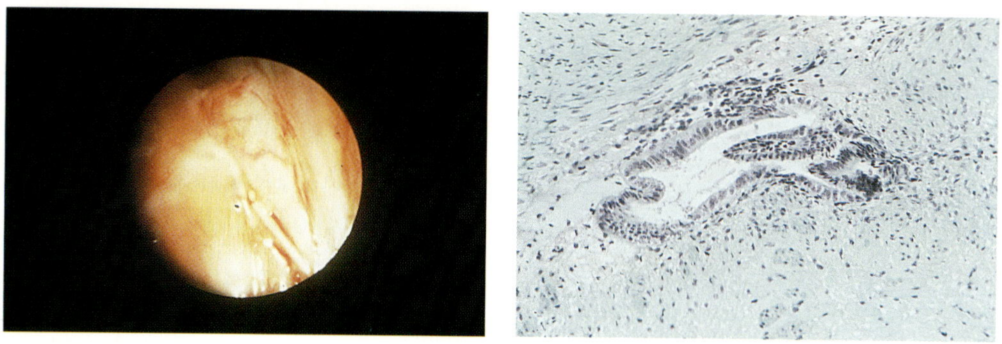 (b)

Plate 3.3 Endometrial peritoneal lesions: white lesion. (a) Laparoscopic aspect; (b) histology: rare retroperitoneal glandular structure and scanty stroma surrounded by fibrotic tissue.

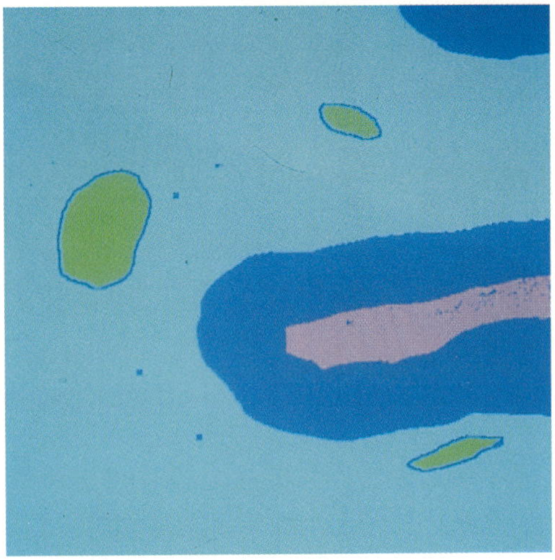

Plate 3.4 Capillaries and glands were drawn moving a cursor. Each different structure was discriminated and grey level images were transferred to binary images.

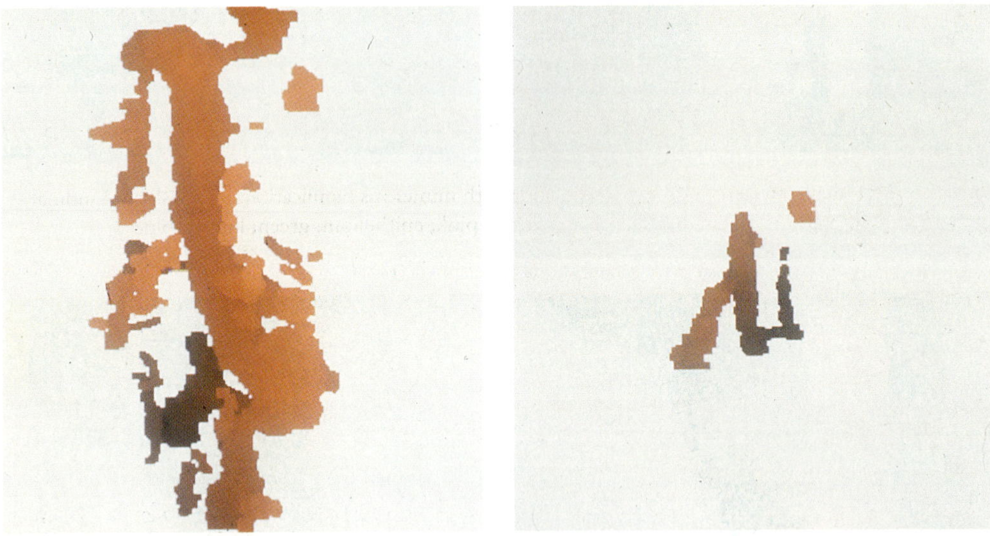

(a)

(b)

Plate 3.5 (a) 3-D evaluation of the capillary network in a red lesion. (b) 3-D evaluation of the capillary network in a white lesion. The network is obviously different from that observed in a red lesion.

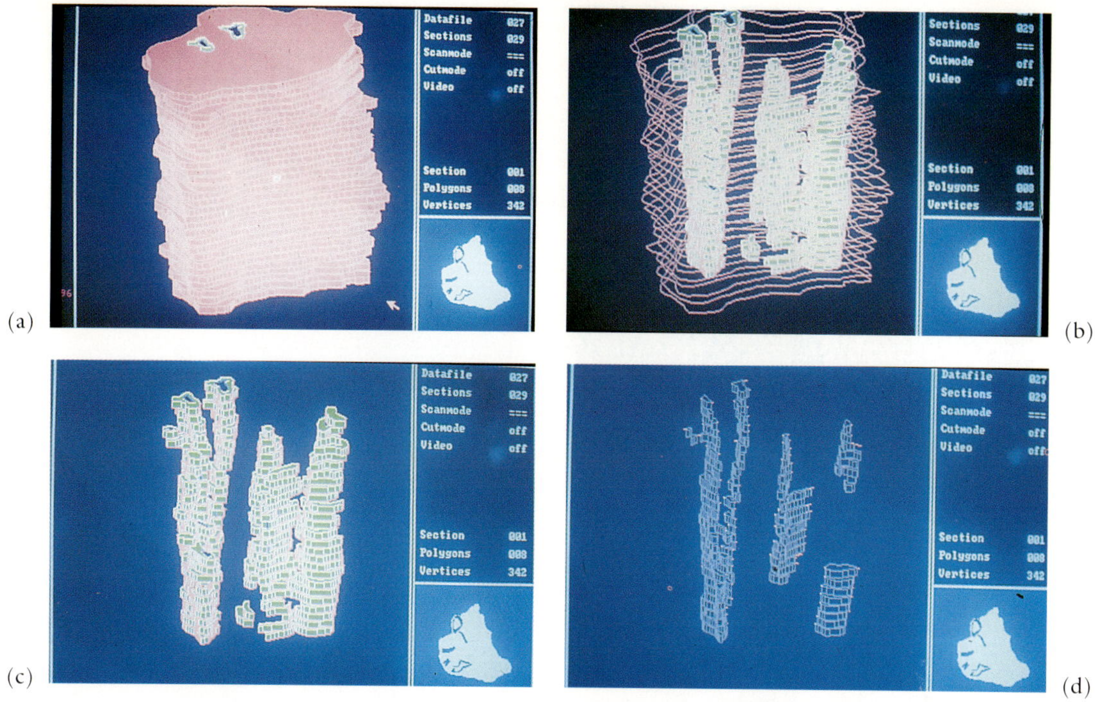

Plate 3.6 3-D image model. Endometriosis glands with numerous ramifications (red lesion). Luminal structures are interconnected with each other (stroma: pink; epithelium: green; lumen: blue).

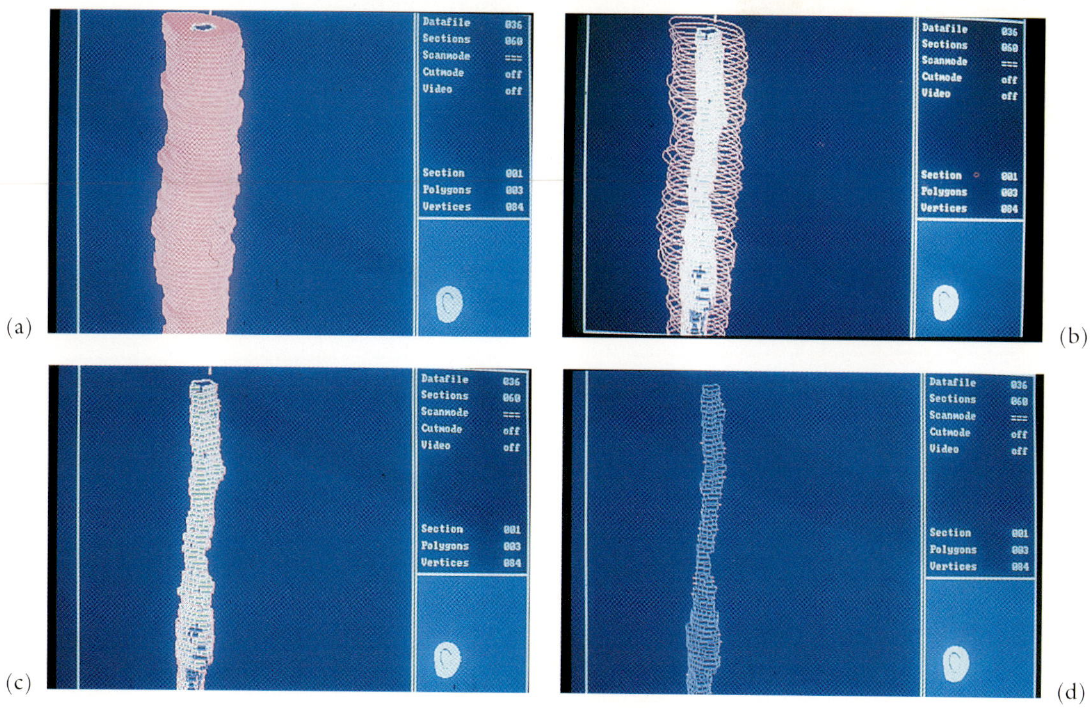

Plate 3.7 3-D image model. Endometriosis cylinder-like gland without ramifications (inactive white lesion).

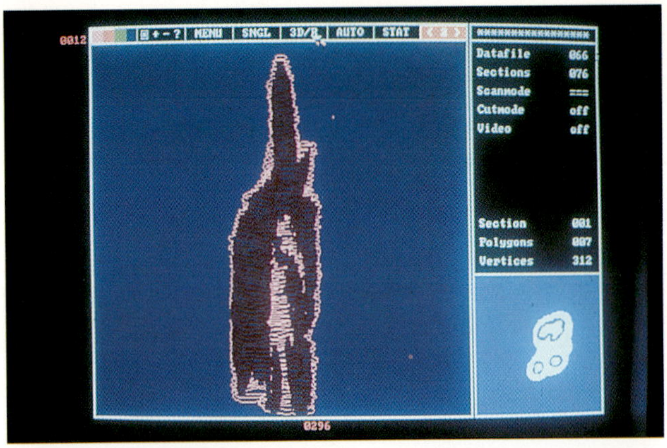

(a)

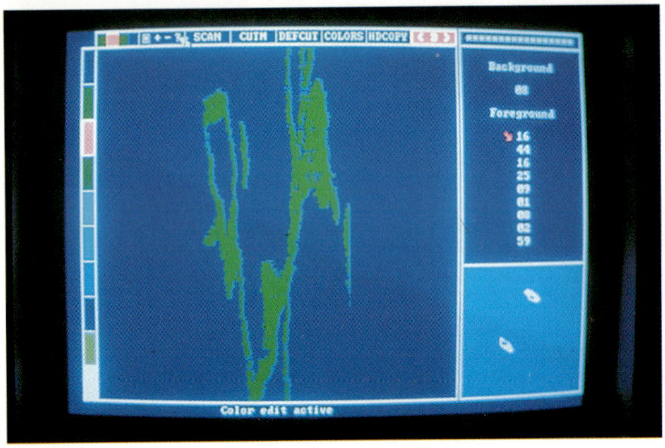

(b)

Plate 3.8 3-D image model. The lumen is narrow when the ramifications are numerous.

progesterone and oestradiol remain relatively low, since the steroid-rich contents of the follicle do not reach the peritoneal cavity. Measurement of these steroids may aid in the diagnosis of LUF cycles [22, 32]. A considerable overlap exists, however, in peritoneal fluid steroid concentrations between normal and LUF cycles.

Prostaglandins

Prostaglandins are biosynthesized from polyunsaturated fatty acids, predominantly arachidonic acid. Arachidonic acid is liberated from cellular phospholipids by the action of phospholipases. After formation of PGG_2 and PGH_2, the prostaglandins PGE_2, PGD_2, $PGF_{2\alpha}$, PGI_2 and thromboxane $(Tx)A_2$ are synthesized. The more stable metabolites of PGI_2 and TxA_2 are 6-keto-$PGF_{1\alpha}$ and TxB_2. Biosynthesis and release of prostaglandins from tissues occur in response to various stimuli. Prostaglandins are rapidly metabolized in the lungs.

The role of prostaglandins in ovulation, corpus luteum function and tubal transport has been reviewed by Chaudhuri [33]. Prostaglandins play a role in the mechanism of ovulation, although the exact mechanism is not yet known. The induction of LUF cycles with prostaglandin synthetase inhibitor drugs has been reported [34]. The exact mechanism and the role of prostaglandins, if any, in luteolysis in humans remain to be elucidated [33]. In the rabbit, the role of prostaglandins in oviductal motility is fairly well established [35]. In the human the role of endogenous and exogenous prostaglandins is less clear [36, 37]. Sources of prostaglandins in peritoneal fluid are the peritoneal macrophages [29], the peritoneum [38] and the ovary by diffusion or at the time of rupture [39, 40]. Besides that, passive diffusion occurs from other organs in the peritoneal cavity. The uterine endometrium can also produce several different prostaglandins [41, 42].

Peritoneal fluid and subfertility in endometriosis

The association between endometriosis and infertility is well established. Reliable figures are hard to find. Before laparoscopy became available, only guesses could be made. A much quoted figure of the incidence of infertility in the presence of endometriosis is 30–40% [43]. This figure is derived from a statement of Rubin in 1933 that the expectation of pregnancy when the disease is present is about one-half that in the general population. Assuming that the usual incidence of infertility approximates 15%, Kistner [43] came to the above-mentioned 30–40%. These figures are based mainly on findings in patients with symptomatic endometriosis.

The association of endometriosis with infertility, to the extent that it compromises tubo-ovarian contact, seems beyond doubt. Disagreement exists on the question whether mild endometriosis adversely affects fertility. Many women with endometriosis are asymptomatic, remain undiagnosed and conceive without treatment. Collins *et al.* [44] showed that, in the absence of treatment, pregnancies occurred in 58% of 49 couples with endometriosis.

The finding of a low prevalence in patients during sterilization laparoscopy, as opposed to the higher prevalence found during laparoscopy in the course of an infertility investigation [45], supports the assumed association between endometriosis and infertility. It has to be emphasized that the data were obtained in a retrospective study and that the difference in parity between the two groups may have influenced the results. Conflicting data arise from the literature on artificial insemination by donor (AID) in patients with endometriosis. Endometriosis was found to reduce monthly fecundability [46–48]. This could not be confirmed by others [49–51].

If mild endometriosis causes subfertility, then we could expect that treatment increases the monthly fecundity rate. However, treatment protocols that have compared hormonal suppression with no treatment did not show benefit of the hormonal treatment regarding achievement of pregnancies [52–57]. Eradication of endometrial implants has not been shown to be more efficacious than hormonal treatment [58].

In summary, the association between endometriosis and subfertility is not a strong one. Wheeler and Malinak [14] have questioned a causal relationship on epidemiological grounds. The presence of endometriosis seems to be an epiphenomenon in patients with otherwise unexplained infertility. The finding that the monthly fecundity rate in these women is below normal is most probably due to age and duration of infertility [59].

Nevertheless, apart from aggressive therapies directed towards eradication of endometrial implants, lots of effort has been spent on elucidating the possible causes of endometriosis by studying the peritoneal environment, in which (peri)conceptional events like folliculogenesis, ovulation, fertilization and tubal transport of spermatozoa, oocytes and pre-implantation embryos take place. Peritoneal fluid volume and changes in peritoneal fluid constituents have been studied to elucidate possible causes of endometriosis-associated infertility, especially in the milder forms of endometriosis, where infertility is not easily explained. The general picture that arises is the presence of an intraperitoneal inflammatory exudate in women with endometriosis without mechanical problems impeding tubo-ovarian relationship. This inflammatory status is manifested by increases in peritoneal fluid volume, leucocyte number, macrophages and macrophage products and prostaglandins (reviews in [9–13]).

Peritoneal fluid volume

Conflicting results have been reported on the influence of endometriosis on peritoneal fluid volume. In the first place, this is due to lack of control for the phase of the cycle studied. Secondly, in some of the studies the control group is composed of patients with unexplained infertility, while in other studies patients with endometriosis are compared with fertile controls without endometriosis. Decreased volumes were noted by Koninckx *et al.* [2] in patients with severe endometriosis in the luteal phase of the cycle. Increased volumes have been reported irrespective of cycle dating [60, 61], in the early follicular phase [2], in the periovulatory phase [23] and in the luteal phase of the cycle [62–64]. Syrop and Halme [11] examined peritoneal fluid volume in 426 patients in a retrospective study. Women with endometriosis had a greater peritoneal fluid volume than fertile controls and patients with adhesive disease or unexplained infertility. The volume in the group with unexplained infertility was higher than that in controls. Several other reports have demonstrated no difference in peritoneal fluid volume between patients with and without endometriosis [65–75], either in the follicular or in the luteal phase of the cycle. If increased peritoneal fluid volume is found, it seems to be associated not only with endometriosis but also with unexplained infertility [76]. These patients with unexplained infertility may be suffering from microscopic endometriosis, not yet discernible to the naked eye. On the other hand, the intra-abdominal inflammatory changes may be due to a factor other than the peritoneal endometrial implants. Most probably the stimulus for these changes is retrograde menstruation [77, 78].

Peritoneal fluid constituents

Macrophages

Normally peritoneal fluid contains 0.5–2.6 × 10^6/ml leucocytes, of which more than 85% are macrophages [23, 25, 26]. Their physiologic function is maintenance of homoeostasis, releasing substances that are involved in tissue remodelling and growth. They are involved in phagocytosis of decaying spermatozoa and removal of blood cells after retrograde menstruation and ovulation.

Haney *et al.* [23] reported an increased total number of macrophages in infertile patients with endometriosis compared with infertile patients without endometriosis. Studying the number of macrophages inside the oviducts, Haney *et al.* [79] found a higher number of oviductal macrophages in endometriosis patients. They suggested that oviductal and peritoneal macrophages in endometriosis patients interfere with fertility by increased sperm phagocytosis. Halme *et al.* [20, 62, 80] published a series of observations on peritoneal macrophages in endometriosis patients. In fertile patients with open Fallopian tubes, they noted a high concentration of macrophages during menstruation, which gradually decreased and remained stable during the rest of the cycle. In contrast, infertile patients with occluded tubes had a low concentration compared with fertile controls and with infertile patients with endometriosis. They concluded that macrophages are attracted by retrograde menstruation [20]. Furthermore, they noted an increased concentration of two proteins, acid phosphatase and neutral protease, in the peritoneal fluid of patients with endometriosis, compared with fertile controls. Additionally, the macrophages in the patients with endometriosis had higher acid phosphatase expression, which is associated with macrophages of a larger size. They concluded that the macrophages of patients with endometriosis were in a more advanced stage of activation, possibly leading to either phagocytosis of gametes or release of active compounds into the surrounding peritoneal fluid [80]. Subsequently they reported on a cyclic activation of macrophages in normal women: the activational status of peritoneal macrophages changes during the cycle, showing an increase toward the luteal phase. This cyclic activation appeared to be more pronounced in patients with endometriosis. They suggested that retrograde menstruation or bleeding from ectopic endometrial implants, acting as irritating agents, could attract macrophages and induce differentiation [62].

Apart from cell number, the activity of peritoneal macrophages has been studied in patients with endometriosis. Muscato *et al.* [26] documented an increased phagocytosis of spermatozoa *in vitro* by the macrophages of the endometriosis patients, compared with those of fertile controls. This could not be confirmed by Awadalla *et al.* [71] in another study involving two large groups of infertile patients with and without endometriosis, nor did they find an increased total count or concentration of macrophages in endometriosis patients. The choice of the control group probably caused this lack of difference. Zeller *et al.* [81] documented that not only peritoneal macrophages but also peripheral monocytes of patients with endometriosis were in an advanced stage of activation. An increased erythrophagocytosis *in vitro* was shown of macrophages of patients with endometriosis [82]. They also showed that these macrophages were in an advanced stage of differentiation. The concept of more advanced macrophages in peritoneal fluid of patients with endometriosis has been supported by the finding of interleukin 1 (IL-1), a product of macrophages in an advanced stage of differentiation, in peritoneal fluid of patients with endometriosis, and not in peritoneal fluid of patients without the disease [83]. IL-1 concentration in the peritoneal fluid and *in vitro* IL-1 production did not differ between 49 patients with and 73 patients without endometriosis [71]. It has to be noted that in this last study both groups consisted of infertile patients.

Olive *et al.* [69] reported that elevated numbers of macrophages are not exclusive to patients with endometriosis but rather correlate with infertility in the absence of endocrinologic or mechanical disorders. They suggested that patients with high macrophage counts represent a distinct group, of which women with endometriosis are only a subset. Syrop and Halme [84] related peritoneal fluid parameters to subsequent pregnancy outcome. They found that peritoneal fluid macrophage count was not a significant predictor variable. It has to be noted that only macrophage count and not macrophage activity was used as parameter.

Steinleitner *et al.* [85] showed in an *in vivo* mouse model that immunomodulation of peritoneal inflammatory cells by pentoxifylline reversed inhibition of fertilization by activated macrophages.

The changes in the peritoneal environment, peritoneal fluid and macrophages and their secretory products may influence ovum pick-up, gametes, fertilization and pre-implantation embryonic development. In advanced cases of endometriosis, disturbances of ovum pick-up due to adhesions and defective tubo-ovarian contact are obvious. Also a peritoneal factor has been implicated: Suginami *et al.* [86] demonstrated that, in contrast to peritoneal fluid of controls, peritoneal fluid of patients with endometriosis inhibited ovum capture by the oviductal fimbriae of the golden hamster *in vitro.*

Phagocytosis of spermatozoa and oocytes by intra-abdominal and intrauterine macrophages has been demonstrated [87–89]. Increased phagocytosis of spermatozoa by tubal and intra-abdominal macrophages and hence a decreased fertilization rate in women with endometriosis has been suggested by Muscato *et al.* [26] and Haney *et al.* [79]. No significant differences were found regarding phagocytic capabilities of macrophages harvested from peritoneal fluid of endometriosis patients versus controls [62]. From these findings the role of increased phagocytosis by peritoneal macrophages was questioned as a mechanism of infertility in endometriosis. On the other hand, especially in those infertile couples where subfertile semen and endometriosis occur together, increased phagocytosis by macrophages in an advanced stage of activation may bring the number of spermatozoa below a certain threshold level.

It has been postulated that secretory products of macrophages in a more advanced stage of activation may affect spermatozoa, oocytes and early embryos. Peritoneal fluid of endometriosis patients has been reported to decrease sperm penetration of oocytes in the hamster [63] or mouse [90], whereas heat-inactivated peritoneal fluid has no effect [90, 91]. Purified cytokines (interferon-γ (IFN) and tumour necrosis factor (TNF)) were shown to affect sperm function in the hamster egg penetration test [92]. Human recombinant TNF did not affect human sperm motility, hamster ovum penetration or mouse *in vitro* fertilization (IVF) and early embryonic development [93]. The number of sperm tightly bound to the zona surface in the hemi-zona assay was significantly reduced in the presence of peritoneal fluid of endometriosis patients [94].

Stone and Himsl [95] determined the rate of sperm recovery at the time of laparoscopy for infertility in 29 patients with and in 77 patients without endometriosis. The number of patients with motile sperm in both groups was similar. The presence of mild endometriosis did not impair sperm motility up to 4 hours after insemination.

A positive influence of peritoneal fluid on sperm viability and motility has been documented [96, 97]. Conversely, an adverse effect of peritoneal fluid of fertile and infertile women with and without endometriosis on sperm motility and velocity has been documented by some [64, 98, 99] but not by others [100]. Soldati *et al.* [101] showed that human peritoneal fluids contain a heat-resistant, protein-bound lipidic component able to rapidly immobilize spermatozoa and to increase acrosome reactions. The adverse effects of peritoneal fluid on sperm velocity have been related to the presence of IFN and TNF. IFN and TNF, products of activated macrophages and present in the abdominal cavity of patients with endometriosis, have been shown to inhibit sperm velocity, while IL-1 did not influence sperm motion parameters. Spermatozoa with a decreased motility would become easier targets for macrophages [102]. If increased sperm phagocytosis is an important factor in endometriosis patients, it is not mediated by peritoneal antisperm antibodies [103, 104].

In vitro studies showed that peritoneal fluid of patients with endometriosis adversely affected mouse embryo cleavage and viability in comparison with peritoneal fluid of controls [105]. This could not be confirmed by others [71, 106]. Recombinant IL-1 was found to be toxic to the growth of two-cell mouse embryos *in vitro* [83]. The embryotoxicity of IL-1 and IL-2 tested in an *in vitro* mouse embryo system, was not confirmed by others [107]. Prough *et al.* [108] showed two-cell mouse embryo growth inhibition by cell-free heat-inactivated peritoneal fluid of endometriosis patients. The greatest inhibition was by the faction of > 100 000 dalton range, coincident with the ovum capture inhibitor presented by Suginami *et al.* [86].

In short, peritoneal fluid of patients with endometriosis possibly has an adverse effect on spermatozoa and pre-implantation embryos. An increased number of intra-abdominal macrophages in an advanced stage of activation may affect fertilization by phagocytosis or by the effect of their secretory products, especially in couples with coincidental male subfertility. It has to be stressed that all the above-mentioned studies, except the one by Stone and

Himsl [95], regard *in vitro* and/or animal experiments with all the related shortcomings.

Prostaglandins

Transport of fertilized ova through the Fallopian tube is effected by both muscular and ciliary activity. Ovarian steroids, adrenergic innervation and prostaglandins interact to influence oviductal contractility. It has been postulated that altered tubal transport is caused by an increased intra-abdominal concentration of prostaglandins; in endometriosis patients prostaglandins may be produced by endometriotic implants [109–111] or macrophages [29]. DeLeon *et al.* [112] demonstrated that peritoneum involved with endometriosis produced significantly more $PGF_{2\alpha}$ and PGE_2 than adjacent normal peritoneum. Vernon *et al.* [111] measured PGF concentration and *in vitro* production by endometriotic implants, endometrium and normal peritoneum. They found that endometriotic implants contained and produced significantly more PGF than normal peritoneum. Endometrium contained twice the amount and exhibited five times the capacity to produce PGF than endometrial implants. They also correlated PGF production with different types of endometrial implants, i.e. petechial, intermediate and powderburn lesions. As judged by PGF production, petechial implants were biochemically more active than intermediate implants, which in turn were more active than powderburn implants.

Initial studies on peritoneal fluid prostaglandins and endometriosis showed increased concentrations of 6-keto-$PGF_{1\alpha}$ and TxB_2 in peritoneal fluid of patients with endometriosis compared with controls [113]. It was suggested that these prostaglandins could alter tubal transport. Altered tubal transport of fertilized ova resulting in an untimely arrival in the uterine cavity, causing implantation failure, has been implicated as a cause of infertility in endometriosis patients [113]. Likewise, peritoneal fluid $PGF_{2\alpha}$ and PGE_2 were found to be significantly increased in patients with endometriosis [114]. DeLeon *et al.* [68] compared peritoneal fluid $PGF_{2\alpha}$, PGE_2, 6-keto-$PGF_{1\alpha}$ and TxB_2 in the proliferative and the secretory phase of the cycle in patients with and without endometriosis. In both phases of the cycle, significantly higher concentrations of all four prostaglandins were found in endometriosis patients. Other studies could not confirm these findings [65–67, 70, 115].

In summary, the available literature on peritoneal fluid prostaglandin concentration in endometriosis patients shows either an increase or no changes compared with patients without the disease. Some of the confusion may be attributed to methodological differences, collection procedures, contamination of peritoneal fluid samples with blood, patient and control group selection and the time of the cycle studied. The presence of 'invisible' microscopic endometriosis may account for high levels of prostaglandins in some patients with unexplained infertility. Within the American Fertility Society (AFS) classification of mild endometriosis, different types of lesions are apparently present [116], characterized by a specific biochemical potential [111]. In view of these conflicting results, a role for prostaglandins in endometriosis-related subfertility is unlikely. Moreover, attempts to modify ovum transport *in vivo* have failed to show that prostaglandins accelerate ovum transport, even in the presence of increased tubal contractility [37]. Finally, accelerated tubal transport resulting in earlier entry of the embryo into the uterine cavity as a cause of infertility is not supported by the clinical results of IVF and embryo transfer.

In conclusion, changes in peritoneal fluid volume and constituents in women with endometriosis are held responsible for the subfertility presumably present in these women. However, despite the numerous reports on peritoneal fluid, endometriosis and subfertility, the available literature seldom correlates changes in peritoneal fluid constituents with the subsequent occurrence of pregnancy. In a retrospective study, Syrop and Halme [84] showed that the occurrence of pregnancy was related to the volume of peritoneal fluid and not to the number of peritoneal cells. In an uncontrolled study, Morita *et al.* [117] documented that treatment of endometriosis by laser irradiation changed the peritoneal fluid volume and its prostanoid content. They suggested that this decrease in prostaglandins correlated with the cumulative pregnancy rate in their patients. Taketani *et al.* [118] showed that the cytokine level of peritoneal fluid dropped significantly in women 3 months after cessation of hormonal treatment for endometriosis. Moreover, peritoneal fluid of treated endometriosis patients was significantly less embryotoxic to mouse two-cell embryos compared with peritoneal fluid of untreated women with endometriosis. They did not give pregnancy rates, however, comparing treated and untreated women.

Haney and Weinberg [77] showed that the parameters of the intraperitoneal inflammatory status, increased peritoneal fluid volume and leucocytes, decreased during anovulation and cessation of retrograde menstruation. They postulated that the changes in the peritoneal environment are secondary to retrograde menstruation rather than to the endometriotic implant. The finding that endometriotic implants in the rabbit, an animal lacking retrograde menstruation, do not impair fecundity supports this contention [119]. It can be argued that endometriosis and infertility are both effects of a third factor, e.g. retrograde menstruation. Following this train of thought, the question '(How) does mild endometriosis cause infertility?' should be replaced by '(How) does retrograde menstruation cause infertility?'. This has major consequences for therapy. In the past, the consequences rather than the cause of the disease have been treated. It seems illogical to expect that destroying or suppressing all visible or even invisible peritoneal implants of endometriosis will affect future fertility, a view corroborated by the available literature on the influence on fertility of medical and surgical treatment of minimal endometriosis. Manipulating amount, contents and/or duration of retrograde menstruation could be far more rewarding in this respect.

Peritoneal fluid and the development of endometriosis

Retrograde menstruation, peritoneal adhesion of shed endometrial tissue and outgrowth of these endometrial cells, glands and stroma are an essential element in the pathogenesis of endometriosis, according to Sampson's classical implantation theory. The reflux implantation theory of Sampson [120] is supported by the distribution of the lesions in the abdominal cavity [121], the demonstration of the viability of shed menstrual endometrium in tissue culture [122], the high prevalence of pelvic endometriosis in girls with congenital menstrual outflow obstruction [123] and animal experiments in which endometriosis was induced by the creation of utero-pelvic fistulas [124]. The theory of endometrial metaplasia of the peritoneal serosa is not contradictory, but may be supplementary [125]. Endometrial cells may stimulate metaplasia after they have been transported to a susceptible tissue. The difference between the implantation and induction theories may be characterized by the statement that the former seeks the origin of endometriosis on the cellular and the latter on the molecular level [125].

Prerequisites for the implantation theory are transtubal regurgitation of viable endometrial tissue, attachment of tissue to the peritoneal mesothelial lining or submesothelial extracellular matrix and outgrowth of this tissue. Retrograde menstruation is seen in the majority of women, with and without endometriotic lesions [126]. Endometrial cells can be found in the peritoneal fluid in patients with and without endometriosis [24, 127]. The factors that regulate the attachment phase and thereafter initiate the ectopic growth are not known. It remains unclear why not all women develop endometriosis, or do they? In 1953 Scott *et al.* [128] stated: 'If serial section of all pelvic tissue were feasible might not all 40 year old women with patent tubes and normal menstrual cycles regardless of parity reveal some endometriosis?'

Nevertheless, the stimuli necessary to provide attachment and outgrowth of endometrial cells after arrival in the peritoneal cavity are unknown. Zhang *et al.* [129] demonstrated that human endometrial stromal cells adhere to peritoneal mesothelial cells *in vitro* and that the cytokine TNF-α promotes this adhesion in a dose-dependent fashion. The relevance of isolated stromal cell culture systems was questioned by Wild *et al.* [130]. They found that isolated stromal cells in coculture with mesothelial cells adhere and form a confluent monolayer. In contrast, whole endometrial fragments cocultured with mesothelial cells adhere to the upper surface of the mesothelial layer and grow along this layer, forming characteristics similar to *in vivo* endometriosis. In this culture system, the complex interaction between stromal and epithelial components in the process of adherence to the mesothelial lining can be studied more precisely. The importance of interactions between stromal and epithelial compartments in cell growth and regulation has been stressed before [131].

Recently it has been shown that cell adhesion molecules – integrins and E-cadherin – are expressed in endometrial tissue recovered from peritoneal fluid, in endometriotic lesions and in the mesothelial peritoneal lining. These cell adhesion molecules potentially play a role in the development of the disease [132].

It has been postulated that endometriosis develops in women with either an increased retrograde menstruation secondary to outflow obstruction or an inability to remove the debris [133]. In order to prevent the endometrial tissue from attaching, growing and developing into endometriosis (or inducing mesothelial cells to transform into endometriosis), the retrograde menstrual debris has to be cleared from the abdominal cavity. Cellular and biochemical components of the peritoneal fluid have been studied in this respect. As mentioned above, the intra-abdominal environment of women with patent tubes is characterized by an inflammatory status secondary to retrograde menstruation, the arrival of spermatozoa, viral and bacterial infections, ovulation and, in women with macroscopical and microscopical endometriosis, the endometrial implants themselves. The concomitant increase in number of peritoneal macrophages in an advanced stage of differentiation has been held responsible for the development of the disease [134, 135]. Macrophages are involved in inflammatory and immunological reactions, in remodelling of tissues and in healing of wounds. In addition to their regulatory functions, macrophages play a central role in the cell-mediated immune response.

The soluble factors produced by macrophages and detectable in peritoneal fluid include growth factors, TNF, fibronectin, immunosuppressive factors and angiogenic factors.

Cellular components

Startseva [136] reported reduced T cell immunity and an increase in B cell reactivity in women with endometriosis, indicating that both cell-mediated and humoral immunity are altered in endometriosis. Dmowski *et al.* [137] found a decrease in the cell-mediated immune response to autologous endometrial antigens in monkeys with spontaneous endometriosis. Steele *et al.* [138] demonstrated that the specific immune response, T-lymphocyte-mediated cytotoxicity, to autologous endometrial cells was significantly reduced in women with endometriosis, suggesting an immunological basis for the development of endometriosis. Wood *et al.* [139] reported that in rhesus monkeys after total body exposure to proton irradiation the prevalence of endometriosis more than doubled compared with normal controls. They suggested that suppression of the immune system facilitated the development of endometriosis.

Hill *et al.* [140] found a significant elevation of total leucocytes, macrophages and helper T lymphocytes in peritoneal fluid of women with stage I and II endometriosis and women with unexplained infertility. They also showed an increased number of natural killer (NK) cells in peritoneal fluid of women with endometriosis. NK cells belong to a subpopulation of lymphocytes that represents the first line of defence against the initiation and spread of tumours *in vivo*. Oosterlynck *et al.* [141] and Vigano *et al.* [142] confirmed defects in the cytotoxicity of peripheral autologous lymphocytes to endometrial target cells in patients with endometriosis. After CO_2 laser excision of the endometrial implants, the decreased NK activity in women with endometriosis persisted [143]. In peritoneal fluid an important NK cell activity was found, and this NK-mediated cytotoxicity was significantly reduced in women with endometriosis [144]. This decrease in NK activity in the peritoneal fluid of women with endometriosis is probably due to a functional deficiency, because Hill *et al.* [140] found an increase in the concentration of NK cells in the peritoneal fluid of women with endometriosis [144]. Furthermore, they demonstrated that the NK activity of lymphocytes pre-incubated with peritoneal fluid of women with endometriosis is decreased compared with the activity of those pre-incubated with peritoneal fluid of fertile women without endometriosis [145]. This immunosuppressive activity of peritoneal fluid in women with endometriosis is most probably the result of soluble factors released by activated macrophages [146].

From these studies the picture arises that a defect in peritoneal fluid NK-cell-mediated cytotoxicity against autologous endometrium in women with endometriosis precedes the development of the disease. This decreased cytotoxicity could facilitate the implantation of endometrial cells. Most probably, many women, if not all, with patent tubes develop a minor, early, subtle form of endometriosis. Outgrowth of these freshly implanted endometrial cells depends on other, soluble factors in the peritoneal fluid.

Biochemical components

The influence of hormones on the development of endometriosis has been postulated by Novak [147]. The probability of hormonal modulation of endometriosis is supported by the presence of oestrogen and progesterone receptors in endometriotic lesions [148–150]. A distinction should be made between the influence of hormones in initiating and in maintaining endometriosis. The initiation of growth of endometriosis in the monkey has been proved to be independent of oestrogens [151, 152]. Scott and Wharton [151] showed that the best growth of endometrial implants in castrated monkeys was achieved when they were treated with constant oestrogen and intermittent progesterone administration. For maintenance of long-term viability of endometrial implants either oestradiol or progesterone, alone or in combination, was required [152]. It should be kept in mind that these studies of the influence of oestrogens and progesterone were performed in an animal model with surgically implanted endometrium.

Brosens *et al.* [4] found a lower concentration of oestradiol and progesterone in the peritoneal fluid of patients with endometriosis, compared with patients without the disease. This lower hormonal content was accompanied by a higher number of LUF in endometriosis patients. They hypothesized that the lower concentration of progesterone allows proliferation and implantation of endometrial cells [5]. In an *in vitro* model, progesterone was shown to inhibit the proliferation of endometriotic cells. The inhibitory effect was completely reversed by the concomitant addition of RU486 (mifepristone) [153]. A high frequency of LUF cycles in patients with endometriosis has not been confirmed by others. The conflicting data on the incidence of LUF cycles mainly depend on the different ways of diagnosing LUF cycles: laparoscopy to detect an ovulation stigma, steroid concentrations of peritoneal fluid or serial ultrasound [6, 32, 154, 155]. Moreover, the concentrations of progesterone and oestradiol in peritoneal fluid are the same in patients with and without endometriosis [68, 73, 156].

Cyclic ovarian hormone secretion seems necessary for the growth or proliferation of ectopic endometrial tissue. The exact mechanisms underlying the proliferation–differentiation of endometrial epithelium, however, are not clear. It is conceivable that the mitogenic effect of oestrogen is modulated by locally produced paracrine and autocrine factors [157]. These and other factors, produced by macrophages, the endometriotic implant or the peritoneum and influencing endometrial growth, have been studied in women with and without endometriosis.

Sampson [158] postulated that the regurgitated menstrual blood acts as an irritant to the peritoneal surfaces and thus facilitates implantation.

Ohtsuka [159] and Malick [160] hypothesized that a change in intra-abdominal fibrinolysis could play an aetiological role in the development of endometriosis and the adhesions seen in this disease. They observed a decreased fibrinolytic activity of the mesothelial cells lining the peritoneal cavity in patients with endometriosis. The fibrin exudate developing as a consequence of peritoneal damage by retrograde menstruation, combined with the decreased fibrinolytic activity, might lead to adhesion formation. In these adhesions endometrial cells might easily implant. Peritoneal fluid fibrinolytic activity in patients with and without endometriosis was shown to be the same [161, 162]. If altered fibrinolysis plays a role in the aetiology of endometriosis, these differences may possibly be found at tissue level rather than in the peritoneal fluid.

Halme *et al.* [134] suggested that the more advanced macrophages found in women with endometriosis, apart from interfering with reproductive events, may produce factors that might facilitate growth of endometrial implants. Peritoneal macrophages of women with endometriosis have been shown *in vitro* to produce fibronectin [163], IL-1 [83], macrophage-derived growth factor [164], TNF [135, 165] and IL-6 [166, 167]. It was suggested that the production of these factors might facilitate the implantation of endometrial cells and their subsequent growth in the pelvis. Besides the documented production of cytokines and growth factors *in vitro* by macrophages, several other soluble substances involved in angiogenesis and in the attraction and proliferation of macrophages and produced by these macrophages have been detected in peritoneal fluid of women with endometriosis: epidermal growth factor [68], TNF [168], human macrophage colony-stimulating factor [169], IL-1β [75], IL-6 [166, 170], the cytokine RANTES [171], a protein in the range of 15–20 kDa with chemotactic activity with regard to macrophages [172], angiogenic factors [173] and IL-8 [174].

It has to be emphasized, however, that the mere presence of these cytokines, growth factors and macrophage attractants and the *in vitro* production of growth-promoting factors by macrophages do not prove their involvement in the development or maintenance of the disease. Besides that, the factors discussed were found in women who had already developed the disease.

The next step in elucidating the role of these substances in the pathogenesis of endometriosis has been their immunohistochemical localization in the target tissues [175–183]. The role of paracrine and autocrine regulation of endometrial growth by local growth factors has been substantiated by these findings.

Finally, the effect of peritoneal fluid and/or growth factors on endometrial stromal cell cultures *in vitro* has been studied, to support the hypothesis that soluble substances released by peritoneal macrophages are instrumental in the development of endometriosis. In most studies, isolated normal endometrial stromal cells in a short-term culture were used. These stromal cells survive more easily in tissue culture conditions than do endometrial epithelial cells [184]. Stromal cell proliferation was greater for cells exposed to endometriosis peritoneal fluid than for those exposed to non-endometriosis peritoneal fluid [184]. Peritoneal fluid from women with and without endometriosis has been shown to contain growth factors that are proteinaceous in nature and capable of stimulating the proliferation of endometrial-like cells and fibroblasts [185]. Koutsilieris *et al.* [186] subsequently purified this protein and suggested that it may be a 25 kDa heparin–sepharose-binding growth factor. In a mouse endometrial stromal cell culture, macrophage-conditioned medium appeared to function as a competence growth factor [187]. Macrophage-conditioned medium from patients with stage III/IV endometriosis demonstrated a mitogenic effect on a carcinoma cell line, while a monoclonal antibody against epidermal growth factor receptor blocked the mitogen effect [188]. The exact nature, however, of these macrophage-derived factors is not known. Several cytokines have been tried for their proliferative effect in endometrial cell cultures. Epidermal growth factor and transforming growth factor-α were mitogenic with regard to an endometrial carcinoma cell line, whereas TNF, IL-1 and platelet-derived growth factor had no effect [188]. In contrast, platelet-derived growth factor stimulated the proliferation of cultured endometrial stromal cells [189]. Epidermal growth factor stimulated the proliferation of cultured endometriotic cells [153]. IL-1 was shown to inhibit growth of endometrial stromal cells [190]. Hammond *et al.* [191] reported on the stromal cell response to a variety of growth factors alone and in combination. They found that epidermal growth factor, transforming growth factor and fibroblast growth factor induce a significant, dose-dependent increase in stromal cell proliferation.

From these observations it can be concluded that steroids and growth factors both play a role in the proliferation of endometrial glands and stroma, the steroidal mitogenic effect being modulated and mediated by locally produced paracrine and autocrine cytokines and growth factors [153, 157, 175, 179].

Conclusion

In conclusion, peritoneal macrophages play a pivotal role in the intra-abdominal environment. Endometrial tissue, after arrival in the peritoneal cavity, is likely to adhere to the mesothelial lining. The adherence may be mediated by cell adhesion molecules and soluble factors produced by peritoneal macrophages in an advanced stage of differentiation. Endometrial tissue can adhere if the regurgitated amount of endometrial tissue is too great or if the capacity of the intra-abdominal cells to clear the abdominal cavity is impaired. After adherence, endometrial tissue growth is promoted by steroids, growth factors and angiogenic factors, present in peritoneal fluid, in a paracrine and autocrine fashion.

Novak's statement in 1931 [147] about progress in understanding endometriosis is equally applicable today, and perhaps even more so, to the study of peritoneal fluid in relation to endometriosis-associated subfertility: 'Investigators have apparently worked themselves into a scientific cul-de-sac from which they can be rescued only by discovery of some new method of attacking the problem.' The progress recently made in peritoneal fluid research regarding the pathogenesis of endometriosis, however, merely sheds new light on the fundamental quandaries of this mysterious disease.

References

1 Maathuis JB, Van Look PFA, Michie EA. Changes in volume, total protein and ovarian steroid concentration of peritoneal fluid throughout the human menstrual cycle. *J Endocrinol* 1978 **76**: 123–133.
2 Koninckx PR, Renaer M, Brosens IA. Origin of peritoneal fluid in women: an ovarian exudation product. *Br J Obstet Gynaecol* 1980 **87**: 177–183.
3 Bouckaert PXJM, Evers JLH, Doesburg WH *et al.* Patterns of changes in proteins in the peritoneal fluid of women during the periovulatory phase of the menstrual cycle. *J Reprod Fert* 1986 77: 329–336.
4 Brosens IA, Koninckx PR, Corveleyn PA. A study of plasma progesterone, oestradiol-17β, prolactin and LH levels and of the luteal phase appearance of the ovaries in patients with endometriosis and infertility. *Br J Obstet Gynaecol* 1978 **85**: 246–250.
5 Koninckx PR, Heyns W, Verhoeven G *et al.* Biochemical characterization of peritoneal fluid in women during the menstrual cycle. *J Clin Endocrinol Metab* 1980 **51**: 1239–1244.
6 Dhont M, Serreyn R, Duvivier P *et al.* Ovulation and concentration of progesterone and estradiol in peritoneal fluid: relation with fertility and endometriosis. *Fertil Steril* 1984 **41**: 872–877.
7 Bouckaert PXJM, Evers JLH, Doesburg WH, Schellekens LA, Rolland R. Patterns of changes in glycoproteins, polypeptides, and steroids in the peritoneal fluid of women during the periovulatory phase of the cycle. *J Clin Endocrinol Metab* 1986 **62**: 293–299.
8 Muse K, Wilson EA. How does mild endometriosis cause infertility? *Fertil Steril* 1982 **38**: 145–152.
9 Walmer DK, Haney AF. Subfertility associated with endometriosis: potential influences of the peritoneal environment. *Sem Reprod Endocrinol* 1988 **6**: 263–267.
10 Bancroft K, Vaughan Williams CA, Elstein M. Minimal/mild endometriosis and infertility: a review. *Br J Obstet Gynaecol* 1989 **96**: 454–460.
11 Syrop CH, Halme J. Cyclic changes of peritoneal fluid parameters in normal and infertile patients. *Obstet Gynecol* 1987 **69**: 416–418.
12 Surrey ES, Halme J. Endometriosis as a cause of infertility. *Obstet Gynecol Clin North Am* 1989 **16**: 79–91.
13 Mahmood TA, Templeton A. Pathophysiology of mild endometriosis: review of the literature. *Human Reprod* 1990 **5**: 765–784.
14 Wheeler JM, Malinak LR. Does mild endometriosis cause infertility? *Sem Reprod Endocrinol* 1988 **6**: 239–249.
15 Gardner E, Gray DJ, O'Rahilly R. *Anatomy: a Regional Study of Human Structure.* 3rd edn, 1969, pp. 387–395, Philadelphia, WB Saunders.
16 Bloom W, Fawcett DW. *A Textbook of Histology*, 9th edn, 1978, pp. 186–187. Philadelphia, WB Saunders.
17 Novak J. Ueber Ursache und Bedeutung des physiologischen Ascites beim Weibe. *Zentralbl Gynaekol* 1922 **21**: 854–858.

18 Bouckaert PXJM. Peritoneumvloeistof. Biochemische veranderingen tijdens de menstruele cyclus (Thesis). 1984, Nijmegen.
19 Lippes J, Gonzales Enders RG, Pragay DA, Bartholomew WR. The collection and analysis of human fallopian tubal fluid. *Contraception* 1972 **5**: 85–103.
20 Halme J, Becker S, Hammond MG, Raj S: Pelvic macrophages in normal and infertile women: the role of patent tubes. *Am J Obstet Gynecol* 1982 **142**: 890–895.
21 Coulam CB, Hill LM, Breekle R. Ultrasonic evidence for luteinization of unruptured preovulatory follicles. *Fertil Steril* 1982 **37**: 524–529.
22 Koninckx PR, De Moor P, Brosens IA. Diagnosis of the luteinized unruptured follicle syndrome by steroid hormone assays in peritoneal fluid. *Br J Obstet Gynaecol* 1980 **87**: 929–934.
23 Haney AF, Muscato JJ, Weinberg JB. Peritoneal fluid cell populations in infertility patients. *Fertil Steril* 1981 **35**: 696–698.
24 Willemsen WNP, Mungyer G, Smets H *et al.* Behavior of cultured glandular cells obtained by flushing of the uterine cavity. *Fertil Steril* 1985 **44**: 92–95.
25 Van Furth R, Raeburn JA, Van Zwet TL. Characteristics of human mononuclear phagocytes. *Blood* 1979 **54**: 485–500.
26 Muscato JJ, Haney AF, Weinberg JB. Sperm phagocytosis by human peritoneal macrophages: a possible cause of infertility in endometriosis. *Am J Obstet Gynecol* 1982 **144**: 503–510.
27 Nathan CF, Murray HW, Cohn ZA. The macrophage as an effector cell. *N Engl J Med* 1980 **303**: 622–626.
28 Adams DO, Hamilton TA. The cell biology of macrophage activation. *Ann Rev Immunol* 1984 **2**: 283–318.
29 Nathan CF. Secretory products of macrophages. *J Clin Invest* 1987 **79**: 319–326.
30 Bonney RJ, Davies P. Possible autoregulatory functions of the secretory products of mononuclear phagocytes. *Contemp Top Immunobiol* 1984 **14**: 199–223.
31 Bursuker I, Goldman R. On the origin of macrophage heterogeneity: a hypothesis. *J Reticuloendo Soc* 1983 **33**: 207–220.
32 Lesorgen PR, Wu CH, Green PJ, Gocial B, Lerner LJ. Peritoneal fluid and serum steroids in infertility patients. *Fertil Steril* 1984 **42**: 237–242.
33 Chaudhuri G. Physiologic aspects of prostaglandins and leukotrienes. *Sem Reprod Endocrin* 1985 **3**: 219–230.
34 Killick S, Elstein M. Pharmacologic production of luteinized unruptured follicles by prostaglandin synthetase inhibitors. *Fertil Steril* 1987 **47**: 773–777.
35 Harper MKJ, Coons LW, Radicke DA, Hodgson BJ, Valenzuela G. Role of prostaglandins in contractile activity of the ampulla of the rabbit oviduct. *Am J Physiol* 1980 **238**: E157–E166.
36 Elder MG, Myatt L, Chaudhuri G. The role of prostaglandins in the spontaneous motility of the Fallopian tube. *Fertil Steril* 1977 **28**: 86–90.
37 Croxatto HB, Ortiz ME, Diaz S, Hess R. Attempts to modify ovum transport in women. *J Reprod Fert* 1979 **55**: 231–237.
38 Herman A, Claeys M, Moncada S, Vane JR. Biosynthesis of prostacyclin PGI_2 and 12-HETE by pericardium, pleura, peritoneum, and aorta of the rabbit. *Prostaglandins* 1979 **18**: 439–446.
39 Ylikorkala O, Tenhunen A. Follicular fluid prostaglandins in endometriosis and ovarian hyperstimulation. *Fertil Steril* 1984 **41**: 66–69.
40 Lenton EA, King H, Thomas EJ *et al.* The endocrine environment of the human oocyte. *J Reprod Fert* 1988 **82**: 827–841.
41 Abel MH, Kelly RW. Differential production of prostaglandins within the human uterus. *Prostaglandins* 1979 **18**: 821–828.

42 Smith SK, Abel MH, Kelly RW, Baird DT. A role for prostacyclin (PGI_2) in excessive menstrual bleeding. Lancet 1981 **i**: 522–524.
43 Kistner RW. Management of endometriosis in the infertile patient. *Fertil Steril* 1975 **26**: 1151–1166.
44 Collins JA, Wrixon W, Janes LB, Wilson EH. Treatment-independent pregnancy among infertile couples. *N Engl J Med* 1983 **309**: 1201–1206.
45 Strathy JH, Molgaard CA, Coulam CB, Melton LJ III. Endometriosis and infertility: a laparoscopic study of endometriosis among fertile and infertile women. *Fertil Steril* 1982 **38**: 667–672.
46 Broekhuizen FF, Haning RV Jr, Shapiro SS. Laparoscopic findings in twenty-five failures of artificial insemination. *Fertil Steril* 1980 **34**: 351–355.
47 Jansen RPS. Minimal endometriosis and reduced fecundability: prospective evidence from an artificial insemination by donor program. *Fertil Steril* 1986 **46**: 141–143.
48 Hammond MG, Jordan S, Sloan CS. Factors affecting pregnancy rates in a donor insemination program using frozen semen. *Am J Obstet Gynecol* 1986 **155**: 480–485.
49 Portuondo JA, Echanojauregui AD, Herran C, Alijarte I. Early conception in patients with untreated endometriosis. *Fertil Steril* 1983 **39**: 22–25.
50 Rodriguez-Escudero FJ, Neyro JL, Corcostegui B, Benito JA. Does mild endometriosis reduce fecundity? *Fertil Steril* 1988 **50**: 522–524.
51 Mahmood TA, Templeton A. The relationship between endometriosis and semen analysis: a review of 490 consecutive laparoscopies. *Human Reprod* 1989 **4**: 782–785.
52 Seibel MM, Berger MJ, Weinstein FG, Taymor ML. The effectiveness of danazol on subsequent fertility in minimal endometriosis. *Fertil Steril* 1982 **38**: 534–537.
53 Hull ME, Moghissi KS, Magyar DF, Hayes MF. Comparison of different treatment modalities of endometriosis in infertile women. *Fertil Steril* 1987 **47**: 40–44.
54 Thomas EJ, Cooke ID. Impact of gestrinone on the course of asymptomatic endometriosis. *Br Med J* 1987 **294**: 272–274.
55 Bayer SR, Seibel MM, Saffan DS, Berger MJ, Taymor ML. Efficacy of danazol treatment for minimal endometriosis in infertile women. *J Reprod Med* 1988 **33**: 179–183.
56 Telimaa S. Danazol and medroxyprogesterone acetate inefficacious in the treatment of infertility in endometriosis. *Fertil Steril* 1988 **50**: 872–875.
57 Fedele L, Parazinni F, Radici E *et al.* Buserelin acetate versus expectant management in the treatment of infertility associated with minimal or mild endometriosis: a randomized clinical trial. *Am J Obstet Gynecol* 1992 **166**: 1345–1350.
58 Chong AP, Keene ME, Thornton NL. Comparison of three modes of treatment for infertility patients with minimal pelvic endometriosis. *Fertil Steril* 1990 **53**: 407–410.
59 Hull MGR. Infertility treatment: relative effectiveness of conventional and assisted conception methods. *Human Reprod* 1992 **7**: 785–796.
60 Drake TS, Metz SA, Grunert GM, O'Brien WF. Peritoneal fluid volume in endometriosis. *Fertil Steril* 1980 **34**: 280–281.
61 Moretuzzo RW, DiLauro S, Jenison E *et al.* Serum and peritoneal fluid lavage fluid CA125 levels in endometriosis. *Fertil Steril* 1988 **50**: 430–433.
62 Halme J, Becker S, Wing R. Accentuated cyclic activation of peritoneal macrophages in patients with endometriosis. *Am J Obstet Gynecol* 1984 **148**: 85–90.
63 Chacho KJ, Stronkowski Chacho M, Andresen PJ, Scommegna A. Peritoneal fluid in patients with and without endometriosis: prostanoids and macrophages and their effect on the spermatozoa penetration assay. *Am J Obstet Gynecol* 1986 **154**: 1290–1299.
64 Oak MK, Chantler EN, Vaughn Williams CA, Elstein M. Sperm survival studies in peritoneal fluid from infertile women with endometriosis and unexplained infertility. *Clin Reprod Fert* 1985 **3**: 297–303.
65 Rock JA, Dubin MH, Ghodgankor RB *et al.* Cul-de-sac fluid in women with endome-

triosis: fluid volume and prostanoid concentration during the proliferative phase of the cycle-days 8 to 12. *Fertil Steril* 1982 **37**: 747–752.

66 Dawood MY, Khan-Dawood, FS, Wilson L Jr. Peritoneal fluid prostaglandins and prostanoids in women with endometriosis, chronic pelvic inflammatory disease, and pelvic pain. *Am J Obstet Gynecol* 1984 **148**: 391–395.

67 Mudge TJ, James MJ, Jones WR, Walsh JA. Peritoneal fluid 6-keto prostaglandin $F_{1\alpha}$ levels in women with endometriosis. *Am J Obstet Gynecol* 1985 **152**: 901–904.

68 DeLeon FD, Vijayakumar R, Brown M *et al.* Peritoneal fluid volume, estrogen, progesterone, prostaglandin, and epidermal growth factor concentrations in patients with and without endometriosis. *Obstet Gynecol* 1986 **68**: 189–194.

69 Olive DL, Weinberg JB, Haney AF. Peritoneal macrophages and infertility: the association between cell number and pelvic pathology. *Fertil Steril* 1985 **44**: 772–777.

70 Rezai N, Ghodgaonkar RB, Zacur HA, Rock JA, Dubin NH. Cul-de-sac fluid in women with endometriosis: fluid volume, protein and prostanoid concentration during the periovulatory period-days 13 to 18. *Fertil Steril* 1987 **48**: 29–32.

71 Awadalla SG, Friedman CI, Haq AU *et al.* Local peritoneal factors: their role in infertility associated with endometriosis. *Am J Obstet Gynecol* 1987 **157**: 1207–1214.

72 Dunselman GAJ, Bouckaert PXJM, Evers JLH. The acute-phase response in endometriosis of women. *J Reprod Fert* 1988 **83**: 803–808.

73 Mahmood TA, Templeton A. Peritoneal fluid volume and sex steroids in the preovulatory period in mild endometriosis. *Br J Obstet Gynaecol* 1991 **98**: 179–183.

74 Moen MH, Hagen B, Onsrud M. CA 125 in peritoneal fluid from patients with endometriosis. *Human Reprod* 1991 **6**: 1400–1403.

75 Mori H, Sawairi M, Nakagawa M *et al.* Expression of interleukin-1 (IL-1) β-messenger ribonucleic acid (mRNA) and IL-1 receptor antagonist mRNA in peritoneal macrophages from patients with endometriosis. *Fertil Steril* 1992 **57**: 535–542.

76 Olive DL, Haney AF, Weinberg JB. The nature of the peritoneal exudate associated with infertility: peritoneal fluid and serum lysozyme activity. *Fertil Steril* 1987 **48**: 802–806.

77 Haney AF, Weinberg JB. Reduction of the intraperitoneal inflammation associated with endometriosis by treatment with medroxyprogesterone acetate. *Am J Obstet Gynecol* 1988 **159**: 450–454.

78 Haney AF, Jenkins S, Weinberg JB. The stimulus responsible for the peritoneal fluid inflammation observed in infertile women with endometriosis. *Fertil Steril* 1991 **56**: 408–413.

79 Haney AF, Misukonis MA, Weinberg JB. Macrophages and infertility: oviductal macrophages as potential mediators of infertility. *Fertil Steril* 1983 **39**: 310–315.

80 Halme J, Becker S, Hammond MG, Raj HMG, Raj S. Increased activation of pelvic macrophages in infertile women with mild endometriosis. *Am J Obstet Gynecol* 1983 **145**: 333–337.

81 Zeller JM, Henig I, Radwanska E, Dmowski WP. Enhancement of human monocyte and peritoneal macrophage chemiluminescence activities in women with endometriosis. *Am J Reprod Immunol Microbiol* 1987 **13**: 78–82

82 Dunselman GAJ, Hendrix MGR, Bouckaert PXJM, Evers JLH. Functional aspects of peritoneal macrophages in endometriosis of women. *J Reprod Fert* 1988 **82**: 707–710.

83 Fakih H, Baggett B, Holtz G *et al.* Interleukin-1: a possible role in the infertility associated with endometriosis. *Fertil Steril* 1987 **47**: 213–217.

84 Syrop CH, Halme J. A comparison of peritoneal fluid parameters of infertile patients and the subsequent occurrence of pregnancy. *Fertil Steril* 1986 **46**: 631–635.

85 Steinleitner A, Lambert H, Kazensky C, Danks P. Peritoneal fluid from endometriosis patients affects reproductive outcome in an *in vivo* model. *Fertil Steril* 1990 **53**: 926–929.

86 Suginami H, Yano K, Watanabe K, Matsuura S. A factor inhibiting ovum capture by the

oviductal fimbriae present in endometriosis peritoneal fluid. *Fertil Steril* 1986 **46**: 1140–1146.

87 Hurst PR, Jefferies K, Eckstein P, Dawson K, Wheeler AG. Leukocytes are consistently associated with degenerating embryos in IUD-bearing rhesus monkeys. *Nature* 1977 **269**: 331–333.

88 Ball RY, Scott N, Mitchinson MJ. Further observations on spermiography by murine peritoneal macrophages *in vitro*. *J Reprod Fert* 1984 **71**: 221–226.

89 London SN, Haney AF, Weinberg JB. Macrophages and infertility: enhancement of human macrophage mediated sperm killing by antisperm antibodies. *Fertil Steril* 1985 **43**: 274–278.

90 Sueldo CE, Lambert H, Steinleiter A, Rathwick G, Swanson J. The effect of peritoneal fluid from patients with endometriosis on murine sperm–oocyte interaction. *Fertil Steril* 1987 **48**: 697–699.

91 Halme J, Hall JL. Effect of pelvic fluid from endometriosis patients on human sperm penetration of zona free hamster ova. *Fertil Steril* 1982 **37**: 573–576.

92 Hill JA, Cohen J, Anderson DJ. The effect of lymphokines and monokines on human sperm fertilizing ability in the zona-free hamster egg penetration test. *Am J Obstet Gynecol* 1989 **160**: 1154–1159.

93 Wincek TJ, Meyer TK, Meyer MR, Kuehl TJ. Absence of a direct effect of recombinant tumor necrosis factor-alpha on human sperm function and murine preimplantation development. *Fertil Steril* 1991 **56**: 332–339.

94 Coddington CC, Oehninger S, Cunningham DS *et al.* Peritoneal fluid from patients with endometriosis decreases sperm binding to the zona pellucida in the hemizona assay: a preliminary report. *Fertil Steril* 1992 **57**: 783–786.

95 Stone SC, Himsl K. Peritoneal recovery of motile and nonmotile sperm in the presence of endometriosis. *Fertil Steril* 1986 **46**: 338–339.

96 Maathuis JB, Houx PCW, Bastiaans LA, Mastboom JL. Some properties of peritoneal fluid obtained by laparoscopy from fertile and infertile women. *J Reprod Fert* 1973 **35**: 630–632.

97 Soldati GA, Piffaretti-Yanez A, Campana A *et al.* Effect of peritoneal fluid on sperm motility and velocity distribution using objective measurements. *Fertil Steril* 1989 **52**: 113–119.

98 Burke RK. Effect of peritoneal washings from women with endometriosis on sperm velocity. *J Reprod Med* 1987 **32**: 743–746.

99 Curtis P, Lindsay P, Jackson AE, Shaw RW. Adverse effect on sperm movement characteristics in women with minimal and mild endometriosis. *Br J Obstet Gynaecol* 1993 **100**: 165–169.

100 Bielfeld P, Graf MA, Jeyendran RS, DeLeon FD, Zaneveld LJD. Effects of peritoneal fluid from patients with endometriosis on capacitated spermatozoa. *Fertil Steril* 1993 **60**: 893–896.

101 Soldati GA, Piffaretti-Yanez A, Medici G, Eppenberger U, Balerna MJ. Purification of a factor from human peritoneal fluid that is able to immobilize spermatozoa. *Human Reprod* 1993 **8**: 428–436.

102 Hill JA, Haimovici F, Politch JA, Anderson DJ. Effects of soluble products of activated macrophages (lymphokines and monokines) on human sperm motion parameters. *Fertil Steril* 1987 **47**: 460–465.

103 Gentry WL, Buster JE, Schriock ED, Carson SA. Failure to demonstrate significant anti-sperm antibodies in peritoneal fluid of patients with endometriosis. *Fertil Steril* 1989 **52**: 949–952.

104 Leach RE, Arneson BW, Ball GD, Ory SJ. Absence of antisperm antibodies and factors influencing sperm motility in the cul-de-sac fluid of women with endometriosis. *Fertil*

Steril 1990 **53**: 351–353.

105 Morcos RN, Gibbons WE, Findley WE. Effect of peritoneal fluid on *in vitro* cleavage of 2-cell mouse embryos: possible role in infertility associated with endometriosis. *Fertil Steril* 1985 **44**: 678–683.

106 Dodds WG, Miller FA, Friedman CI *et al.* The effect of preovulatory peritoneal fluid from cases of endometriosis on murine *in vitro* fertilization, embryo development, oviduct transport, and implantation. *Am J Obstet Gynecol* 1992 **166**: 219–224.

107 Schneider EG, Armant DR, Kupper TS, Polan ML. Absence of a direct effect of recombinant interleukins and cultured peritoneal macrophages on early embryonic development in the mouse. *Biol Reprod* 1989 **40**: 825–833.

108 Prough SG, Aksel S, Gilmore SM, Yeoman RR. Peritoneal fluid fractions from patients with endometriosis do not promote two-cell mouse embryo growth. *Fertil Steril* 1990 **54**: 927–930.

109 Moon YS, Leung PCS, Ho Yuen B, Gomel V. Prostaglandin F in human endometriotic tissue. *Am J Obstet Gynecol* 1981 **141**: 344–345.

110 Ylikorkala O, Viinikka L. Prostaglandins and endometriosis. *Acta Obstet Gynecol Scand* 1983 **113**: 105–107.

111 Vernon MW, Beard JS, Graves K, Wilson EA. Classification of endometriotic implants by morphologic appearance and capacity to synthesize prostaglandin F. *Fertil Steril* 1986 **46**: 801–806.

112 DeLeon FD, Vijayakuma R, Rao CV, Yussman MA. Production of prostaglandin (PG) $F_{2\alpha}$ and PGE_2 by peritoneum involved with and without endometriosis (Abstract). *Soc Gyn Invest* 1983 **30**: 161.

113 Drake TS, O'Brien WF, Ranwell PW, Metz SA. Peritoneal fluid thromboxane B_2 and 6-keto-prostaglandin $F_{1\alpha}$ in endometriosis. *Am J Obstet Gynecol* 1981 **140**: 401–404.

114 Badawy SZA, Marshall L, Gabal AA, Nusbaum ML. The concentration of 13,14-dihydro-15-keto prostaglandin $F_{2\alpha}$ and prostaglandin E_2 in peritoneal fluid of infertile patients with and without endometriosis. *Fertil Steril* 1982 **38**: 166–170.

115 Sgarlata CS, Hertelendy F, Mikhail G. The prostanoid content in peritoneal fluid and plasma of women with endometriosis. *Am J Obstet Gynecol* 1983 **147**: 563–565.

116 Vasquez G, Cornillie F, Brosens IA. Peritoneal endometriosis: scanning electron microscopy and histology of minimal pelvic endometriotic lesions. *Fertil Steril* 1984 **42**: 696–703.

117 Morita M, Yano Y, Otaka K, Kojima E, Momose K. Minimal and mild endometriosis: Nd:YAG laser treatment and changes in prostaglandin concentrations in peritoneal fluid. *J Reprod Med* 1990 **35**: 621–624.

118 Taketani Y, Kuo TM, Mizuno M. Comparison of cytokine levels and embryo toxicity in peritoneal fluid in infertile women with untreated or treated endometriosis. *Am J Obstet Gynecol* 1992 **167**: 265–270.

119 Dunselman GAJ, Dumoulin JC, Land JA, Evers JLH. Lack of effect of peritoneal endometriosis on fertility in the rabbit model. *Fertil Steril* 1991 **56**: 340–342.

120 Sampson JA. The development of the implantation theory for the origin of peritoneal endometriosis. *Am J Obstet Gynecol* 1940 **40**: 549–557.

121 Jenkins S, Olive DL, Haney AF. Endometriosis: pathogenetic implications of the anatomic distribution. *Obstet Gynecol* 1986 **67**: 355–338.

122 Keettel WC, Stein RJ. The viability of the cast-off menstrual endometrium. *Am J Obstet Gynecol* 1951 **61**: 440–442.

123 Sanfilippo JS, Wakin NG, Schikler KN, Yussman MA. Endometriosis in association with uterine anomaly. *Am J Obstet Gynecol* 1986 **154**: 39–43.

124 TeLinde RW, Scott RB. Experimental endometriosis. *Am J Obstet Gynecol* 1950 **60**: 1147–1173.

125 Levander G, Normann P. The pathogenesis of endometriosis: an experimental study. *Acta Obstet Gynecol Scand* 1955 **34**: 366–398.
126 Halme J, Hammond MG, Hulka JF, Raj SG, Talbert LM. Retrograde menstruation in healthy women and in patients with endometriosis. *Obstet Gynecol* 1984 **64**: 151–154.
127 Bartosik D, Jacobs SL, Kelly LJ. Endometrial tissue in peritoneal fluid. *Fertil Steril* 1986 **46**: 796–800.
128 Scott RB, Te Linde RW, Wharton LR Jr. Further studies on experimental endometriosis. *Am J Obstet Gynecol* 1953 **66**: 1082–1099.
129 Zhang R, Wild RA, Ojago JM. Effect of tumor necrosis factor-alpha on adhesion of human endometrial stromal cells to peritoneal mesothelial cells: an *in vitro* system. *Fertil Steril* 1993 **59**: 1196–1201.
130 Wild RA, Zhang R, Medders D. Whole endometrial fragments form characteristics of *in vivo* endometriosis in a mesothelial cell co-culture system: an *in vitro* model for the study of the histogenesis of endometriosis. *J Soc Gynecol Invest* 1994 **1**: 65–68.
131 Cunha GR, Bigsby RM, Cooke PS, Sugimura Y. Stromal–epithelial interactions in adult organs. *Cell Differentiation* 1985 **17**: 137–148.
132 Van der Linden PJQ, De Goeij AFPM, Dunselman GAJ *et al.* Expression of integrins and E-cadherin in cells from menstrual effluent, endometrium, peritoneal fluid, peritoneum, and endometriosis. *Fertil Steril* 1994 **61**: 85–90.
133 Olive DL, Henderson DY. Endometriosis and Müllerian anomalies. *Obstet Gynecol* 1987 **69**: 412–415.
134 Halme J, Becker S, Haskill S. Altered maturation and function of peritoneal macrophages: possible role in pathogenesis of endometriosis. *Am J Obstet Gynecol* 1987 **156**: 783–789.
135 Halme J. Release of tumor necrosis factor-alpha by human peritoneal macrophages *in vivo* and *in vitro*. *Am J Obstet Gynecol* 1989 **161**: 1718–1725.
136 Startseva NV. Clinico-immunological aspects in genital endometriosis. *Akush Ginekol* 1980 **3**: 23–26.
137 Dmowski WP, Steele RN, Baker GF. Deficient cellular immunity in endometriosis. *Am J Obstet Gynecol* 1981 **141**: 377–383.
138 Steele RW, Dmowski WP, Marmer DJ. Immunologic aspects of endometriosis. *Am J Reprod Immunol* 1984 **6**: 33–36.
139 Wood DH, Yochmowitz MG, Salmon YL, Eason RL, Boster RA. Proton irradiation and endometriosis. *Aviat Space Environ Med* 1983 **54**: 718–724.
140 Hill JA, Faris HMP, Schiff I, Anderson DJ. Characterization of leukocyte subpopulations in the peritoneal fluid of women with endometriosis. *Fertil Steril* 1988 **50**: 216–222.
141 Oosterlynck DJ, Cornillie FJ, Waer M, Vandeputte M, Koninckx PR. Women with endometriosis show a defect in natural killer activity resulting in a decreased cytotoxicity to autologous endometrium. *Fertil Steril* 1991 **56**: 45–51.
142 Vigano P, Vercellini P, DiBlasio AM *et al.* Deficient antiendometrium lymphocyte-mediated cytotoxicity in patients with endometriosis. *Fertil Steril* 1991 **56**: 894–899.
143 Oosterlynck DJ, Waer M, Koninckx PR, Vandeputte M. CO_2 laser excision of endometriosis does not improve the decreased natural killer activity. *Acta Obstet Gynecol Scand* (in press).
144 Oosterlynck DJ, Meuleman C, Waer M, Vandeputte M, Koninckx PR. The natural killer activity of peritoneal fluid lymphocytes is decreased in women with endometriosis. *Fertil Steril* 1992 **58**: 290–295.
145 Oosterlynck DJ, Meuleman C, Waer M, Koninckx PR, Vandeputte M. Immunosuppressive activity of peritoneal fluid in women with endometriosis. *Obstet Gynecol* 1993 **82**: 206–212.
146 Oosterlynck DJ, Meuleman C, Waer M, Vandeputte M, Koninckx PR. Transforming growth factor-β in peritoneal fluid of women with endometriosis. *Obstet Gynecol* (in press).

147 Novak E. Pelvic endometriosis: spontaneous rupture of endometrial cysts, with a report of three cases. *Am J Obstet Gynecol* 1931 **22**: 826–837.
148 Jänne O, Kaupilla A, Kokko E *et al.* Estrogen and progestin receptors in endometriosis lesions: comparison with endometrial tissue. *Am J Obstet Gynecol* 1981 **141**: 562–566.
149 Lessey BA, Metzger DA, Haney AF, McCarty KS Jr. Immunohistochemical analysis of estrogen and progesterone receptors in endometriosis: comparison with normal endometrium during the menstrual cycle and the effect of medical therapy. *Fertil Steril* 1989 **51**: 409–415.
150 Bergqvist A, Ljungberg O, Skoog L. Immunohistochemical analysis of oestrogen and progesterone receptors in endometriotic tissue and endometrium. *Human Reprod* 1993 **8**: 1915–1922.
151 Scott RB, Wharton LR Jr. The effect of estrone and progesterone on the growth of experimental endometriosis in rhesus monkeys. *Am J Obstet Gynecol* 1957 **74**: 852–865.
152 DiZerega GS, Barber DL, Hodgen GD. Endometriosis: role of ovarian steroids in initiation, maintenance and suppression. *Fertil Steril* 1980 **33**: 649–653.
153 Taketani Y, Mizuno M. Hormonal regulation of endometriotic cell growth in primary cell culture system. *Arch Gynecol Obstet* 1992 **251**: 127–132.
154 Donnez J, Langerock S, Thomas K. Peritoneal fluid volume, 17β-estradiol and progesterone concentrations in women with endometriosis and/or luteinized unruptured follicle syndrome. *Gynecol Obstet Invest* 1983 **16**: 210–220.
155 Thomas EJ, Lenton EA, Cooke ID. Follicle growth patterns and endocrinological abnormalities in infertile women with minor degrees of endometriosis. *Br J Obstet Gynaecol* 1986 **93**: 852–858.
156 Ylikorkala O, Koskimies A, Laatkainen T, Tenhunen A, Viinikka L. Peritoneal fluid prostaglandins in endometriosis, tubal disorders and unexplained infertility. *Obstet Gynecol* 1984 **63**: 616–620.
157 Tabibzadeh SS, Satyaswaroop PG, Rao PN. Antiproliferative effect of interferon-γ in human endometrial epithelial cells *in vitro*: potential local growth modulatory role in endometrium. *J Clin Endocrinol Metab* 1988 **67**: 131–138.
158 Sampson JA. Metastatic or embolic endometriosis due to menstrual dissemination into the venous circulation. *Am J Pathol* 1927 **3**: 93–109.
159 Ohtsuka N. Study on pathogenesis of adhesions in endometriosis. *Acta Obstet Gynaec Jpn* 1980 **32**: 1758–1766.
160 Malick JE. The etiology of endometriosis. *J A O A* 1982 **81**: 407–412.
161 Batzofin JH, Holmes SD, Gibbons WE, Buttram VC Jr. Peritoneal fluid plasminogen activator activity in endometriosis and pelvic adhesive disease. *Fertil Steril* 1985 **44**: 277–279.
162 Dunselman GAJ, Bouckaert PXJM, van Wersch JWJ, Brommer EJP, Evers JLH. Fibrinolytic properties of peritoneal fluid in endometriosis of women. *Gynecol Obstet Invest* 1988 **26**: 302–307.
163 Kauma S, Clark MR, White C, Halme J. Production of fibronectin by peritoneal macrophages and concentration of fibronectin in peritoneal fluid from patients with or without endometriosis. *Obstet Gynecol* 1988 **72**: 13–18.
164 Halme J, White C, Estes J, Haskill S. Peritoneal macrophages from patients with endometriosis release growth factor activity *in vitro*. *J Clin Endocrinol Metab* 1988 **66**: 1044–1049.
165 Buyalos RP, Rutanen EM, Tsui E, Halme J. Release of tumor necrosis factor alpha by human peritoneal macrophages in response to toxic-shock syndrome toxin-1. *Obstet Gynecol* 1991 **78**: 182–186.
166 Rier SE, Parsons AK, Becker JL. Altered interleukin-6 production by peritoneal leukocytes from patients with endometriosis. *Fertil Steril* 1994 **61**: 294–299.

167 Keenan JA, Chen TT, Eaton NL, Torry DS, Caudle MR. Interferon gamma (IFN-γ) and interleukin-6 (IL-6) in peritoneal fluid (PF) and macrophage conditioned media (MCM) of women with and without endometriosis (Abstract). *Proc Soc Gynecol Invest* 1994 213.

168 Eisermann J, Gast MJ, Pineda J, Odem RR, Collins JL. Tumor necrosis factor in peritoneal fluid of women undergoing laparoscopic surgery. *Fertil Steril* 1988 **50**: 573–579.

169 Weinberg JB, Haney AF, Ramakrishan S. Peritoneal fluid and plasma levels of human macrophage colony-stimulating factor in relation to peritoneal fluid macrophage content. *Blood* 1991 **78**: 513–516.

170 Boutten A, Dehoux M, Edelman P *et al.* IL6 and acute phase plasma proteins in peritoneal fluid of women with endometriosis. *Clin Chim Acta* 1992 **210**: 187–195.

171 Khorram O, Taylor RN, Ryan IP, Schall TJ, Landers DV. Peritoneal fluid concentrations of the cytokine RANTES correlate with the severity of endometriosis. *Am J Obstet Gynecol* 1993 **169**: 1545–1549.

172 Leiva MC, Hasty LA, Pfeifer S, Mastroianni L Jr, Lyttle CR. Increased chemotactic activity of peritoneal fluid in patients with endometriosis. *Am J Obstet Gynecol* 1993 **168**: 592–598.

173 Oosterlynck DJ, Meuleman C, Sobis H, Vandeputte M, Koninckx PR. Angiogenic activity of peritoneal fluid from women with endometriosis. *Fertil Steril* 1993 **59**: 778–782.

174 Ryan IP, Tseng JF, Schriock ED *et al.* Interleukin (IL)-8 concentrations are elevated in peritoneal fluid of women with endometriosis (Abstract). *Proc Soc Gynecol Invest* 1994 214.

175 Haining REB, Cameron IT, van Papendorp C *et al.* Epidermal growth factor in human endometrium: proliferative effects in culture and immunohistochemical localization in normal and endometriotic tissues. *Human Reprod* 1991 **6**: 1200–1205.

176 Melega C, Balducci M, Bulletti C *et al.* Tissue factors influencing growth and maintenance of endometriosis. *Ann N Y Acad Sci* 1991 **662**: 256–268.

177 Simms JS, Chegini N, Williams RS, Rossi AM, Dunn WA Jr. Identification of epidermal growth factor, transforming growth factor-alpha, and epidermal growth factor receptor in surgically induced endometriosis in rats. *Obstet Gynecol* 1991 **78**: 850–857.

178 Prentice A, Thomas EJ, Weddell A *et al.* Epidermal growth factor receptor expression in normal endometrium and endometriosis: an immunohistochemical study. *Br J Obstet Gynaecol* 1992 **99**: 395–398.

179 Chegini N, Rossi MJ, Masterson BJ. Platelet-derived growth factor (PDGF), epidermal growth factor (EGF), and EGF and PDGF β-receptors in human endometrial tissue: localization and *in vitro* action. *Endocrinology* 1992 **130**: 2373–2385.

180 Zhang Z, Krause M, Davis DL. Epidermal growth factor receptors in porcine endometrium: binding characteristics and the regulation of prostaglandin E and $F_{2\alpha}$ production. *Biol Reprod* 1992 **46**: 932–936.

181 Ferriani RA, Charnock-Jones DS, Prentice A, Thomas EJ, Smith SK. Immunohistochemical localization of acidic and basic fibroblast growth factors in normal human endometrium and endometriosis and the detection of their mRNA polymerase chain reaction. *Human Reprod* 1993 **8**: 11–16.

182 Sahakian V, Anners J, Haskill S, Halme J. Selective localization of interleukin-1 receptor antagonist in eutopic endometrium and endometriotic implants. *Fertil Steril* 1993 **60**: 276–279.

183 Chegini N, Gold LI, Williams RS. Localization of transforming growth factor β-isoforms TGF-β1, TGF-β2, and TGF-β3 in surgically induced endometriosis in the rat. *Obstet Gynecol* 1994 **83**: 455–461.

184 Surrey ES, Halme J. Effect of peritoneal fluid from endometriosis patients on endometrial stromal cell proliferation *in vitro*. *Obstet Gynecol* 1990 **76**: 792–797.

185 Koutsilieris M, Allaire-Michaud L, Fortier M, Lemay A. Mitogen(s) for endometrial-like

cells can be detected in human peritoneal fluid. *Fertil Steril* 1991 **56**: 888–893.
186 Koutsilieris M, Niklinski W, Frenette G, Lemay A. Heparin–sepharose binding growth factors in peritoneal fluid of women with endometriosis. *Fertil Steril* 1993 **59**: 93–97.
187 Olive DL, Montoya I, Riehl RM, Schenken RS. Macrophage-conditioned media enhance endometrial stromal cell proliferation *in vitro*. *Am J Obstet Gynecol* 1991 **165**: 953–958.
188 Zhang R, Wild RA, Medders D, Gunupudi SR. Effects of peritoneal macrophages from patients with endometriosis on the proliferation of endometrial carcinoma cell line ECC-1. *Am J Obstet Gynecol* 1991 **165**: 1842–1846.
189 Surrey ES, Halme J. Effect of platelet-derived growth factor on endometrial stromal cell proliferation *in vitro*: a model for endometriosis? *Fertil Steril* 1991 **56**: 672–679.
190 Van Le L, Oh ST, Anners JA, Rinehart CA, Halme J. Interleukin-1 inhibits growth of normal endometrial stromal cells. *Obstet Gynecol* 1992 **80**: 405–409.
191 Hammond MG, Oh ST, Anners J, Surrey ES, Halme J. The effect of growth factors on the proliferation of human endometrial stromal cells in culture. *Am J Obstet Gynecol* 1993 **168**: 1131–1138.

Chapter 5
Immune System

D.H. BARLOW AND S. FERNÁNDEZ-SHAW

Introduction

Endometriosis is a multifactorial disorder. Sampson's theory [1] suggests that retrograde menstruation may be necessary for endometriosis. However, retrograde menstruation occurs in at least 90% of women [2] and is much more prevalent than endometriosis, suggesting that it is not by itself sufficient to originate the disease. This raises the question of what circumstances might favour the development of endometriosis. The host response to ectopic endometrium has been considered as an aetiological factor. This chapter addresses the issues of changes in specific and non-specific immunity and in humoral and cell-mediated immune responses that have been associated with endometriosis.

General outline of immune system

The immune system aims at the recognition and disposal of foreign material which enters the body, protecting us from a variety of diseases while maintaining an indifferent stance to self-components. Four major cell types are involved in the immune responses: macrophages or monocytes, natural killer (NK) cells, T lymphocytes (T cells) and B lymphocytes (B cells). Macrophages and NK cells are characteristic of non-specific or innate immune responses while T and B cells are active in specific or adaptive immune responses. The macrophages' main function is to take up and digest particles, cells or organisms. They also produce soluble molecules that mediate inflammatory responses, leading to the classic symptoms of pain, heat, redness and swelling. NK cells can destroy certain virally infected, embryonic or tumour cells. They are capable of spontaneous cytotoxic activity without a prior sensitization; their reactivity is not restricted by the major histocompatibility complex (MHC).

B lymphocytes mediate humoral immune responses. Surface receptors on B lymphocytes bind foreign antigens, which results in their transformation and clonal expansion into plasma cells, which produce specific antibodies. These antibodies bind to free or soluble antigen and, if the binding is on a cell surface, this is followed by activation of the complement cascade, with resulting damage to the target cell and opsonization of the target cell for phagocytosis by inflammatory cells.

T lymphocytes are responsible for the cell-mediated immune responses. They respond to cell surface antigens when those antigens are processed by antigen-presenting cells and presented in association with either class I or II MHC antigens. The MHC antigens in humans are designated as human leucocyte antigens (HLA). T cells are involved in antiviral immunity, as well as the graft-versus-host reaction and graft rejection. Different T cell subsets with regulatory or effector functions interact to stimulate or suppress immune responses. They kill specific target cells by a cytolytic mechanism (T_c, cytotoxic T cell). They also suppress (T_s, suppressor T cell) and promote (T_h, helper T cell) immune responses through interactions with lymphocytes and accessory cells.

Macrophages and lymphocytes, as well as many other nucleated cell types, produce cytokines. They have multiple effects, including the regulation of the differentiation, growth and function of haematopoietic and many other cell types. It was generally believed that cytokines were produced as part of inflammatory processes or else as part of the host response to infection or immune challenge, but it is now known that they also have a role in the normal physiology of various tissues [3]. In contrast to hormones, cytokines usually act over short distances as autocrine and paracrine intercellular signals within tissues and only occasionally spill over into the circulation and initiate systemic reactions [4]. Cytokines include interleukins (IL-1 to IL-11), macrophage and granulocyte colony-stimulating factors (M-, G- and GM-CSF), tumour necrosis factors (TNF; alpha and beta), interferons (IFN; alpha, beta and gamma), transforming growth factors (TGF; alpha and beta), activin, inhibin, chemotactic factors and epidermal, fibroblast, insulin-like, nerve and platelet-derived growth factors.

Humoral and immune cell immune responses can be linked. The immune cells interact with themselves and one another to protect the host from disease, from infectious diseases to neoplasia. In endometriosis, relevant events are likely to be the retrograde spill of endometrial tissue and its processing by phagocytic cells (probably occurring in most women); the presence of endometriotic implants with their associated tissue damage and inflammatory reaction. These create many possibilities for immune system activation by autoantigen presentation after retrograde spill or tissue damage or by the secretion of cytokines by the implants, in association with the peritoneal inflammation, and by the activated macrophages.

Cellular immune changes in endometriosis

Several authors have suggested that some aspects of cell-mediated immunity may be altered in women with endometriosis. Dmowski *et al.* [5] observed decreased *in vivo* reactivity to intradermal injection of autologous endometrial antigens (measured as intensity of perivascular lymphocytic infiltration), and decreased *in vitro* lymphocyte proliferation in response to the same autologous antigens, in monkeys with endometriosis compared with controls. In other studies, T-cell-mediated cytotoxicity to autologous endometrial antigens was significantly decreased in women with endometriosis [6–8], this effect being more significant in women with severe endometriosis [6]. Other tests for non-specific immune function, such as lymphocyte stimulation response to the mitogen phytohaemagglutinin, were similar in women with endometriosis and in controls [6]. In contrast to these reports, some studies have described increased concentrations of T and B lymphocytes in the peritoneal fluid (PF) and serum of women with endometriosis [9], while others found no differences between patients and controls [10].

Macrophages

Many investigators have confirmed an increase in the number of macrophages in PF of women with endometriosis, although there is some debate as to whether their concentration is also increased [11, 12]. As well as increasing in number, peritoneal macrophages have been reported to be more activated in endometriosis. This higher level of activation has been measured by cellular enlargement; by capping or segregation of specific membrane receptors at one pole of the cell; by increases in enzymes such as acid phosphatase, myeloperoxidase and leucine aminopeptidase; by increases in chemiluminescence; and by *in vitro* phagocytic activity. Many studies, but not all, have confirmed an activation of peritoneal macrophages in the PF of women with endometriosis using at least one of the above criteria (reviewed by [11, 12]. Once activated, macrophages may release products such as cytokines, prostaglandins, complement components and hydrolytic enzymes, regulating events in the peritoneal cavity. Macrophages can remove red blood cells, damaged tissue fragments and, most probably, endometrial cells that gain access to the peritoneal cavity. The monocyte/macrophage system in the peritoneal cavity is, by some, thought to be part of a 'disposal system', meaning the first line of cellular immune response to the presence of endometrial cells inside the peritoneal cavity [13]. Endometriosis may develop when the 'disposal system' is overwhelmed by high levels of retrograde menstruation [13] or when a defective peritoneal 'disposal system' permits implantation and growth of the endometrial cells or fragments [14]. Other authors have suggested that the alterations in peritoneal macrophages may predate the development of endometriosis, rather than being a consequence [15]. Using a rabbit model, Johnson *et al.* [15] were unable to observe a significant increase in macrophage number or activation in the peritoneal cavity of those rabbits in which endometrium was surgically implanted in the peritoneum. Whether present before or as a consequence of the disease, Dmowski [13] suggested that the cytotoxic activities of peritoneal macrophages in endometriosis may be suppressed, especially in severe endometriosis (unpublished data), the inefficiency of the 'disposal system' leading to the changes in humoral immunity. The higher number and activation of macrophages in the peritoneal cavity is also likely to be accompanied by an increase in macrophage-derived cytokines. Some of these cytokines may, as suggested by Dmowski [13], stimulate the proliferation and differentiation of T cells, and subsequently T-cell-derived factors may play a critical role in the activation of B cells, leading to the development of an autoimmune reaction. Moreover, it is also possible that these cytokines may affect other cells present in the peritoneal cavity, such as the ectopic endometrial cells.

An alternative explanation for the activation of macrophages and increase in autoantibodies in endometriosis has been suggested. The expression of HLA-DR (an MHC class II antigen) can be found in mature B cells, macrophages and activated T cells but, in general, is not observed in non-immunocompetent cells. However, it is known that HLA-DR expression is positive in glandular epithelium, lymphocytes and vascular endothelial cells in uterine endometrium [16]. Ota and Igarashi [17] found, by immunohistology, that there was an increased expression of HLA-DR antigen in the glandular cells in uterine and ectopic endometrium in women with endometriosis compared with uterine endometrium from control women. They suggested that this aberrant expression may be deeply involved in antigen presentation and the subsequent immune reactions. Ectopic endometrium could be recognized by macrophages that would in turn activate T_h cells and stimulate B cells to produce antibodies. In fact, increased expression of HLA-DR has been observed in the target organs of several autoimmune diseases [18, 19].

Cytokines

Peritoneal macrophage-derived growth factors are produced in higher amounts by macrophages from patients with endometriosis than from controls, and it has been proposed that these factors could enhance the ectopic growth of endometrial cells in the peritoneal cavity [20]. There is evidence suggesting that platelet-derived growth factor (PDGF) is identical to the major macrophage-derived growth factor [21].

Other cytokines known to be secreted by macrophages, particularly activated macrophages, and present in peritoneal fluid are IL-1, TNF, IL-6 and M-CSF. IL-1 activity and IL-1β expression have been found to be elevated in PF of patients with stage I and II endometriosis [22, 23] or in all stages of the disease [24]. PF controls had either no detectable IL-1 activity [22] or had IL-1β as a normal constituent [23]. In culture, macrophages from the PF of endometriosis patients have been shown to produce more IL-1 than those of controls [22]. In contrast, Awadalla *et al.* [25] found no difference in PF IL-1 activity between patients with and without endometriosis. There are, however, several physiological and pathological effects attributed to IL-1 which could relate to endometriosis. IL-1 induces the synthesis of prostaglandins; it stimulates fibroblast proliferation, collagen deposition and fibrinogen formation, which could contribute to the fibrosis and adhesion formation associated with endometriosis; and it stimulates B cell proliferation and antibody production, which could be related to the autoantibodies associated with the disease [22].

Increased levels of TNF have also been found in PF of women with endometriosis. TNF-α is made by a wide variety of cells, including fibroblasts, macrophages and T and B cells, whereas TNF-β is a product predominantly of lymphocytes [26]. Patients with pelvic adhesions and those with minimal and mild endometriosis have elevated TNF activity (α and β) in PF, but only those with moderate or severe endometriosis had significantly higher levels compared with women with normal pelvic anatomy ($P < 0.01$) [27]. The concentration of peritoneal macrophages in women with endometriosis was not correlated with the presence or level of PF TNF, which suggests that macrophages may not be the only source of TNF in PF [27].

IL-6 has also been found in PF. IL-6 could be secreted by macrophages in response to a variety of substances found in the PF, including IL-1 and TNF [28–30]. However, when measured in PF of women with endometriosis, IL-6 levels were similar to those of controls, the concentration being higher, though, in PF of women with pelvic inflammatory disease (PID) [31]. Similarly, M-CSF has been found in PF, with no significant differences found between PF levels in women with endometriosis, peritoneal adhesions and PID and in controls [32].

Although it is not known whether macrophages produce epidermal growth factor (EGF), monoclonal anti-EGF-receptor antibody caused > 50% inhibition of the mitogenic activity (on an endometrial epithelial carcinoma cell line) of media conditioned with peritoneal macrophages from women with stage III/IV endometriosis [33], suggesting that EGF activity is higher in those patients. However, levels of EGF directly measured in PF of women with endometriosis (stages I, II and III) were found to be the same as those in controls [34]. In both groups, though, there was a significant increase in PF EGF levels in secretory as opposed to proliferative phase ($P < 0.05$) [34].

Natural killer cells

Recent studies have reported a defect in NK activity resulting in a decreased cytotoxicity to autologous endometrium [7, 35]. There is no consensus, however, on whether there is also a general impairment of NK functions, since the radioisotope release assay performed in the K562 cell line was significantly different in controls and endometriosis women for some [35] but not for others [7]. NK cell activity has been reported to be decreased in the peripheral blood and PF of women with endometriosis [36, 37]. The decrease in NK cell activity was significantly related to an increase in disease stage [37, 38]. Garzetti *et al.* [38] observed an inverse relationship between NK activity and serum E_2 (oestradiol) levels. In contrast, Oosterlynck *et al.* [37] found that the PF NK activity was significantly decreased in the follicular phase of the cycle compared with the postovulatory phase, which they suggested might be important pathophysiologically since that is the moment when endometrial cells reach the peritoneal cavity. The defect found in PF in women with endometriosis was 2.4-fold greater than the defect found in peripheral blood [37]. In a recent paper, Oosterlynck *et al.* [39] found that lymphocytes preincubated with the PF from women with severe endometriosis had a decreased cytotoxicity toward K562 target cells compared with lymphocytes preincubated with the PF of women without endometriosis, suggesting the presence of a suppressive factor in PF. There was no significant difference between the effect on lymphocytes of sera of women with or without endometriosis, suggesting that the suppressive effect of PF was local [39].

These experiments have given rise to the NK theory of endometriosis, which presupposes that endometriotic cells are natural NK target cells, and that impaired clearance of ectopic endometrium by NK cells in the peritoneal cavity may contribute to the development of the disease. However, it can still be argued that alterations in NK activity associated with endometriosis can be a cause or an effect of the disease. Aberrant NK cell activity may be the result of an imbalance in the immune response to a chronic antigenic stimulus, such as ectopic endometrium, or to a previously initiated autoimmune event unrelated to endometriosis [40]. Kikuchi *et al.* [41] suggested that changes in the differentiation of NK cells were the consequence of the presence of endometriotic implants. In contrast with previous reports [37], they found that the percentage and absolute numbers of moderately differentiated NK cells in peripheral blood were significantly lower in patients with endometriosis than in controls. After the resection of endometriotic lesions, levels of immature NK cells significantly decreased and the number of moderately differentiated NK cells significantly increased in number and percentage [41].

Immune cell population in ectopic endometrium

Immune cell populations in uterine endometrium from women with and without endometriosis have been compared and immune cells in ectopic endometrium studied to obtain information on the local cellular immune response. The number and composition of the bone-marrow-derived population in uterine endometrium vary through the cycle. In the proliferative phase 10–15% cells in stroma are positive for the leucocyte common antigen (CD45) and the number increases in the late secretory/premenstrual phase (20–25% of the stroma) [16, 42]. The major leucocyte populations are T cells and macrophages. T cells are most often found in dense lymphocyte aggregates within the deeper layers of the endometrium, and macrophages are found scattered throughout the endometrium. The numbers of macrophages and T cells in endometrium are more or less constant throughout the menstrual cycle, apart from an increased density of macrophages during menstruation [16, 43]. Other cells, such as B cells, are limited in stroma and in nodules and they are very low throughout the cycle [16]. There is an additional population of phenotypically unusual lymphocytes, which are unique to the endometrium and early pregnancy decidua [16]. These lymphocytes are an unusual subset of large granular lymphocytes (LGLs) expressing high levels of CD56. In the latter half of the menstrual cycle, the number of $CD56^+$ cells increases sharply and they become the dominant cell type among the bone-marrow-derived cells [16]. Most endometrial LGLs are strongly positive for CD56 but negative for CD16. A minor subset of endometrial LGLs is negative or only mildly positive for CD56 but positive for CD16. These cells resemble the major type of NK cells in peripheral blood. The precise role of immune cells in endometrium is unknown, although they may be a source of cytokines and the LGLs in particular are believed to play a role in pregnancy success [16].

We have studied immune cells in uterine endometrium from women with and without endometriosis and found they are similar in number and distribution (unpublished results). Ectopic endometrium, like uterine endometrium, contains macrophages, T and B cells, LGLs and $CD16^+$ cells (unpublished results). The distribution of these bone-marrow-derived cells in ectopic endometrium is similar to that of uterine endometrium. There is less variation with the phase of the menstrual cycle in which the tissues were collected, but a greater variability between the tissues. The most striking finding is the presence in ectopic endometrial stroma of $CD56^+$ LGLs. Bone-marrow-derived cells in endometriotic tissue may have been there at the time of implantation, or, more probably, were attracted in by a specific stimulus of uterine endometrium that, reproduced by the ectopic endometrium, attracted the cells from the bloodstream and formed an extremely similar pattern to uterine endometrium. These two circumstances are not mutually exclusive. T cells and LGLs can proliferate *in situ* [44,45]. Macrophages, however, are end-stage cells and they do not normally divide in tissues, although occasional divisions may be seen as a completion of a division process started before the cell entered the tissue [46]; therefore they are likely to have been attracted in. The presence of LGLs in ectopic endometrium can be attributed, as in uterine endometrium [47], to a direct influx from the blood, or to a differentiation from bone-marrow-derived immature precursors. The lower levels of bone-marrow-derived cells in the tissues surrounding the implants (i.e. ovary and peritoneum) and the total lack of endometrial LGLs in those tissues suggest that the presence of bone-marrow-derived cells in ectopic endometrium corresponds to the high degree of differentiation of the endometriosis process and not to a cytotoxic immune cell infiltration, although this might have taken place before our tissues were collected.

Humoral immune changes in endometriosis

The interest in changes in humoral immunity in women with endometriosis centres on the observations that women with endometriosis may have higher than normal levels of circulating autoantibodies. There are two types of changes in humoral immunity reported in endometriosis cases. Firstly, a broad range of antibodies to cell components are more common in endometriosis, which implies polyclonal B cell activation. Secondly, there are reports that autoantibodies against specific tissues, particularly endometrium, are more common in endometriosis. Adverse reproductive performance has been attributed to either type of antibody.

The activation of B cells to produce antibodies which react with the subject's own tissue cells or cell components is well recognized and such autoantibodies can be present in serum without causing disease. The term 'autoimmune disease' is appropriate when there is a clinical syndrome in association with detectable autoantibodies. Many examples are known, particularly in the field of connective tissue disease. In general, the link between the autoantibodies and the disease is ill defined and in most examples the levels of antibody do not correlate with disease severity. It is possible that in some cases the autoantibodies are an epiphenomenon.

The tendency to produce autoantibodies can be due to several interacting mechanisms. The mechanisms include polyclonal B cell activation, abnormalities in the activation and regulation of lymphocyte activity, including defective Fc signalling, as well as possible cross-reactivity between foreign antigens and 'self' antigens [48]. Polyclonal activation and specific immune response against selected autoantigens can be combined so that an intrinsic hyper-responsiveness to polyclonal activators initiates the activation and differentiation of B lymphocytes [49].

Autoantibodies to cell components

The major contribution to this aspect of the problem has been from Gleicher's group. In 1987 they reported the finding of a range of autoantibodies in 59 laparoscopically staged endometriosis cases [10]. Twenty-nine per cent were antinuclear-factor-positive; 46% were lupus-anticoagulant-positive and, in a subgroup of 31 cases tested for various autoantibodies, the positive immunoglobulin G (IgG) results ranged from 13% to 42% for phospholipids, 0% to 26% for histones and 3% to 19% for polynucleotides. It was common for women to have several of the autoantibodies, suggesting polyclonal B cell activation, which is a feature of systemic lupus erythematosus (SLE), a disease which has been associated with endometriosis [50]. We showed elevated anticardiolipin antibodies in women with endometriosis, but at levels that were significantly lower than in women with SLE [51]. However, Kilpatrick *et al.* [52] found no significant difference (SD) in anticardiolipin levels in women with endometriosis and controls. They argued that finding a small number of women with endometriosis and levels >4 SD may be explained coincidentally as coexisting subclinical connective tissue disease or recent non-specific infection [52]. They suggested that polyclonal B cell activation would explain the findings but, although there was a trend to higher immunoglobulin levels in the endometriotics than in controls, only IgG levels were significantly elevated. The occurrence of the autoantibodies in the control group was not given in that report [53] but in a subsequent paper they defined autoantibody levels in a series of 200 'healthy' female and 200 male blood donors who gave no history suggestive of autoimmune disease [54]. They tested for antibodies against phospholipids, histones and polynucleotides, using an enzyme-linked immunosorbent assay (ELISA) method. In this 'normal' population, for each of the 15 antibodies tested, 1–3% of subjects showed abnormal elevation of the level of that antibody.

A further study compared total immunoglobulin levels and levels of autoantibodies in 20 endometriosis cases who received either danazol or a gonadotrophin-releasing hormone (GnRH) agonist as therapy with those in control female blood donors (n = 200) and in fertile women who had no pelvic disease at laparoscopic sterilization (n = 50) [53]. No significant difference was found in total immunoglobulin levels or in the levels of the autoantibodies. It was noted, however, that, with nine of the 45 autoantibody isotypes tested, treatment with danazol produced a significant reduction in the autoantibody titre.

Although the non-endometriotic control groups have not been matched with the endometriotics, the suggestion has been a trend towards higher levels of autoantibodies against cellular components, from which it has been suggested that endometriosis might be an autoimmune disease [10] and might contribute to reproductive autoimmune failure [55, 56], which will be discussed below.

Antiendothelial antibodies

Our finding [57] of antibodies against vascular endothelium in the serum of some women with endometriosis, by immunohistology, adds to the spectrum of autoantibodies described in the disease and supports the hypothesis that generalized autoimmunity may be involved in some cases of endometriosis [10]. The antiendothelial antibodies were not specific to endometrium, thus indicating a possible multiorgan involvement. The finding that the reaction of antiendothelial antibodies was stronger with tissues from women with endometriosis than those from controls suggests that the antigen(s) recognized may be up-regulated in endometriosis, perhaps as part of a general inflammatory response.

Antiendothelial cell antibodies are frequently found in diseases, such as SLE [58], systemic sclerosis [59], rheumatoid vasculitis [60], microscopic polyarteritis [61] and insulin-dependent diabetes mellitus [62], in which vascular damage is prominent.

Autoantibodies to tissues – ovary

Antibodies to ovary, theca cells and granulosa cells have been found in sera of women with endometriosis, using passive haemagglutination and immunofluorescence. Control sera from 'normal', healthy, age-matched, non-pregnant women had significantly lower levels of antiovarian antibodies compared with women with endometriosis [63]. The presence of antiovarian antibodies did not directly relate to endometriotic lesions involving the ovary or to the severity of the disease. Mathur *et al.* [63] suggested that antiovarian antibodies in some patients with endometriosis may be relevant to the reported association of endometriosis with anovulation or with inadequate corpus luteum function.

Autoantibodies to tissues – endometrium

Before considering antiendometrial antibodies, it is necessary to define the current understanding of the immunoglobulin content of endometrium, since assays for the binding of circulating antibodies to endometrium should take account of the baseline state of normal endometrium. In 1979 Kelly and Fox [64] used immunoperoxidase staining and concluded that endometrium lacked a true local secretory immune system but compensated by using secretory component (SC) to extract IgA from the circulation. IgA and SC were found in the epithelial component of the endometrium and only a small amount of IgA was found in the stroma. Staining was lowest during the proliferative phase of the cycle and increased in the secretory phase.

Endogenous immunoglobulin (IgG) has been found in the stromal interstitium in uterine and ectopic endometrium by immunofluorescence [65, 66] and immunoperoxidase staining [57, 64, 67], and it was found in many glandular secretions [57, 68, 69]. Some reports describe patchy staining in the proliferative and maximal staining in the secretory phase [64, 69]. Endogenous IgG has also been found in the stroma of the ovary and the peritoneum in which ectopic endometrium is implanted. This IgG, as that of the endometrium, is probably the result of passive diffusion of serum IgG [69]. Some authors, however, have suggested that the presence of stromal endogenous IgG is indicative of an autoimmune response [70–72] as they found endogenous IgG more often in the endometrium of women with than without endometriosis. IgG could be identified in endometrial stroma in 40–60% of non-endometriotics and in 75–100% of endometriotics and in endometrial glands in 30–40% and 65–75%, respectively [70].

Weed and Arquembourg [73] had reported finding complement in endometrium only in endometriosis but in 1987 it was reported [74] that complement was present in many endometria in women with and without the disease, complement C3 and/or C4 being detected in 66% of endometriotics and in 67% of controls. This does not negate the possibility that the complement is fixed by the presence of immunoglobulins in endometrium are a feature of both normal and endometriotic endometria. In our experience, positive staining for IgG can be demonstrated consistently in endometria, using immunohistochemcial methods [57, 67], as well as in most other tissues.

Study of the antiendometrial antibody binding has localized the binding to the gland epithelium [67, 75], both in uterine and in ectopic endometrium [57]. This indicates that in endometriosis the endometriotic implants could be both the immunogen stimulating the production of autoantibodies and their target, as had been suggested by Weed and Arquembourg [73]. The ensuing autoimmune reaction could contribute to the peritoneal inflammation associated with the disease.

Antiendometrial antibodies recognize components of normal endometrium, as described using passive haemagglutination [76, 77], immunofluorescence [78] and immunohistochemistry [57]. Moreover, it has been suggested that there are several different antigens involved, and that the spectrum of antigens is different in control and normal tissues. In two reports, Mathur *et al.* [72, 79] using Western blots, showed that there are some antigens in normal uterine endometrium that are commonly recognized by antibodies in the serum of all women (19, 31, 38 and 42 kDa MW). There are other antigens, however, that are only recognized by serum of women with endometriosis; some of these antigens are normally present in endometrium (26 and 34 kDa MW), but others are only found in the endometrium of women with endometriosis (82, 94, 100 and 120 kDa MW) [72]. Mathur *et al.* [79] suggested that the reaction of antibodies in control sera against 'normal' antigens may help to activate the macrophages for clearing the reproductive tract of unwanted menstrual debris.

There have been many positive reports on the presence of antiendometrial antibodies in the serum of women with endometriosis [63, 67, 71, 75–78, 80–83], including a comparison with CA-125 in the detection of endometriosis [84]. Weighed against this is a report which questions whether an association of endometrial autoimmunity with endometriosis is established [66].

Direct detection of immunoglobulins has been employed [63, 71] but most studies have used indirect techniques to test the binding of serum antibodies to endometrium, either from the patients themselves [80], to 'normal' endometrium [67, 76, 78, 81] or to an endometrial carcinoma cell line [82, 84]. There has been considerable variation in the techniques used. These include immunofluorescence [63, 71, 78, 82, 84], immunodiffusion [80], immunoelectrophoresis [80], haemagglutination [76, 77], double-antibody immunohistochemistry [57, 67] and ELISA [81]. The nature of the control group has been another source of variation. In some studies the controls included men [67, 76, 81] or women who had been laparoscoped so that the absence of endometriosis had been confirmed [57, 71, 76–78, 80, 82, 84], but in one the absence of endometriosis was assumed [63].

In one study there was a clear-cut difference between endometriotics and controls because binding was absent in the controls but present in the endometriosis cases [63]. In other studies immunoglobulin could be detected in the sera of some subjects in each group tested and the difference was therefore one of degree [67, 71, 76, 78, 81, 82, 84]. In a recent study using laparoscoped infertile women as controls [77] antiendometrial antibodies were detected in 88% of the controls; however, the mean titre was still significantly higher in the infertile endometriosis cases.

Switchenko *et al.* [66] attempted to replicate experiments that had detected antiendometrial antibodies using immunofluorescence [78], passive haemagglutination [76], ELISA [81] and Western blotting [79]. Their data contradicted all previous findings: there were no significant differences in the results obtained from endometriosis patients and controls, which included women with normal laparoscopic findings. These authors concluded that the case for specific antiendometrial antibodies remained unproved.

In our recent studies ELISA [81] has been developed further in an effort to improve its discrimination. Endometrial gland cells were purified and their cytosolic proteins extracted with saline. A pool of extracts from 10 women without endometriosis was used to coat ELISA wells. With this quantitative assay endometriotic women have higher levels of antiglandular antibodies than cord blood and adult male controls. There is, however, no discrimination between women with and without endometriosis, both groups showing a wide scatter of results (unpublished data).

Our recent studies using the double-binding immunohistological method [57] indicate that the specific endometrial sample used to test for binding from serum is of great importance since differing responses can be obtained under the same conditions, testing the same serum samples but using endometrial sections from different women. The importance of the particular tissue sample used in the testing for antiendometrial antibodies is exemplified by our results with sera from women with Rokitansky syndrome. These women have a congenitally absent uterus and their immune system has therefore never been exposed to endometrium. We have tested sera from these women and most of the sera did not show significant binding to endometrium, but some did bind to two particular tissue samples (unpublished data). Exposure to endometrium is clearly not a prerequisite for the presence of antibodies which will bind to endometria.

We have recently been unable to detect any difference in antibody levels in the sera of women with endometriosis before and after 6 months of medical treatment, either by immunohistology or with ELISA, in contrast to previous studies by passive haemagglutination [76] or by ELISA [81]. And, in common with others, we observed no correlation between the presence of antiendometrial antibodies and the severity of the disease [76, 77, 81, 82].

The controversy about antiendometrial antibodies in endometriosis [66, 85] and our findings may be explained by the variation of antigenicity between tissue samples, and the suggested low affinity of autoantibodies [66]. Furthermore, endogenous immunoglobulin in normal endometrium complicates the detection of additional binding from endometriotic sera to a considerable extent. The very wide range of results observed in the groups studied hinders discrimination between groups, particularly when it can be shown that different 'normal' endometria can give different binding responses. The Rokitansky syndrome data indicate that some endometria express antigens recognized by serum antibodies which are unlikely to be specific to endometrium. In addition, it is not possible to know whether the published literature on antiendometrial antibodies, almost all of which demonstrate positive findings, includes any publication bias, which it is recognized acts to deter the publication of studies which fail to demonstrate positive findings [86].

In summary, antiendometrial antibodies are probably produced as a response to retrograde menstruation, which is a common event. Levels of antiendometrial antibodies may be higher in women with endometriosis, probably as a response to implantation and an increased proliferation of endometrium in the peritoneal cavity. However, these antibodies may be of low affinity and are not likely to be functionally important. Normal endometrium is probably, at the same time, a tissue with low antigenicity. This is not surprising. Endometrium is the only tissue which is shed regularly, on a monthly cycle, with parts of it reaching sites in the body distant from its normal location. The peritoneum may not reject the implantation of what is effectively an 'autograft', or transplantation from one part of the body to another in the same individual, where no immunological rejection takes place [87].

Antiendometrial antibodies for the diagnosis of endometriosis

Detection of circulating antibodies to endometrium as a non-invasive method of diagnosing and monitoring endometriosis is appealing. To date, several attempts have been made to use a passive haemagglutination assay [66, 76, 77], indirect immunofluorescence [66, 82] or an ELISA [66, 81] to measure the levels of antiendometrial antibodies in serum. Detecting antiendometrial antibodies in serum rather than in PF is preferable because of the easy availability of serum compared with PF. In addition, it has been reported that levels of antiendometrial antibodies, measured by passive haemagglutination, are higher in serum than in PF of patients with endometriosis [77]. Moreover, Halme and Mathur [88] reported no increase in antiendometrial antibodies in mild endometriosis, compared with controls, in PF. The identification of the best source of antigen(s) is, however, controversial.

The complexity of the reaction of antiendometrial antibodies with endometrium shown by immunohistological studies [57] is the main problem in considering it as a possible diagnostic tool. Several endometria reacted with some sera but not with others, and, at the same time, some sera reacted with some tissue but not with others, suggesting a variability both in the antibodies in sera and in the antigens in the tissue. This marked variability would make it difficult to develop a specific and sensitive diagnostic method for endometriosis based on the immunohistological reaction.

Detection of antiendometrial antibodies by immunofluorescence has been compared with detection of circulating CA-125 as a diagnostic test for endometriosis [84]. It was found that indirect immunofluorescence appeared to be more sensitive (83% against 27%) but not more specific (78% against 82%) than the determination of circulating CA-125 antigen, for detecting endometriosis [84]. The disadvantage of immunofluorescence is the subjective interpretation of the results. This, and the different choice of antigen(s) source, could explain why Wild *et al.* [82] (with an endometrial carcinoma cell line as antigen) found significant differences between sera of women with and without endometriosis, whereas Switchenko *et al.* [66] (using isolated endometrial epithelial cells as antigen) did not.

Passive haemagglutination assay is more objective than immunofluorescence and, to date, all studies have chosen whole endometrial extracts as the antigen source, which makes them comparable. Antiendometrial antibodies were diagnosed to be significantly higher in women with endometriosis than in controls [76, 77], with a 74% sensitivity and 100% specificity, but, for some, the false negative rate was still 38% [76]. However, Switchenko *et al.* [66] again failed to demonstrate any difference between patients and control women sera, despite using the same method as Chihal *et al.* [76], casting doubts upon the suitability of the method as a non-invasive diagnostic tool.

An antiendometrial antibody ELISA is the latest method attempted for the diagnosis of endometriosis. While Kennedy *et al.* [81] found that the levels of antiendometrial antibodies were significantly higher in women with endometriosis than in male controls ($P < 0.001$), Switchenko *et al.* [66], using a different ELISA protocol, did not. Our recent ELISA work has failed to detect any difference in the levels of antiendometrial antibodies in women with and without endometriosis. We concluded that the possible cross-reaction or presence of low levels of antiendometrial antibodies in sera of women without clinical symptoms of endometriosis, the high variability in the detected levels of autoantibodies in endometriosis and, in general, the complexities of the immunological reaction in endometriosis are likely to defeat the development of a reliable method to measure antiendometrial antibodies as a diagnostic tool for the disease, unless a more specific antigen is found for this purpose. This may explain the confusing and contradictory data obtained by others.

The clinical relevance of autoantibodies in endometriosis

The immunological changes in endometriosis are thought to be related to the infertility associated with the disease; however, no study to date has demonstrated a causal relationship between them. Antiendometrial and antiendothelial antibodies might affect the capacity of the endometrium to be receptive to the embryo. It is also likely that changes in the PF might be related to the aetiology of infertility. Experimental data have demonstrated that PF from women with endometriosis does not affect sperm motility [89] but is detrimental to mouse sperm–ova interaction [90] and toxic to the growth and development of mouse embryos [91]. This has been attributed to increased levels of macrophages and macrophage-derived factors that may interfere with ovulation, sperm motility, oocyte pick-up and early embryo survival [12]. IL-1 in concentrations similar to those present in PF has been found to be toxic to mouse embryo development [22] and women with primary infertility have increased levels of PF TNF [27], which suggests that IL-1 and TNF may play a role in the infertility associated with endometriosis.

Given the present level of knowledge, the most rational approach to the issue is to consider autoantibody abnormalities that have been detected in endometriosis patients an epiphenomenon until the evidence proves otherwise.

References

1 Sampson JA. Peritoneal endometriosis, due to menstrual dissemination of endometrial tissue into peritoneal cavity. *Am J Obstet Gynecol* 1927 **14**: 422–469.

2 Halme J, Hammond MG, Hulka JF, Raj SG, Talbert LM. Retrograde menstruation in healthy women and in patients with endometriosis. *Obstet Gynecol* 1984 **64**: 151–154.

3 Semer D, Reisler K, MacDonald PC, Casey ML. Responsiveness of human endometrial stromal cells to cytokines. *Ann N Y Acad Sci* 1991 **622**: 99–110.

4 Oppenheim JJ. Foreword. In: Thomson A (ed.). *The Cytokine Handbook*, 1991. London, Academic Press.

5 Dmowski WP, Steele RW, Baker GF. Deficient cellular immunity in endometriosis. *Am J Obstet Gynecol* 1981 **141**: 377–383.

6 Steele RW, Dmowski WP, Marmer DJ. Immunologic aspects of human endometriosis. *Am J Reprod Immun* 1984 6: 33–36.

7 Vigano P, Vercellini P, Di Blasio AM *et al.* Deficient antiendometrium lymphocyte-mediated cytotoxicity in women with endometriosis. *Fertil Steril* 1991 **56**: 894–899.

8 Gilmore SM, Aksel S, Hoff C, Peterson RDA. *In vitro* lymphocyte activity in women with endometriosis – an altered immune response? *Fertil Steril* 1992 **58**: 1148–1152.

9 Badawy SZA, Cuenca V, Stizel A, Tice D. Immune rosettes of T- and B-lymphocytes in infertile women with endometriosis. *J Reprod Med* 1987 **32**: 194–197.

10 Gleicher N, El-Roely A, Confino E, Friberg J. Is endometriosis an autoimmune disease? *Obstet Gynecol* 1987 **70**: 115–122.

11 Burns WN, Schenken RS. Pathophysiology. In: Schenken RS (ed.). *Endometriosis: Contemporary Concepts in Clinical Management*, 1989, pp. 83–106. Philadelphia, J.B. Lippincott.

12 Hurst BS, Rock JA. The peritoneal environment in endometriosis. In: Thomas EJ, Rock JA (eds). *Modern Approaches to Endometriosis*, 1991, pp. 79–95. Dordrecht, Kluwer Academic Publishers.

13 Dmowski WP. Etiology and histogenesis of endometriosis. *Ann N Y Acad Sci* 1991 **622**: 236–241.

14 Olive DL, Montoya I, Riehl RM, Schenken RS. Macrophage-conditioned media enhance endometrial stromal cell proliferation *in vitro*. *Trans Am Gynecol Obstet Soc* 1991 **9**: 15–20.

15 Johnson JV, Rozek M, Moreno AC, Olive DL, Schenken RS. Surgically induced endometriosis does not alter peritoneal factors in the rabbit model. *Fertil Steril* 1991 **56**: 343–348.

16 Starkey PM, Clover LM, Rees MPC. Variation during the menstrual cycle of immune cell populations in human endometrium. *Eur J Obstet Gyneaecol Reprod Biol* 1991 **39**: 203–207.

17 Ota H, Igarashi S. Expression of major histocompatibility complex class II antigen in

endometriotic tissue in patients with endometriosis and adenomyosis. *Fertil Steril* 1993 **60**: 834–838.

18 Hanafusa T, Fujino-Kurihara H, Miyazaki A *et al.* Expression of class II major histocompatibility complex antigens on pancreatic B cells in the NOD mouse. *Lancet* 1983 **ii**: 1111–1115.

19 Bottazzo GF, Dean BM, McNally JM *et al. In situ* characterization of autoimmune phenomena and expression of HLA molecules in the pancreas in diabetic insulitis. *N Engl J Med* 1985 **313**: 353–360.

20 Halme J, White C, Kauma S, Estes J, Haskill S. Peritoneal macrophages from patients with endometriosis release growth factor activity *in vitro. J Clin Endocrinol Metab* 1988 **66**: 1044–1049.

21 Shimokado K, Raines EW, Madtes DK *et al.* A significant part of macrophage-derived growth factor consists of at least two forms of PDGF. *Cell* 1985 **43**: 277–286.

22 Fakih H, Baggett B, Holtz G *et al.* Interleukin-1: a possible role in the infertility associated with endometriosis. *Fertil Steril* 1987 **46**: 213–217.

23 Mori H, Itoh N, Sawairi M *et al.* Expression of interleukin-1 beta messenger ribonuclic acid and IL-1 receptor antagonist mRNA in peritoneal macrophages from patients with endometriosis. *Fertil Steril* 1992 **57**: 535–542.

24 Hill JA, Anderson DJ. Lymphocyte activity in the presence of peritoneal fluid from fertile women and infertile women with and without endometriosis. *Am J Obstet Gynecol* 1989 **161**: 861–864.

25 Awadalla SG, Friedman CI, Haq AU *et al.* Local peritoneal factors: their role in infertility associated with endometriosis. *Am J Obstet Gynecol* 1987 **157**: 1207–1214.

26 Ruddle NH, Turetskaya RL. Tumour necrosis factor beta. In: Thomson A (ed.). *The Cytokine Handbook*, 1991, pp. 257–268. London, Academic Press.

27 Eisermann J, Gast MJ, Pineda J, Odem RR, Collins JL. Tumor necrosis factor in peritoneal fluid of women undergoing laparoscopic surgery. *Fertil Steril* 1988 **50**: 573–579.

28 Bauer J, Ganter U, Geiger T *et al.* Regulation of interleukin 6 expression in cultured human blood monocytes and monocyte-derived macrophages. *Blood* 1988 **72**: 1134–1140.

29 Sironi M, Breviario F, Proserpio P *et al.* IL1 stimulates IL6 production in endothelial cells. *J Immunol* 1989 **142**: 549–553.

30 Ray A, Tatter SB, Santhanam U *et al.* Regulation of expression of interleukin 6. *Ann N Y Acad Sci* 1989 **557**: 353–361.

31 Buyalos RP, Funari VA, Azziz R, Watson JM, Martinez-Maza O. Elevated interleukin-6 levels in peritoneal fluid of patients with pelvic pathology. *Fertil Steril* 1992 **58**: 302–306.

32 Weinberg JB, Haney AF, Ramakrishnan S. Peritoneal fluid and plasma levels of human macrophage colony-stimulating factor in relation to peritoneal fluid macrophage content. *Blood* 1991 **78**: 513–516.

33 Zhang R, Wild RA, Medders D, Gunupudi SR. Effects of peritoneal macrophages from patients with endometriosis on the proliferation of endometrial carcinoma cell line ECC-1. *Am J Obstet Gynecol* 1991 **165**: 1842–1846.

34 DeLeon FD, Vijayakumar R, Brown M *et al.* Peritoneal fluid volume, estrogen, progesterone, prostaglandin, and epidermal growth factor concentrations in patients with and without endometriosis. *Obstet Gynecol* 1986 **68**: 189–194.

35 Oosterlynck DJ, Cornillie FJ, Waer M, Vandeputte M, Koninckx PR. Women with endometriosis show a defect in natural killer activity resulting in a decreased cytotoxicity to autologous endometrium. *Fertil Steril* 1991 **56**: 45–51.

36 Tanaka E, Sendo F, Kawagoe S, Hiroi M. Decreased natural killer cell activity in women with endometriosis. *Gynecol Obstet Invest* 1992 **34**: 27–30.

37 Oosterlynck DJ, Vandeputte M, Meuleman C, Koninckx PR, Waer M. The natural killer

activity of peritoneal fluid lymphocytes is decreased in women with endometriosis. *Fertil Steril* 1992 **58**: 290–295.
38 Garzetti G, Ciavattini A, Provinciali M *et al.* Natural killer cell activity in endometriosis: correlation between serum estradiol levels and cytotoxicity. *Obstet Gynecol* 1993 **81**: 665–668.
39 Oosterlynck DJ, Meuleman C, Waer M, Koninckx PR, Vandeputte M. Immunosuppressive activity of peritoneal fluid in women with endometriosis. *Obstet Gynecol* 1993 **82**: 206–212.
40 Hill JA. Immunology and endometriosis. *Fertil Steril* 1992 **58**: 262–264.
41 Kikuchi Y, Ishikawa N, Hirata J *et al.* Changes of peripheral blood lymphocyte subsets before and after operation of patients with endometriosis. *Acta Obstet Gynecol Scand* 1993 **72**: 157–161.
42 Kamat BR, Isaacson PG. The immunocytochemical distribution of leukocytic subpopulations in human endometrium. *Am J Pathol* 1987 **127**: 66–73.
43 King A, Wellings V, Gardner L, Loke YW. Immunocytochemical characterization of the unusual large granular lymphocytes in human endometrium throughout the menstrual cycle. *Human Immunol* 1989 **24**: 195–205.
44 Pace D, Morrison L, Bulmer JN. Proliferative activity in endometrial stromal granulocytes throughout menstrual cycle and early pregnancy. *J Clin Pathol* 1989 **42**: 35–39.
45 Tabibzadeh S. Proliferative activity of lymphoid cells in human endometrium throughout the menstrual cycle. *J Clin Endocrinol Metab* 1990 **70**: 437–443.
46 Auger MJ, Ross JA. The biology of the macrophage. In: Lewis CE, McGee JO (eds). *The Macrophage*, 1992, pp. 1–74. Oxford, IRL Press.
47 Starkey PM. Natural killer cells/large granular lymphocytes in pregnancy. In: Lewis CE, McGee JO (eds). *The Natural Killer Cells.* 1992, pp 206–240. Oxford, IRL Press.
48 Sinclair NR, Panoskaltsis A. The immunoregulatory apparatus and autoimmunity. *Immunol Today* 1988 **9**: 260–265.
49 Dziarski R. Autoimmunity: polyclonal activation or antigen induction? *Immunol Today* 1988 **9**: 340–342.
50 Grimes DA, LeBolt SA, Grimes KR, Wingo PA. Systemic lupus erythematosus and reproductive function: a case–control study. *Am J Obstet Gynecol* 1985 **153**: 179–186.
51 Kennedy SH, Nunn B, Cederholm Williams SA, Barlow DH. Cardiolipin antibody levels in endometriosis and systemic lupus erythematosus. *Fertil Steril* 1989 **52**: 1061–1062.
52 Kilpatrick DC, Haining RE, Smith SS. Are cardiolipin antibody levels elevated in endometriosis? *Fertil Steril* 1991 **55**: 436–437.
53 el-Roeiy A, Dmowski WP, Gleicher N *et al.* Danazol but not gonadotropin-releasing hormone agonists suppresses autoantibodies in endometriosis. *Fertil Steril* 1988 **50**: 864–871.
54 el-Roeiy A, Gleicher N. Definition of normal autoantibody levels in an apparently healthy population. *Obstet Gynecol* 1988 **72**: 596–602.
55 Gleicher N, el-Roeiy A, Confino E, Friberg J. Reproductive failure because of autoantibodies: unexplained infertility and pregnancy wastage. *Am J Obstet Gynecol* 1989 **160**: 1376–1380.
56 Gleicher N, El-Roeiy A. The reproductive autoimmune failure syndrome. *Am J Obstet Gynecol* 1988 **159**: 223–227.
57 Fernandez-Shaw S, Hicks BR, Yudkin PL *et al.* Anti-endometrial and anti-endothelial autoantibodies in women with endometriosis. *Hum Reprod* 1993 **8**: 310–315.
58 Cines DB, Lyss AP, Reeber M, Bina M, DeHoratius RJ. Presence of complement fixing anti-endothelial cells antibodies in systemic lupus erythematosus. *J Clin Invest* 1984 **73**: 611–625.
59 Holt CM, Lindsey N, Moult J *et al.* Antibody-dependent cellular cytotoxicity of vascular endothelium: characterization and pathogenic associations in systemic sclerosis. *Clin Exp Immunol* 1989 **78**: 359–365.

60 Heurkens AHM, Hiemstra PS, Lafeber GJM, Daha MR, Breedveld FC. Anti-endothelial cell antibodies in patients with rheumatoid arthritis complicated with vasculitis. *Clin Exp Immunol* 1989 **78**: 7–12.
61 Ferraro G, Meroni PL, Tincani A *et al.* Anti-endothelial cell antibodies in patients with Wegener's granulomatosis and micropolyarteritis. *Clin Exp Immunol* 1990 **79**: 47–53.
62 Wangel AG, Kontiainen S, Scheinin T *et al.* Anti-endothelial cell antibodies in insulin-dependent diabetes mellitus. *Clin Exp Immunol* 1992 **88**: 410–413.
63 Mathur S, Peress MR, Williamson HO *et al.* Autoimmunity to endometrium and ovary in endometriosis. *Clin Exp Immunol* 1982 **50**: 259–266.
64 Kelly JK, Fox H. The local immunological defence system of the human endometrium. *J Reprod Immunol* 1979 **1**: 39–45.
65 Tourville DR, Ogra SS, Lippes J, Tomasi TB. The human female reproductive tract: immunohistological localization of IgA, IgC, IgM, secretory 'piece', and lactoferrin. *Am J Obstet Gynecol* 1970 **108**: 1102–1108.
66 Switchenko AC, Kauffman RS, Becker M. Are there antiendometrial antibodies in sera of women with endometriosis? *Fertil Steril* 1991 **56**: 235–241.
67 Kennedy SH, Sargent IL, Starkey PM, Hicks BR, Barlow DH. Localization of anti-endometrial antibody binding in women with endometriosis using a double-labelling immunohistochemical method. *Br J Obstet Gynaecol* 1990 **97**: 671–674.
68 Yaneva H. La sécrétion d'immunoglobulines par l'endomètre humain normal: étude immuno-histochimique. *Pathol Biol* 1974 **22**: 607–610.
69 Bulmer JN, Hagin SV, Browne CM, Billington WD. Localization of immunoglobulin-containing cells in human endometrium in the first trimester of pregnancy and throughout the menstrual cycle. *Eur J Obstet Gynecol Reprod Biol* 1986 **23**: 31–44.
70 Saifuddin A, Buckley CH, Fox H. Immunoglobulin content of the endometrium in women with endometriosis. *Int J Gynecol Pathol* 1983 **2**: 255–263.
71 Kreiner D, Fromowitz FB, Richardson DA, Kenigsberg D. Endometrial immunofluorescence associated with endometriosis and pelvic inflammatory disease. *Fertil Steril* 1986 **46**: 243–246.
72 Mathur S, Garza DE, Smith LF. Endometrial autoantigens eliciting immunoglobulin (Ig)G, IgA, and IgM responses in endometriosis. *Fertil Steril* 1990 **54**: 56–63.
73 Weed JC, Arquembourg PC. Endometriosis: can it produce an autoimmune response resulting in infertility? *Clin Obstet Gynecol* 1980 **23**: 895–900.
74 Bartosik D, Damjanov I, Viscarello RR, Riley JA. Immunoproteins in the endometrium: clinical correlates of the presence of complement fractions C3 and C4. *Am J Obstet Gynecol* 1987 **156**: 11–15.
75 Wild RA, Satyaswaroop PG, Shivers AC. Epithelial localization of antiendometrial antibodies associated with endometriosis. *Am J Reprod Immunol Microbiol* 1987 **13**: 62–65.
76 Chihal HJ, Mathur S, Holtz GL, Williamson HO. An endometrial antibody assay in the clinical diagnosis and management of endometriosis. *Fertil Steril* 1986 **40**: 408–411.
77 Badawy SZA, Cuenca V, Freliech H, Stefanu C. Endometrial antibodies in serum and peritoneal fluid of infertile patients with and without endometriosis. *Fertil Steril* 1990 **53**: 930–932.
78 Wild RA, Shivers CA. Antiendometrial antibodies in patients with endometriosis. *Am J Reprod Immunol Microbiol* 1985 **8**: 84–86.
79 Mathur S, Garza DE, Chihal HJ *et al.* Endometrial antigens involved in the autoimmunity of endometriosis. *Fertil Steril* 1988 **50**: 860–863.
80 Badawy SZA, Cuenca V, Stitzel A, Jacobs RDB, Tomar RH. Autoimmune phenomena in infertile patients with endometriosis. *Obstet Gynecol* 1984 **63**: 271–275.
81 Kennedy SH, Starkey PM, Sargent IL, Hicks BR, Barlow DH. Anti-endometrial antibodies in endometriosis measured by an enzyme-linked immunoabsorbent assay before and after

treatment with danazol and nafarelin. *Obstet Gynecol* 1990 **75**: 914–918.
82 Wild RA, Hirisave V, Podczaski ES *et al.* Autoantibodies associated with endometriosis: can their detection predict presence of the disease? *Obstet Gynecol* 1991 77: 927–931.
83 Confino E, Harlow BS, Gleicher N. Peritoneal fluid and serum autoantibody levels in patients with endometriosis. *Fertil Steril* 1990 **53**: 242.
84 Wild RA, Podczaski ES, Hirisave V, Demers LM, Bianco A. Endometrial antibodies versus CA-125 for the detection of endometriosis. *Fertil Steril* 1991 **55**: 90–94.
85 Mathur S, Chihal HJ. Antiendometrial antibodies? *Fertil Steril* 1992 **57**: 704–705.
86 Chalmers I. Underreporting research is scientific misconduct. *JAMA* 1990 **263**: 1405–1408.
87 Sell S. *Immunology, Immunopathology and Immunity*, 1987, p. 170. New York, Elsevier.
88 Halme J, Mathur S. Local autoimmunity in mild endometriosis. *Int J Fertil* 1987 **32**: 309–311.
89 Muse KN, Estes S, Vernon M, Zavos P, Wilson EA. Effect of endometriosis on sperm motility in peritoneal fluid *in vitro*. *Fertil Steril* 1986 **46** (Suppl.): 99.
90 Sueldo C, Lambert H, Steinleitner AJ, Swanson JA. Effect of peritoneal fluid on murine sperm ova interaction. *Fertil Steril* 1986 **46**: 8.
91 Morcos RN, Gibbons WE, Findley WE. Effect of peritoneal fluid on *in vitro* cleavage of 2-cell embryos: possible role in infertility associated endometriosis. *Fertil Steril* 1985 **44**: 678–683.

Part 2
Clinical Features

Chapter 6
Ovarian Endometriosis

I.A. BROSENS

History of the identification

The first case of ovarian endometriosis was described by W.W. Russel in 1899 in a woman of premenopausal age operated for a cystic adenocarcinoma of the left ovary who had 'the right ovary enveloped in adhesions of the posterior face of the broad ligament' [1]. On microscopic examination, Russel was 'astonished to find areas which were an exact prototype of uterine glands and interglandular connective tissue'. In spite of the precision of the description, Russel considered the 'tumour' as due to the presence of 'aberrant portions of the Müllerian duct' in the ovary. Another case which can be recognized as ovarian endometriosis is that of Casler [2], who described the presence of 'uterine mucosa in remaining ovary' after hysterectomy. In the discussion that followed Casler's presentation to the American Gynecological Society, Norris [3] reported a case of a 29-year-old woman operated for severe pelvic pain. At gross examination the 'ovary showed a number of adhesions' and on histological examination an area of endometrium about 6–7 mm in diameter was found. The endometrium of the ovary was similar to that removed from the uterus by curettage and was of the same periodicity.

In spite of the accurate description it took several decades before the pathogenesis of the cysts, which were described as 'haemorrhagic cysts or haematomas of the ovary', became elucidated. Cullen [4] was the first to suggest that, in cases of adenomyosis of the rectovaginal septum, the glands in the ovarian cyst were of uterine origin. The escape of chocolate-coloured fluid during the relief of the ovary from adhesions and the identification of the site of perforation in the adhesions made Sampson [5] believe that perforation of these cysts – which he gave the expressive name of chocolate cyst – was a frequent phenomenon, leading to spilling, adhesions and spreading of peritoneal endometriosis (Fig. 6.1). The original paper of Sampson on this condition, in which he coined the word 'endometriosis', was a discussion of the leaking or ruptured endometrial cyst spreading endometriosis by 'seeding' the adjacent peritoneal surfaces and structures with these viable Müllerian cells. The idea that the ovarian endometrioma has a great tendency for perforation and adhesion formation has persisted in recent publications. However, in 1957 Hughesdon [6] demonstrated on serial sectioning of

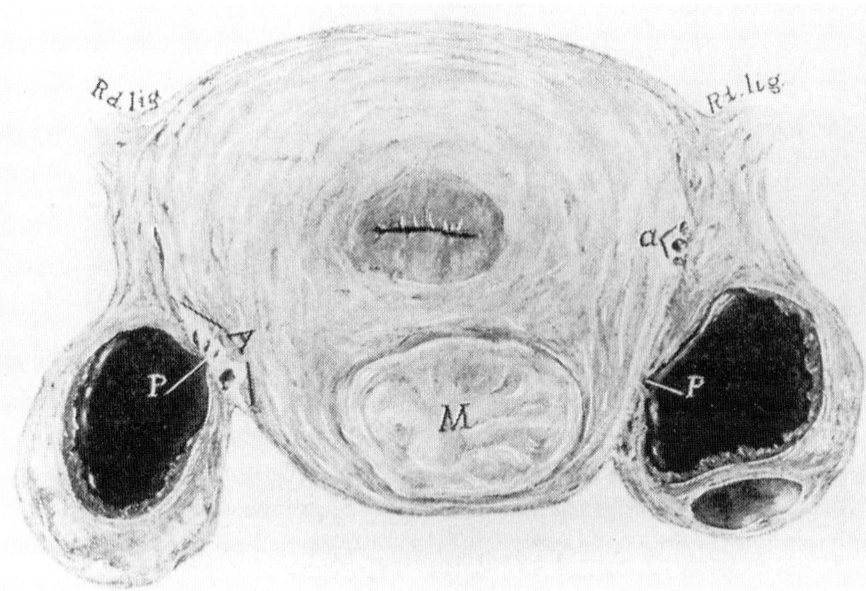

Fig. 6.1 Sampson's [5] illustration of the site of perforation and adhesions. This observation made him believe that the chocolate cyst of the ovary had a great tendency to perforate and seed endometrial tissue on the adjacent peritoneal surfaces.

ovaries containing an endometrioma that 90% of the typical endometriomas are formed by invagination of the cortex (Fig. 6.2). The so-called site of perforation, as described by Sampson [5] represents the stigma of invagination. At this site, small but very active mucosa-type implants of endometriosis can be found. These findings contradict Sampson's hypothesis [5] and suggest that adhesions are not the consequence but the cause of endometrioma formation by sealing off active superficial implants. In 1962 Nieminen [7] showed that, in contrast to nodular, enclosed implants, the free superficial implants respond during the menstrual cycle as superficial eutopic endometrium, with vascular necrosis and bleeding at the time of menstruation.

Pathogenesis

The pathogenesis of the typical ovarian endometrioma has now been clarified as a process originating from a free superficial implant which is in contact with the ovarian surface and is sealed off by adhesions. The pseudocyst is formed by accumulation of menstrual debris from shedding and bleeding of the small implant, resulting in a progressive invagination of the ovarian cortex. Ovulation and collapse of the cortex may favour the process of invagination and explain why the ovary is a preferred site for endometrioma formation.

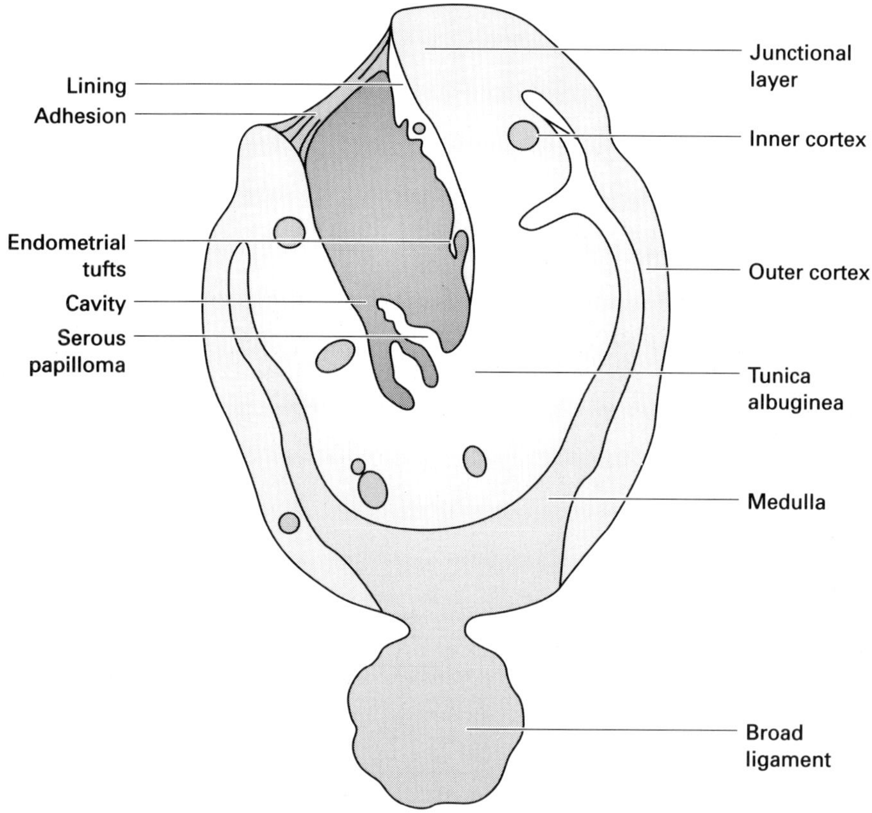

Fig. 6.2 Section through an ovary with typical endometrioma (after [6], from [47], with permission).

Fibroreactive tissue progressively thickens the inverted cortex, and outgrowths of the endometrial epithelium with or without stroma extend over the surface or become embedded in the fibroreactive tissue covering the wall of the pseudocyst.

The pathogenesis explains the typical features of the endometrioma, such as the frequent location of the cyst and the adhesions on the anterior side of the ovary opposing the posterior side of the parametrium, the presence of the adhesions and/or the scarification on the ovarian surface, the frequent spilling by freeing the adhesions, the lining of the cyst by cortical or fibroreactive tissue and the paucity of endometrial tissue in the wall of the cyst. In a few cases, however, a different pathogenesis is not excluded, such as development from Müllerian remnants in the ovary, or implantation of endometrial tissue in a ruptured follicle or through differentiation of the coelomic epithelium in the ovary. Germinal inclusion cysts are often mistaken for endometrial glands and therefore the diagnosis of endometrial tissue should rely on the presence of additional features such as stroma, haemorrhage or pigment-laden macrophages.

Clinical appearance

The ovary is a frequent site for the development of endometriosis [8]. Redwine [9] has shown that peritoneal endometriosis precedes the appearance of ovarian endometriosis by several years (Table 6.1). The red haemorrhagic lesions are the predominant type in adolescents [10]. These lesions have been shown to represent the most active type of peritoneal endometriosis [11]. The subtle early lesions, such as the vesicles and haemorrhagic blisters, appear and disappear on the peritoneal surface, giving early endometriosis a changing appearance, like mushrooms in a field [12]. Ovarian endometriomas rarely occur in the adolescent, but occurrence increases with age [13].

Table 6.1 Age-related frequency of common endometriosis sites

	Frequency of involvement (%)				
Site of lesion	16–20 years (*n* = 14)	21–25 years (*n* = 22)	26–30 years (*n* = 52)	31–35 years (*n* = 25)	36–52 years (*n* = 19)
Ovarian lesions					
Right ovary	0	8.7	11.3	21.4	16.0
Left ovary	0	13.0	9.6	17.9	24.0
Peritoneal lesions					
Cul-de-sac	78.6	78.3	52.8	56.0	52.6
Right broad ligament	57.1	43.5	32.1	39.3	20.0
Left broad ligament	35.7	39.1	35.8	25.0	12.0
Right uterosacral ligament	57.1	39.1	43.4	25.0	12.0
Left uterosacral ligament	42.9	52.2	32.1	25.0	20.0

Adapted from [9] with permission.

Functional luteal or follicular cysts were frequently found by Nezhat *et al.* [14] in association with large ovarian endometriomas in women not using oral contraceptives. The authors suggest that large endometriomas may develop as a result of secondary involvement of functional ovarian cysts by the endometriosis process. They noted a lack of development of large endometriomas in patients on ovulation suppressive therapy despite the development of small surface implants.

Diagnosis

The clinical presentation of ovarian endometriosis is by either pelvic pain, infertility, the finding of a pelvic mass at gynaecological examination or sonography or, rarely, its complications, such as rupture or infection. In the absence of typical symptoms, the detection and characterization of ovarian masses by imaging techniques is a continuing challenge. The laparoscopy, however, remains the gold standard for diagnosis.

Sonography

Sonography fails to demonstrate superficial implants and small endometriomas. Endometriomas present different sonographic patterns, such as purely cystic, cystic with few septations or minimal debris, complex combinations of cystic and solid elements and largely solid [15, 16]. The sensitivity and specificity of ultrasonographic diagnosis is reported as 75% and 75% respectively [17]. Due to the non-specificity of the ultrasound examination, the mass has to be differentiated from haemorrhagic ovarian cysts and occasionally from a cystadenoma or tubo-ovarian abscess. It is, however, useful in identifying the presence and location of endometriomas and may also be helpful in following the size of endometriomas in response to therapy. Aspiration of the cyst under ultrasound can reveal the chocolate content but a similar chocolate-coloured haemorrhagic content may be found in some follicle haematomas or even in cystadenomas.

Magnetic resonance imaging

Ultrasonography continues to be the initial modality of choice for evaluating adnexal masses, but magnetic resonance imaging (MRI) is increasingly used for problem-solving when further characterization is needed. MRI has a higher accuracy than ultrasonography and appears to be the most accurate method of differentiating an endometrioma from other gynaecologic masses [18]. The haemorrhagic cyst can be accurately distinguished from the non-haemorrhagic cyst by MRI. The blood element of a chronic-stage haematoma exhibits a hyperintense signal on both T1- and T2-weighted images and the thick viscous content is likely to explain the shading of the signal intensity of the fluid. The signal intensity typical of acute haematomas (intermediate intensity on T1-weighted masses) and subacute haematomas (hyperintensity with a distinct central area of hypointensity on T1-weighted images) allows differentiation from chronic bleeding in the endometrial cyst [19, 20]. In addition, MRI can reflect some specific macroscopic features of an endometrioma, such as the anatomical localization of the adhesions, by the indistinct interface and the irregular lining of the wall in this area (Fig. 6.3). The multilocularity or the presence of two or more hyperintense cysts communicating with each other or adhering to each other or to neighbouring organs can be visualized. The overall diagnostic sensitivity, specificity and accuracy for MRI diagnosis of endometrial cyst are reported as 90%, 98% and 96%, respectively [18]. Given the 96% accuracy, MRI is an acceptable and useful technique for the diagnosis of the endometrioma. The direct evaluation of the content and the detection of cyst in the presence of extensive adhesions provide additional information which cannot be provided by laparoscopy.

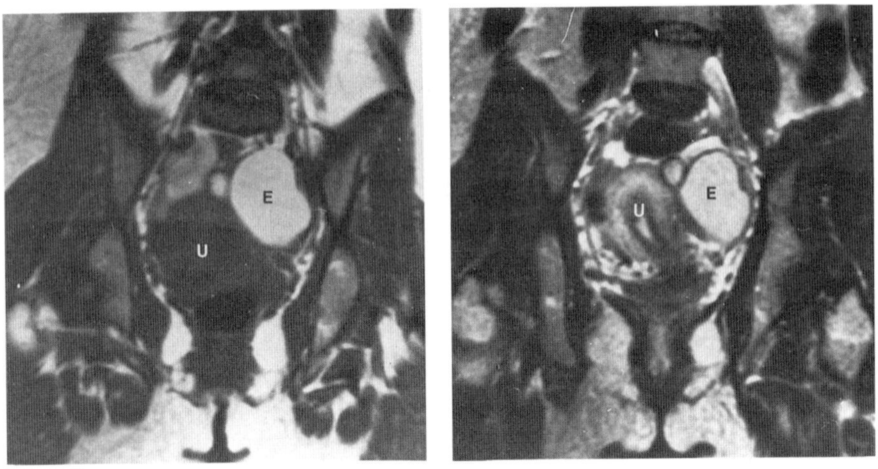

(a) (b)

Fig. 6.3 Endometrioma. Coronal T1-weighted (a) and T2-weighted (b) images. On the T1-weighted image, the endometrioma (E) is of high signal intensity consistent with haemorrhage. The endometrioma demonstrates multilocularity and an indistinct interface with the adjacent uterus (U). From [48] with permission.

Laparoscopy

The visual diagnosis of a typical endometrioma demonstrates a sensitivity, specificity and accuracy of 97%, 95% and 96% respectively [21]. The laparoscopic features of a typical endometrioma include: (i) ovarian cysts not greater than 12 cm in diameter; (ii) adhesions to the pelvic side wall and/or the posterior broad ligament; (iii) 'powderburns' and minute red or blue spots with adjacent puckering on the surface; and (iv) tarry, thick chocolate-coloured fluid content.

Random biopsies

Recommendations to biopsy the endometrioma are made on the priority of excluding malignancy and detecting epithelial atypia [22]. However, random biopsies and even resected specimens frequently fail to reveal endometriotic tissue [23].

Aspiration and examination of the content

In the absence of typical features, a deep cyst or a cyst obscured by dense adhesions can be detected by aspiration of chocolate-coloured content [24], but there is a need for histological confirmation. The diagnosis of an endometrioma should not be based on inspection of the aspirate alone. As in most ovarian cysts, cytology of the aspirate does not contribute to the diagnosis because of the poor yield of cells. CA-125 and steroid hormone assays have been suggested to be helpful in the differential diagnosis between an endometrioma and a functional cyst [25], but the multiplicity of endometriomas and lutein cysts may confuse the results.

Ovarian cystoscopy and guided biopsies

Ovarian cystoscopy has recently been proposed as a useful additional technique for the diagnosis of the endometrioma and the localization of implants for biopsy [26]. The technique, as described by Brosens and Puttemans [27] uses a second optic, such as a 4 mm 30° rigid Hamou II hysteroscope with an operating channel (Karl Storz Endoscope, Tüttlingen, Germany), which is introduced through a secondary suprapubic port. After careful inspection of the pelvis and in the absence of signs suspicious of malignancy, the cyst is first punctured and an aspiration sample is obtained. The cyst is subsequently flushed abundantly, using a suction irrigator with sterile saline at body temperature until the fluid becomes clear. After introduction of the optic through the small hole, a saline infusion is allowed to run freely to distend the cyst. The 30° angle of the optic allows a nearly complete visualization of the wall of the cyst.

The technique allows identification of the characteristics of the wall of the cyst, particularly in cases when the laparoscopic inspection fails to reveal typical features. Recurrent chocolate cysts after previous surgery were found to be functional haemorrhagic cysts in 73% of the cases [26]. Follicular and serous cysts are characterized by a smooth undulating or flat surface with a fine, retinal network of vascularization (Fig. 6.4). Lutein cysts present a uniform, yellow appearance with discrete vascularization. The typical features of the endometrioma cyst are the concentric retraction of the wall and the presence of haemorrhagic foci at the site of external adhesions or scarification and the irregular pattern of superficial vascularization and red implants (Fig. 6.5). The colour of the wall appears pearl-white, like normal ovarian cortex,

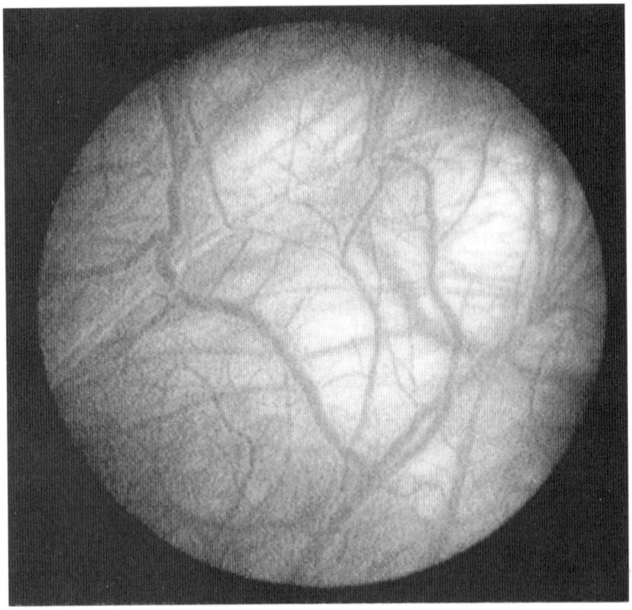

Fig. 6.4 Ovarian cystoscopy of a functional cyst: note the retinal pattern of vascularization covered by an undulating epithelium.

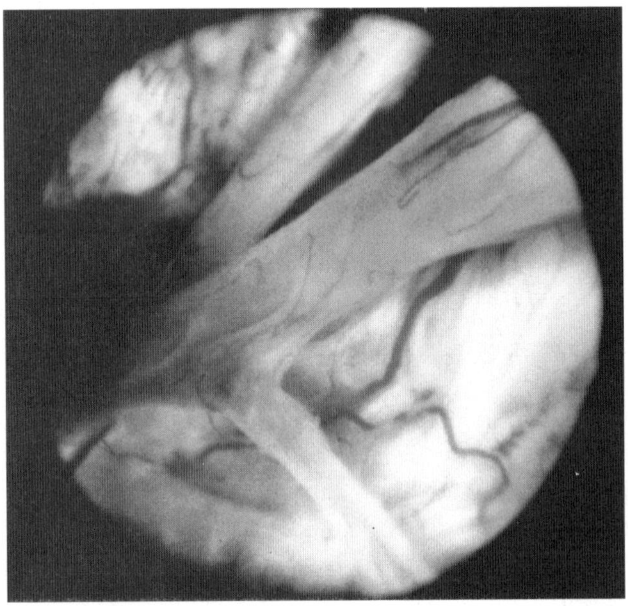

Fig. 6.5 Ovarian cystoscopy of an endometrioma: note the retraction of the cortex, the vascularization overlying the cortex and the small haemorrhagic implant at the site of inversion in an endometrioma.

yellow-pigmented or dark fibrotic depending on the age of the endometrioma. Red, haemorrhagic foci with an irregular network of vascularization cover the surface of the wall and are easily dislodged from the surface by manipulation. At histology the red, haemorrhagic foci are frequently found to be endometrial tissue or non-specific haemorrhage [28]. At the site of retraction small foci of full-thickness endometrial mucosa can be found (Fig. 6.6), while at a distance only surface epithelium with or without stroma is found, suggesting a progressive outgrowth of endometrial tissue over the inverted cortex from the site of invagination. Biopsies from the pearl-white surface confirm the presence of cortex with or without primordial follicles, while pigmented and dark areas represent progressive fibrosis infiltrated with haemosiderin-loaded macrophages. Luteinized follicles are also seen as red areas in early endometriomas, but in contrast to the endometrial implants they are located in the wall and are not detachable. Microbiopsies of 1–2 mm in size obtained under ovarioscopic guidance produce more representative endometriosis tissue than large at random biopsies or even resected specimens. The location of small endometrial implants at the site of adhesions and inversion stigma explains the failure of some authors [23] to detect any endometriosis in resected specimens.

In situ cystoscopy before surgery of the endometrioma has the advantage

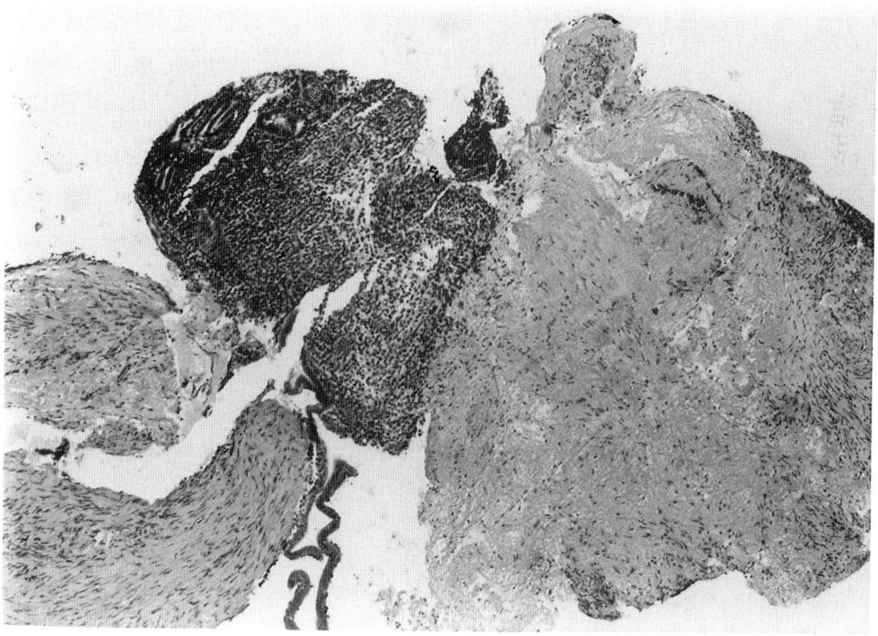

Fig. 6.6 Microbiopsy from the site of inversion: a small mucosa-type implant of endometriosis is seen in the inversion stigma (courtesy of Dr Joëlle Wallon).

of detecting the site of inversion, which is otherwise destroyed by adhesiolysis and excision. The wall can be inspected before the vision is blurred by collapse and haemorrhage, and distension by fluid allows inspection while the tissue covering the wall is floating, enhancing the identification of endometrial tissue.

Histopathology

Biopsies of the wall of endometriomas can reveal mucosal endometrium, columnar epithelium with or without stroma, cortex with or without oocytes, primordial follicles, luteinized follicles or fibroreactive tissue with haemosiderin-loaded macrophages. All these findings are diagnostic or compatible with the diagnosis of a haemorrhagic pseudocyst or endometrioma. Nuclear atypia in the epithelium can be seen but its significance is not always clear as it may represent a chronic reactivity. However, the small implants can show the same cyclicity as eutopic endometrium and it is therefore not surprising to see reactivation during hormonal replacement therapy [29] or the occurrence of premalignant and malignant changes after long-term continuous oestrogen therapy [30, 31].

Pathophysiology

Symptoms

Ovarian endometriosis is known to be associated with symptoms of infertility and pelvic pain. There is now ample experimental [32] and clinical evidence that endometriosis associated with distortion of the tubo-ovarian structures is associated with infertility. Rupture of endometriomas is described to occur around the time of menstruation but the association remains controversial [33]. The symptoms of an acute or subacute abdomen are likely to regress spontaneously. It has always been assumed that spilling of the content, or so-called perforation, was the cause of adhesion formation, but recent experimental studies have failed to induce adhesions by the endometrioma content [34]. This observation is in agreement with the pathogenesis that adhesions enclosing an active implant are the cause of endometrioma formation.

Multiplicity or multilocularity of endometriomas is a frequent phenomenon. The observed combined occurrence of endometriomas and haemorrhagic corpora lutea or lutein cysts, particularly in large cysts, is of no surprise as the ovarian cortex is involved in the formation of the wall of the cyst. Luteinization of the unruptured follicle has been associated with pelvic endometriosis [35, 36].

Torsion

The rare occurrence of torsion of an ovarian endometrioma is readily explained by the frequent occurrence of adhesions with surrounding pelvic structures. Ovarian endometriosis can be tightly fixed on pelvic supportive structures, such as the uterosacral ligament or ovarian ligament. These structures can show nodular endometriosis, which is characterized by fibromuscular hyperplasia and infiltration of glandulostromal tissue. Such nodules are known to be frequently associated with pelvic pain.

Response to hormone therapy

Ovarian endometriosis has been shown to respond poorly to hormonal therapy [37], to be less in phase with corresponding endometriosis [38] and to have fewer oestrogen receptors than the endometrium [39]. The differences between ovarian endometriosis and eutopic endometrium can be explained by several hypotheses, such as the degree of fibrosis, the differentiation of the cell and different cell-regulating mechanisms. However, the selection of the site of biopsy is likely to be most important for detecting the active implant in an endometrioma. In our study we have observed remarkable inactivation of mucosa-type implants after 3 months gonadotrophin-releasing hormone (GnRH) agonist therapy.

Classification

The terminology of deep endometriosis used in the American Fertility Society (AFS) revised classification of endometriosis [40] is inappropriate for the typical endometrioma in the sense that endometriosis does not invade the inside of the ovary but remains largely on the outside [41]. Endometriosis has a great capacity to deform the ovarian structure. It can also be questioned whether the ovarian endometrioma represents progressive disease or, rather, a complication, as the pseudocyst is caused by the adhesions in much the same way as a haematometra is caused by cervical occlusion.

The size of the cyst also has little bearing on the operability in reconstructive surgery. The most important criterion of operability is the extent of adhesion formation [42]. Studying the incidence of bilateral adnexal disease and dense adhesions, Canis *et al.* [43] suggested that a stage V needs to be considered in the AFS classification.

Principles of treatment

The logical treatment of the typical endometrioma is primarily the surgical release of the adhesions and fibrosis at the site of invagination and the eversion of the invaginated cortex. The surgical procedure is performed in much the same way as a salpingostomy (Fig. 6.7). It is not surprising that puncture, whether or not followed by GnRH agonist, has no beneficial effect on the endometrioma [44].

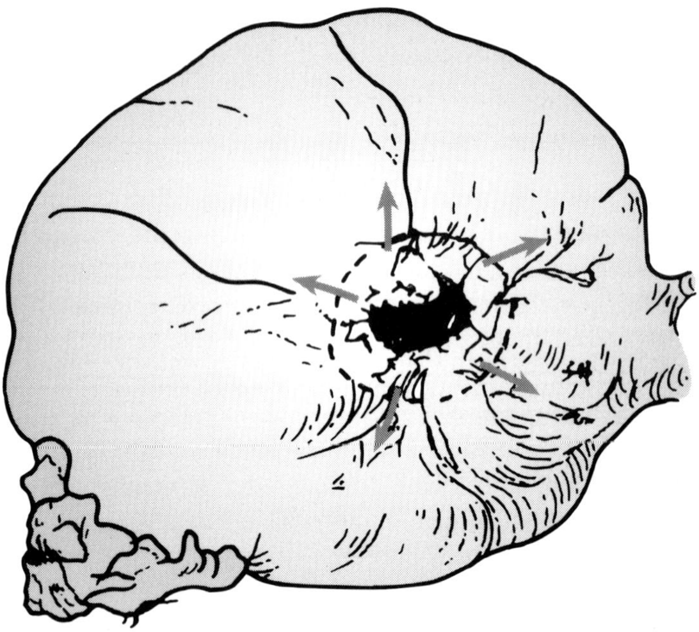

Fig. 6.7 Reconstructive surgery of an endometrioma: the inversion stigma is excised and the pseudocyst is everted by incisions along the lines of retraction.

The second principle is the destruction of the active implants. In the non-fibrotic endometrioma, excisional techniques should be avoided, as the active implants are located on the surface of normal ovarian cortex and can be easily destroyed with electrosurgery or laser. On the other hand, fibrotic endometriomas have a thickened capsule, which is more likely to be removed effectively by excisional techniques.

The third principle is the prevention of postoperative ovarian adhesion formation. Postoperative adhesion formation is the major complication of ovarian surgery for endometriomas [45]. Primary prevention is achieved by avoiding unnecessary surgery such as the excision of functional cysts. The use of atraumatic surgical techniques is essential, as there is no compensation by adhesion-preventive methods for bad surgery. The second efficient technique for adhesion prevention is second-look adhesiolysis. In large endometriomas,

3 months GnRH agonist therapy preceding second-look laparoscopy has the advantage of allowing the involution of the ovarian distension and suppressing the presence of functional cysts at the time of surgery [46].

References

1 Benagiano G, Brosens I. The history of endometriosis: identifying the disease. *Human Reprod* 1991 7: 963–968.
2 Casler DB. A unique, diffuse uterine tumor, really an adenomyoma, with stroma, but no glands: menstruation after complete hysterectomy due to uterine mucosa remaining in the ovary. *Trans Am Gynecol Soc* 1919 **44**: 69–84.
3 Norris CC. Ovary containing endometrium. *Am J Obstet Gynecol* 1921 **1**: 831–834.
4 Cullen TS. The distribution of adenomyoma containing uterine mucosa. *Arch Surg* 1920 **1**: 215–283.
5 Sampson JA. Perforating haemorrhagic (chocolate) cysts of the ovary. *Arch Surg* 1921 **3**: 245–323.
6 Hughesdon PE. The structure of endometrial cysts of the ovary. *J Obstet Gynaecol Br Emp* 1957 **44**: 481–487.
7 Nieminen U. Studies on the vascular pattern of ectopic endometrium with special reference to cyclic changes. *Acta Obstet Gynecol Scand* 1962 **41** (Suppl. 3): 1–81.
8 Jenkins S, Olive DL, Haney AF. Endometriosis: pathogenic implications of the anatomic distribution. *Obstet Gynecol* 1986 **67**: 335–338.
9 Redwine DB. The distribution of endometriosis in the pelvis by age groups and fertility. *Fertil Steril* 1987 **47**: 173–175.
10 Davis GD, Thillet E, Lindemann J. Clinical characteristics of adolescent endometriosis. *J Adolesc Health* 1993 **14**: 362–368.
11 Nisolle M, Casanas-Roux F, Anaf V, Mine JM, Donnez J. Morphometric study of the stromal vascularization in peritoneal endometriosis. *Fertil Steril* 1993 **59**: 681–684.
12 Wiegerinck MAHM, Van Dop PA, Brosens IA. The staging of peritoneal endometriosis by the type of active lesion in addition to the revised American Fertility Society classification. *Fertil Steril* 1993 **3**: 461–464.
13 Hoshiai H, Ishikawa M, Sawatari Y, Noda K, Fukaya T. Laparoscopic evaluation of the onset and progression of endometriosis. *Am J Obstet Gynecol* 1993 **169**: 714–719.
14 Nezhat F, Nezhat C, Allan CJ, Metzger DA, Sears DL. A clinical and histologic classification of endometriomas: implications for a mechanism of pathogenesis. *J Reprod Med* 1992 **37**: 771–776.
15 Athey PA, Diment DD. The spectrum of sonographic findings in endometriomas. *J Ultrasound Med* 1989 **8**: 487–491.
16 Fried AM, Rhodes RA, Morehouse IR. Endometrioma: analysis and sonographic classification of 51 documented cases. *South Med J* 1993 **86**: 297–301.
17 Mais V, Guerriero S, Ajossa S *et al.* The efficiency of transvaginal ultrasonography in the diagnosis of endometrioma. *Fertil Steril* 1993 **60**: 776–780.
18 Togashi K, Nishimura K, Kimura I *et al.* Endometrial cysts: diagnosis with MR imaging. *Radiology* 1991 **180**: 73–78.
19 Sugimura K, Takemori M, Sugiura M *et al.* The value of magnetic resonance relaxation time in staging ovarian endometrial cysts. *Br J Radiol* 1992 **65**: 502–506.
20 Sugimura K, Okizuka H, Imaoka I *et al.* Pelvic endometriosis: detection and diagnosis with chemical shift MR imaging. *Radiology* 1993 **188**: 435–438.
21 Vercellini P, Vendola N, Bocciolone L *et al.* Reliability of the visual diagnosis of ovarian endometriosis. *Fertil Steril* 1990 **53**: 1198–1200.

22 Barbieri RL. Visual diagnosis of endometriosis – reliability? (Letter). *Fertil Steril* 1992 **58**: 221–222.

23 Fayez JA, Vogel MF. Comparison of different treatment methods of endometriomas by laparoscopy. *Obstet Gynecol* 1991 **78**: 660–665.

24 Candiani GB, Vercellini P, Fedele L. Laparoscopic ovarian puncture for correct staging of endometriosis. *Fertil Steril* 1990 **53**: 994–997.

25 Koninckx PR, Muyldermans M, Moerman P *et al.* CA 125 concentrations in ovarian 'chocolate' cyst fluid can differentiate an endometriotic cyst from a cystic corpus luteum. *Hum Reprod* 1992 7: 1314–1317.

26 Brosens IA, Puttemans PJ, Deprest J. The endoscopic localization of endometrial implants in the ovarian chocolate cyst. *Fertil Steril* 1994 (in press).

27 Brosens IA, Puttemans PJ. Double-optic laparoscopy: salpingoscopy, ovarian cystoscopy and endo-ovarian surgery with the argon laser. *Baillière's Clin Obstet Gynaecol* 1989 **3**: 595–608.

28 Martin DC, Berry JD. Histology of chocolate cysts. *J Gynecol Surg* 1990 **6**: 43–46.

29 Goh JT, Hall BA. Postmenopausal endometrioma and hormonal replacement therapy. *Austr NZ J Obstet Gynaec* 1992 **32**: 384–385.

30 DePriest PD, Banks ER, Powell DE *et al.* Endometrioid carcinoma of the ovary and endometriosis: the association in postmenopausal women. *Gynec Oncol* 1992 **47**: 71–75.

31 Vercellini P, Parazzini F, Bolis G *et al.* Endometriosis and ovarian cancer. *Am J Obstet Gynecol* 1993 **169**: 181–182.

32 Kaplan CR, Eddy CA, Olive DL, Schenken RS. Effects of ovarian endometriosis on ovulation in rabbits. *Am J Obstet Gynecol* 1989 **160**: 40–44.

33 Ranney B. Endometriosis. II. Emergency operations due to hemoperitoneum. *Am J Obstet Gynecol* 1970 **36**: 437–442.

34 Kennedy SH, Cederholm-Williams SA, Barlow DH. The effect of injecting endometriotic 'chocolate' cyst fluid into the peritoneal cavity of mice. *Hum Reprod* 1992 **9**: 1329.

35 Brosens I, Koninckx PR, Corveleyn P. A study of plasma progesterone, oestradiol-17β, prolactin and LH levels, and of the luteal phase appearance of the ovaries in patients with endometriosis and infertility. *Br J Obstet Gynaec* 1978 **85**: 250–264.

36 Mio Y, Toda T, Harada T, Terakawa N. Luteinized unruptured follicle in the early stages of endometriosis as a cause of unexplained infertility. *Am J Obstet Gynecol* 1992 **167**: 271–273.

37 Nisolle-Pochet M, Casanas-Roux F, Donnez J. Histologic study of ovarian endometriosis after hormonal therapy. *Fertil Steril* 1988 **3**: 423–426.

38 Metzger DA, Szpak CA, Haney AF. Histologic features associated with hormonal responsiveness of ectopic endometrium. *Fertil Steril* 1993 **58**: 83–88.

39 Bergqvist A, Fernoe M. Estrogen and progesterone receptors in endometriotic tissue and endometrium: comparison according to localization and recurrence. *Fertil Steril* 1993 **60**: 63–68.

40 American Fertility Society. Revised American Fertility Society classification of endometriosis. *Fertil Steril* 1985 **43**: 351–352.

41 Brosens IA. Classification of endometriosis revisited. *The Lancet* 1990 **341**: 630.

42 Canis M, Mage G, Wattiez A *et al.* Second-look laparoscopy after laparoscopic cystectomy of large ovarian endometriomas. *Fertil Steril* 1992 **58**: 617–619.

43 Canis M, Pouly JL, Wattiez A *et al.* Incidence of bilateral adnexal disease in severe endometriosis (revised American Fertility Society (AFS), stage IV): should a stage V be included in the AFS classification? *Fertil Steril* 1992 **57**: 691–692.

44 Vercellini P, Vendola N, Bocciolone L *et al.* Laparoscopic aspiration of ovarian endometriomas: effect with postoperative gonadotropin releasing hormone agonist treatment. *J Reprod Med* 1992 **37**: 577–580.

45 Wood C, Maher P, Hill D. Diagnosis and surgical management of endometriomas. *Austr NZ J Obstet Gynaecol* 1992 **32**: 161–163.
46 Donnez J, Nisolle M, Clerckx F *et al.* The ovarian endometrial cyst: the combined (hormonal and surgical) therapy. In: Brosens I, Jacobs HS, Runnebaum B (eds). *LHRH-Analogues in Gynaecology*, 1990, pp.165–175. Carnforth, Parthenon Publishing.
47 Brosens IA, Gordon H. *Tubal Infertility*, 1989. London, Gower Medical Publishing.
48 Popovick MJ, Hricak H. The role of magnetic resonance imaging in the evaluation of gynecologic disease. In: Callen B (ed.). *Ultrasonography in Obstetrics and Gynecology*, 3rd edn, 1994. WB Saunders, New York.

Chapter 7
Pelvic Pain and Endometriosis

C.M. MACLAVERTY AND R.W. SHAW

Introduction

Pain is perhaps the cardinal symptom of endometriosis. Various types of pain are associated with the disease; dysmenorrhoea, deep dyspareunia as well as pelvic pain unrelated to intercourse or menstruation. Pelvic pain is the second most commonly presenting symptom: as can be seen from Table 7.1 [1–4] pelvic pain occurs in 30–50% of patients. However, an earlier series of 717 Australian women with endometriosis studied by O'Connor [5], in which the chief complaint only in each woman was recorded, revealed dysmenorrhoea to be the commonest presenting symptom, closely followed by dyspareunia and then pelvic pain. (Table 7.2).

Pelvic pain is arguably the symptom causing the most misery amongst endometriosis sufferers and is more distressing than infertility. The discovery of infertility in an individual, where fertility is desired, is similar to a loss event and reactive depression may ensue, but usually the individual or couple recovers and adapts. Chronic pelvic pain, however, as with other forms of pain, often produces serious long-term detrimental effects on personality, and affect working, social and marital life. Dysmenorrhoea often occurs with pelvic pain but patients commonly describe a background of constant dragging/aching pain which may be exacerbated by the menses but is often a

Table 7.1 Frequency of the more common symptoms in endometriosis patients

Symptom	Likely frequency (%)
Dysmenorrhoea	60–80
Pelvic pain	30–50
Infertility	30–40
Dyspareunia	25–40
Menstrual irregularities	10–20
Cyclical dysuria/haematuria	1–2
Dyschesia	1–2
Rectal bleeding (cyclic)	< 1

Adapted from [1–4] with permission.

Table 7.2 Frequency distributions of symptoms of endometriosis

Symptom	Number	Percentage ($n = 717$)
Dysmenorrhoea	227	32
Dyspareunia	188	26
Pelvic pain	114	16
Infertility	64	9
Asymptomatic	155	22

Adapted from [5] O'Connor.

different type of pain from the typical cramping of spasmodic dysmenorrhoea and often in a different site.

Whilst the symptoms of dysmenorrhoea, dyspareunia and pelvic pain can occur with other gynaecological pathologies, it is the cyclical and menstrually related component of several symptoms which should alert the clinician to the potential diagnosis of endometriosis. It is probably helpful in this chapter considering pain in endometriosis to outline the female pelvic anatomy and innervation before discussion of pain pathways and surgical intervention.

Innervation of the female pelvis

All the internal reproductive organs as well as the pelvic peritoneum have solely autonomic innervation with no somatic supply. The autonomic nerves carry sensory and motor fibres, both adrenergic and cholinergic. Visceral branches generally arise from the spinal cord at a high level and then descend steeply to form visceral plexuses [6–8].

Sympathetic

Visceral branches or splanchnic nerves containing sympathetic fibres arising from T5 to L1 sympathetic ganglia pass down from the coeliac plexus through the intermesenteric (aortic) plexus to lie retroperitoneally below the bifurcation of the abdominal aorta, forming the superior hypogastric plexus. This plexus was formerly known as the presacral nerve, which is a misnomer, firstly, since it is a plexus, not a nerve and, secondly, since it is prelumbar, not presacral, lying as it does just above the sacral promontory (Fig. 7.1).

The superior hypogastric plexus gives rise to two main chains, the hypogastric nerves, which run downwards and outwards on the pelvic side wall to join the two inferior hypogastric plexuses, also known as pelvic plexuses.

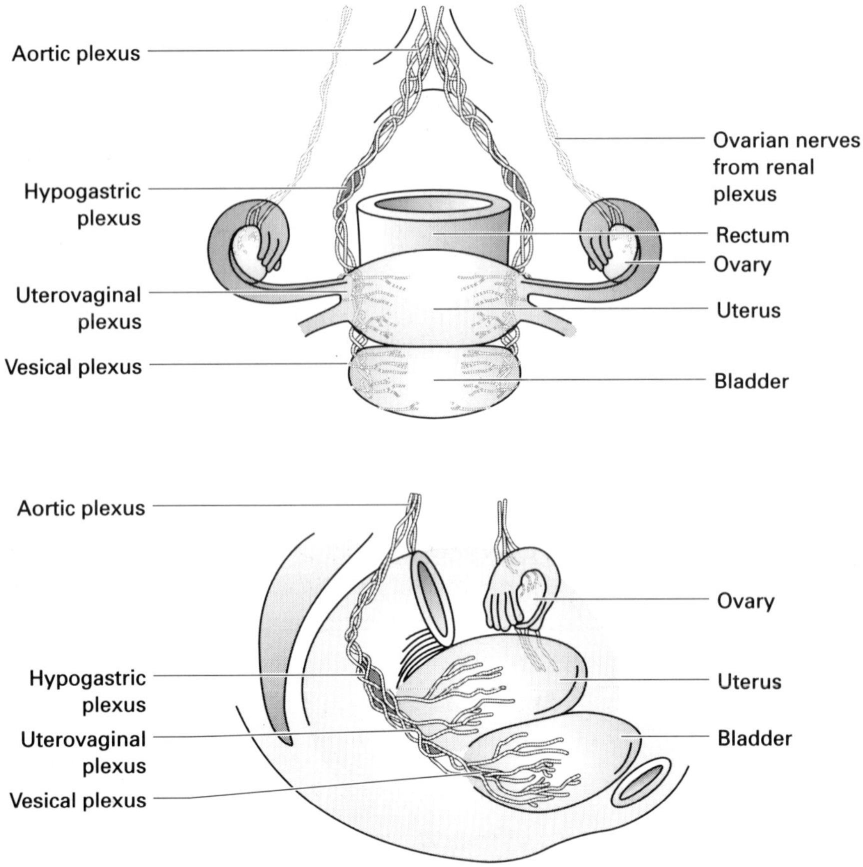

Fig. 7.1 Pelvic autonomic plexus and nerves. Redrawn from [9] with permission.

These two plexuses lie on either side of the rectal ampulla and extend anteriorly beneath the uterosacral and broad ligaments and superior to the transverse cervical ligament. This forward extension of the pelvic plexus or inferior hypogastric plexus is also referred to as the Lee–Frankenhauser plexus or the uterovaginal plexus (Fig. 7.2).

Parasympathetic

The inferior hypogastric plexus also receives parasympathetic fibres from S2–S5 nerve roots. These probably carry sensation from the cervix and the lower part of the uterus and thus cause lower backache as referred pain from the cervix if it is inflamed or traumatized.

Macroscopically the inferior hypogastric plexus is a coarse meshwork of myelinated and unmyelinated nerves containing paracervical and other ganglia. It measures 5 cm anteroposteriorly and 2 cm superoinferiorly. It

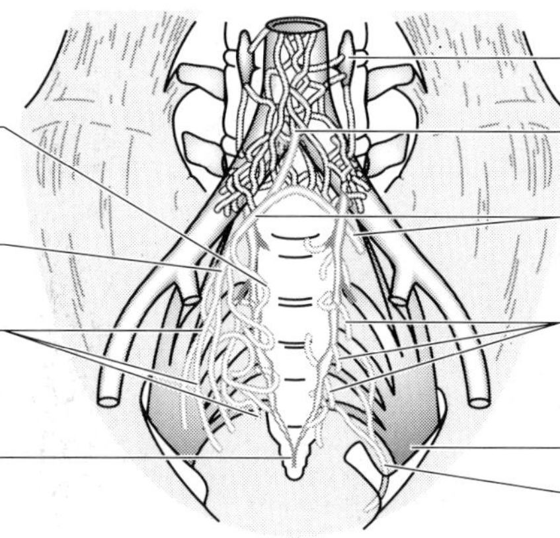

Fig. 7.2 Dissection of a median section of a female pelvis showing the autonomic nerves Redrawn from [8] with permission of Williams and Wilkins, Baltimore, MD.

supplies sympathetic and parasympathetic nerves to all the pelvic organs, including bladder and bowel. Those fibres passing to the cervix and uterus pass through the paracervical ganglia in the base of the broad ligament.

Uterine innervation

This is largely from the uterovaginal plexus (forward extension of the inferior hypogastric), which gives sympathetic fibres passed from the superior hypogastric plexus and parasympathetic fibres from the pelvic splanchnic nerves. Afferent fibres ascend through the inferior hypogastric plexus and enter the cord via T10–L1 spinal nerves. The uterine fundus probably receives some fibres from nerves accompanying the ovarian vessels.

Pain sensation from the cervix uteri is carried via the pelvic splanchnics and referred to the sacral region, where it is experienced as lower back pain. Dysmenorrhoea and labour pain sensation is carried via the sympathetic fibres to T10-L1 and pain is referred to these periumbilical dermatomes. Abolition of all uterine sensation requires transection of the cord above the level of T10 or division of all uterine nerves in the hypogastric plexuses. In both these situations, labour proceeds normally.

Ovary

Sympathetic fibres reach the ovary with the ovarian arteries. The cell bodies lie in the T10 and T11 segments of the cord. Pain is again referred to the periumbilical dermatomes as with pain of internal origin. Parasympathetic fibres are fewer in number and arrive from the inferior hypogastric plexuses.

Fallopian tubes

Unlike the uterine body and cervix, the Fallopian tubes are sensitive to heat, distension, compression and cutting. Their nerve supply is partly via the ovarian plexus via the ovarian arteries and partly via the uterovaginal plexus. The different fibres are found in T11–L1 nerve roots.

Vagina

The upper part is supplied by the uterovaginal plexus and thus fibres arise from the inferior hypogastric plexus and the pelvic splanchnic nerves.

Nociception

Nociception or pain perception is produced in response to mechanical distortion or thermal stimuli, if great enough, or in response to the release of chemical substances (serotonin, bradykinin, prostaglandins, substance P) [10,11]. A polymodal nociceptor responds to many forms of stimulation, whereas a mechanosensitive nociceptor responds to only mechanical stimulation.

There are two types of nociceptor; those connected to A-delta fibres (also known as group III fibres) and those connected to C fibres (also known as group IV afferents). The C fibres are polymodal nociceptors, whereas the A-delta fibres are mechanosensitive. Pain sensation is conducted from the nociceptor in the tissues via these small-diameter myelinated fibres (A-delta) and large-diameter unmyelinated fibres (C fibres), which enter the dorsal root of the spinal column in most cases. It is thought that about half of all afferent fibres entering the dorsal roots are nociceptive. Some nociceptors may also enter the spinal cord via the ventral roots.

Not all A-delta and C fibres have nociceptive functions. In these fibre classes there are also low-threshold mechanoreceptors. Knowledge of nociceptors in the viscera is much less advanced than that of cutaneous nociceptors, and no clear differentiation is possible between nociceptors and receptors which serve other functions in the viscera. The A-delta nociceptors are said to be situated mostly in the skin, parietal peritoneum and muscle. Stimulation of these leads to a sharper, more well-focused pain of more rapid outset. C nociceptors are distributed more widely, particularly in viscera, deep muscle and peritoneum. Stimulation of innervation results in a more poorly focused, dull pain or ache, of slower onset, typical of that experienced in endometriosis.

The nociceptor fibres synapse in the grey matter of the dorsal horn of the same segment or in adjacent segments. These nociceptor impulses are relayed to fibres ascending in the contralateral spinothalamic tract to the reticular formation and thalamic nuclei, and thence to the somatosensory cortex. There is no single pain perception centre in the brain and it is likely that many other areas of the brain are involved, not merely the somatosensory cortex, which is just the cognitive area. Other areas receiving nociceptive information are recognized to be: the limbic system, which is responsible for effective and motivational components of pain behaviour; the basal ganglia and cerebellum, which are responsible for motor activity or programming related to pain behaviour; the hypothalamus, which stimulates release of pituitary hormones; and the brainstem, which effects changes in circulation and respiration in response to pain.

Nociceptive impulses may be modified at all levels within the pain pathway, from initiation to final recognition or perception. Modifying influences at initiation could be the presence of analgesic drugs, such as acetylsalicylate (aspirin) or other prostaglandin synthetase inhibitors, which decrease the amount of noxious prostaglandin to inhibit initial timing of the receptor. Inhibition at the level of the spinal cell body could be via continuous stimulation from A-beta fibres, which are non-nociceptive-sensitive mechanoreceptors. These fibres synapse with the same spinal neurons as the A-delta and C nociceptive fibres, but the overriding stimulus is not noxious and so the pathway which would otherwise have been used for nociception is blocked.

Opiate receptors may inhibit spinal neurons either locally in the dorsal horns or via descending inhibitory pathways if the opiate receptors in the periaqueductal grey matter in the midbrain are stimulated (Fig. 7.3).

Visceral and somatic pain localization

It is striking that there is so much similarity in pain descriptors used by patients suffering from the pelvic pain associated with endometriosis. The site is usually lower abdominal, often in either iliac fossa or suprapubic. The patient usually describes the pain as aching, constant, dull, deep, dragging, tiring and debilitating. When asked to indicate the site of their pain, the patient will usually rub a general area and rarely uses a finger to indicate a specific area. These characteristics of poor localization and the aching, dull, deep nature of the pain are typical of visceral pain. It usually has a relatively longer period of outset.

Somatic pain is characterized by more superficial, precise localization and a sharp or stabbing nature and is often of more rapid onset. Somatic pain does not demonstrate cyclical or irregular variations in intensity, as visceral pain may do [12–14].

Autonomic phenomena, such as sweating, nausea, vomiting, tachypnoea

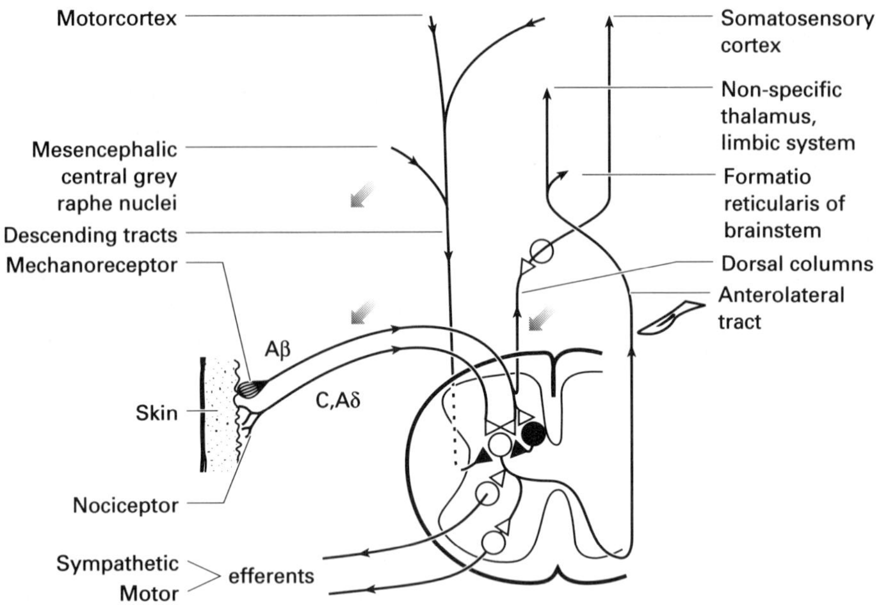

Fig. 7.3 Highly schematic diagram of the dorsal horn neuron. Afferent fibres synapse on to dorsal horn neurons, which conduct their impulses to segmental motor and sympathetic efferents and to ascending tracts. The dorsal horn neuron can be inhibited: inhibitory synapses and neurons denoted by filled circles and triangles. Voltage arrows indicate sites where stimulation can produce inhibition of the dorsal horn neuron. The scalpel indicates cordotomy for pain relief. Redrawn from [10] with permission.

and tachy- or bradycardia, are not characteristic of either type of pain but may serve as indicators of severity.

Cervero [12] suggested that pain could be classified into three types according to the embryological origin of the tissue concerned. Using this approach, pain in tissues of ectodermal origin (skin and mucous membranes) would show characteristics of good localization and sharpness. Tissues of mesodermal origin (muscles, ligaments, bones and joints) would be manifest as deeper pain, with slightly less accurate localization and not as sharp. Tissues of endodermal origin, i.e. the viscera, would give rise to painful sensations which were the most ill-localized, most dull and most aching.

Very much more is known about cutaneous nociceptors and nociception than about visceral nociception, since most of our knowledge has been obtained from studies involving the application of noxious stimuli to cutaneous areas. It has been possible to trace the central nervous system (CNS) connections of these nociceptor fibres anatomically and functionally. It is clearly not possible to apply the same techniques to viscera, leaving the rest of the body undisturbed.

Afferent and sensory visceral innervation

Some viscera, particularly the parenchymatous viscera, such as the liver, kidney and spleen, are relatively insensitive and a disease process taking place in these organs will only become painful when the capsule or parietal peritoneum becomes affected or distended. Other viscera when affected by a disease process seem more readily to produce painful stimuli, e.g. bowel and uterus.

Practically all internal organs have an afferent innervation, but the activation of many visceral receptors does not impinge on consciousness, e.g. the process of respiration, blood-pressure changes, normal peristalsis. When these receptors do impinge on consciousness, the sensation usually ranges from one of mild discomfort to a definite pain. In this case, the afferent innervation has become a sensory innervation. The answer to the question 'How does an afferent stimulus become a noxious one?' could be either that receptors for visceral pain have an increased rate of impulses firing which actually produces pain in response to the pain-producing stimulus, but under normal circumstances and under normal firing rates no pain is produced or there may be specific nociceptors which respond only to noxious stimuli.

Specific nociceptors have been discovered in the heart and the lungs and the biliary system, but it is thought that there is no evidence for specific visceral receptors in other intra-abdominal viscera.

Visceral pain pathways

The theory for visceral pain pathways explains both the dull, ill-localized nature of visceral pain and also the occurrence of referred pain which may be a feature of ovarian inflammation. Referred pain is characterized by pain being perceived in a site some distance from the affected organ, poor localization of the pain and pain characteristics of an aching and constant nature. As early as 1893, Head [15] assumed that this pain referral was due to the convergence of visceral and cutaneous nerves on to the same spinal cord neurons and this stimulation was misinterpreted by the brain as pain originating from a cutaneous site. Ruch [16] in 1946 proposed a comprehensive hypothesis called the convergence–projection theory, which explained all clinical manifestations of visceral pain:

> Visceral afferent fibres converge with cutaneous pain afferents to end upon the same neurones in the same sensory pathways. The resulting impulses, on reaching the brain, are interpreted as having come from the skin, an interpretation which has been learned from previous experience in which the same pathways were stimulated by cutaneous afferent nerves.

Visceral activation is diffuse and intermittent and more inconsistent than cutaneous input to spinal neurons, and it is this pattern of stimulation of spinal cord neurons which explains its characteristics, together with the fact that nociceptive C fibres outnumber A-delta fibres in afferent bundles for the viscera, whereas the situation is reversed for cutaneous nociceptors. C fibres, being of broader diameter and unmyelinated, produce a more dull pain of slower onset than small-diameter, rapidly conducting A-delta fibres.

Perhaps our general lack of understanding of the precise nature of innervation and types of receptors in the peritoneum and pelvic organs explains our poor understanding of pain of endometriosis.

Mechanisms of pelvic pain in endometriosis

Mechanisms of causation of pelvic pain may generally be divided either according to whether somatic or visceral pathways are employed or according to whether the pain is caused directly by endometriotic deposits (early) or consequent on the scarring and ensuing fibrotic reaction (late).

Somatic afferent fibres are found in the skin, muscles and parietal peritoneum. Sympathetic and parasympathetic fibres, as already discussed, innervate the pelvic organs as well as the visceral peritoneum.

Postulated mechanisms of pain in endometriosis could be:

1 Implantation on to peritoneum causing an inflammatory reaction, with consequent release of chemical mediators of pain (prostaglandins, histamine, kinins).

2 Deep infiltrating endometriosis may lead to tissue damage and nerve damage with nerve activation (see Fig. 7.4).

3 Endometrioma rupture may cause acute pain with a chemical peritonitis. Slow leakage may cause a more chronic episode of pain and this may continue until the capsule of the endometrioma becomes sealed over with superficial endometriosis of the ovary.

4 Scarring, retraction, fibrosis and adhesions cause tethering of tissues and may lead to pain on exercise, standing and ovulation, due to tension on tissues and organs and distortion of normal contours.

5 Bowel fixity due to adhesions and scarring with retraction may lead to pain on distension at the time of defecation (dyschesia). Fixity of bowel may also lead to deep dyspareunia.

6 Fixed uterine retroversion and tethering of the ovaries in the pouch of Douglas may cause dyspareunia, as may modularity and scarring of the uterosacral ligaments.

7 Fixity of bowel may also lead to colicky abdominal pain on distension, which explains why the symptoms of irritable bowel syndrome and endometriosis overlap.

Correlation between severity of endometriosis and severity of pain

There appears to be little correlation between sites involved by endometriosis and symptoms complained of. Various 'types of symptoms' can, however, to some degree be related to the system involved (Table 7.3) [17]. However, these do not correlate with the sites of deposits (Table 7.4). Reasons for this may be multiple and partially explained by the anatomical and type of pain innervation of the pelvis.

It has long been cited as a further supporting piece of evidence in the enigmatic and puzzling features of the disease that there is little correlation between the severity of the disease and the severity of the pain symptoms, as well as the disease site. Buttram in 1979 [2], using both the Acosta *et al.* [18] and their own more detailed classification, could not find any significant correlation between the severity of the endometriosis and the severity of the pelvic pain symptoms of dysmenorrhoea and dyspareunia in their series of 206 women. A decade later, two studies, by Fedele *et al.* [19] and Mahmood and Templeton [20], also failed to relate severity of pelvic pain symptoms to disease severity, using the revised American Fertility Society (RAFS) classification system [21]. Nor did these recent studies relate severity of pelvic pain symptoms to the disease site.

There are several reasons for this apparent paradox. Firstly, although the RAFS system is a classification system used for endometriosis whether the

Table 7.3 Symptoms of endometriosis in relationship to site of endometriotic implants

Site	Symptoms
Female reproductive tract	Dysmennorhoea Lower abdominal and pelvic pain Dyspareunia Infertility Menstrual irregularity Rupture/torsion endometrioma Low back pain
Gastrointestinal tract	Cyclical tenesmus/rectal bleeding Diarrhoea Colonic obstruction
Urinary tract	Cyclical haematuria/pain Ureteral obstruction
Surgical scars, umbilicus	Cyclical pain and bleeding
Lung	Cyclical haemoptysis

From [17] with permission.

Table 7.4 Frequency of location of endometriotic implants in the pelvis (from review of 500 consecutive cases, many individuals having multiple sites of involvement)

Site	Percentages
Uterosacral ligaments	63
Ovaries	
Superficial	56
Deep (endometrioma)	19.5
Ovarian fossae	32.5
Anterior vesicle pouch	21.5
Pouch of Douglas	18.5
Broad ligament	7.5
Intestines	5.0
Fallopian tube	
Mesosalpinx	4.5
Salpingitis isthmica nodosa	3.0
Uterus	4.5

From [17] with permission.

presenting complaint is infertility or pain, it was primarily designed as a prognostic tool for fertility. Thus superficial endometriosis affecting the ovary receives an increased weighting (higher score) than superficial endometriosis affecting the peritoneum, although the above studies have not shown that pain severity is greater in the presence of ovarian rather than peritoneal endometriosis.

Secondly, deeply infiltrating endometriosis is very strongly associated with the presence and severity of pelvic pain [22] but is not recognized as an entity in the RAFS system of classification. The histology, morphology and activity of deeply infiltrating endometriosis were investigated by Cornillie *et al.* [23]. They showed that disease activity was increased (as gauged by histological appearance) in superficial (< 1 mm) and deep (> 5 mm) implants, but was more quiescent in intermediate implants (2–4 mm). Cornillie *et al.* postulated that this was due to the relative concentrations of oestradiol and progesterone in the peritoneal fluid bathing the superficial implants and in the circulating serum in closer proximity to the deeper endometriosis than the intermediate endometriosis. This study [23] and another conducted by Koninckx *et al.* [22] demonstrated that deep endometriosis is strongly associated with pelvic pain. The superficial and often innocuous appearance of deep infiltrating endometriosis belie its extent of invasion, as the diagrams illustrate (Fig. 7.4). The Allen–Masters syndrome is the presence of a circular peritoneal defect,

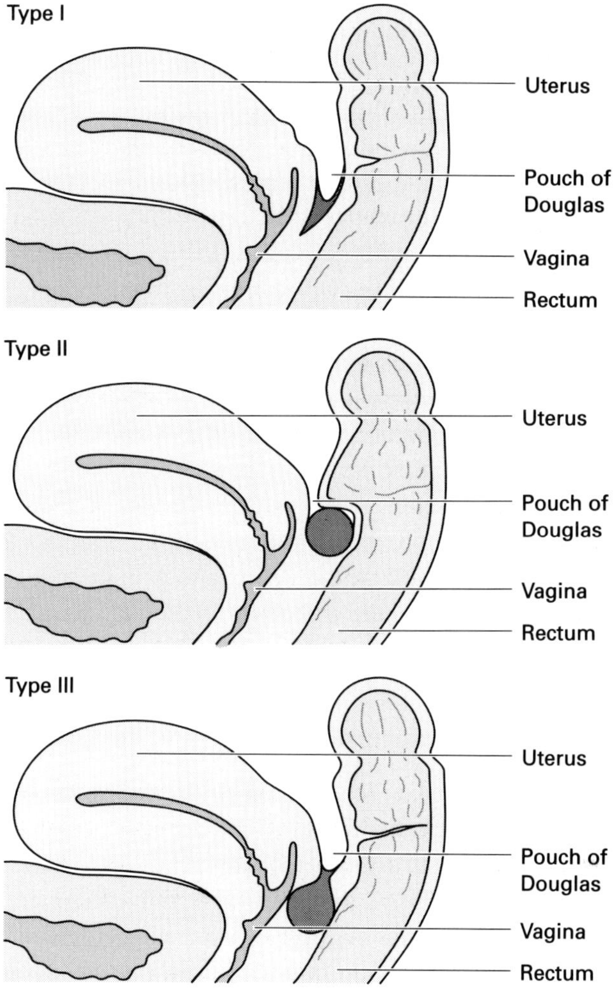

Fig. 7.4 Deeply infiltrating endometriosis. (a) Type I is infiltration. (b) Type II is retraction. (c) Type III is adenomyosis externa. Redrawn from [24] Atlas of Endometriosis, by Dan C Martin, Wolfe Medical Publishing an imprint of Times Mirror International Publishers Ltd., London, UK, 1992.

which is formed by incomplete reperitonealization over the base of an endometriotic implant. It is represented by type II infiltrating endometriosis.

Thirdly, minimal superficial non-pigmented endometriosis has the capacity to produce more prostaglandin F (PGF) than pigmented classical powderburn lesions. PGF is implicated in pain causation [25].

Jansen and Russell [26] identified endometriosis histologically in a large percentage of peritoneal lesions which were non-pigmented. They identified three new types of lesions macroscopically which were very likely to be proved to be endometriotic histologically: (i) white opacified lesions; (ii) red flame-like lesions; and (iii) glandular lesions. These non-pigmented lesions are now erroneously referred to as atypical.

Redwine [27] found that these non-pigmented lesions were more commonly present in younger than in older women. Conversely the classical, easily recognized powderburn lesions and puckered scarred lesions were more commonly found in older women. He postulated convincingly an age-related change in the colour of endometriotic lesions. This suggestion of younger, more active initial disease was supported by Vernon *et al.* [25], who found that the non-pigmented lesions had more capacity to synthesize PGF than the powderburn (possibly older) lesions.

Thus, in its earlier less florid, less well-recognized stages, before it has become destructive and more easily recognized, the disease may be producing large amounts of PGF and hence a greater severity of pain. The type of the pain may alter with the disease progression, with constant pain and exacerbation with the menses present initially in the disease, and later pain due to scarring, retraction and infiltration predominating. A detailed correlation between visual and histological type of lesion and pain has not been made. A further complication is that there are often several different types of lesion present at any one time.

Methods of pain measurement

Pain is defined as an unpleasant sensory and emotional experience with actual or potential tissue damage or described in terms of tissue damage [28]. Huskisson [29] stated that pain is a personal psychological experience and an observer can play no legitimate part in its direct measurement. Therefore, most methods of pain measurement rely on the subject's reporting of pain, not on an observer's interpretation of pain-related behaviour.

It is obviously very useful to measure pain in an individual with endometriosis, both to establish baseline pain and to monitor progression and regression of this symptom with the natural course of the disease or to evaluate efficacy of treatment. If the same method of pain measurement is used, then responses of different populations and different treatment options can be studied.

Diverse methods of pain assessment can be used, ranging from the simplest verbal rating scale (VRS) to visual analogue use or multidimensional pain scoring systems, with concomitant personality questionnaires, depression inventories and psychological assessments. While the latter, more sophisticated questionnaires provide a very useful insight into the patient's psyche and the effect of depression on the patient's pain or vice versa, they are probably too complicated to use practically if one is attempting to assess the efficacy of a particular treatment of pain on a large group of women. These methods are useful in scientific research but not as a general tool for clinical assessment.

The simpler methods of pain assessment gauge only pain intensity and no other aspect. These methods consist of VRS, numerical rating scales and visual analogue scales.

Verbal rating scales

At its simplest, a VRS consists of a three-point scale of increasing pain, e.g. mild, moderate or severe. Usually VRS consist of five or six points, ranging from mild to very severe or excruciating. The advantage of a VRS is that it is simple to explain and to understand. Its disadvantages are that it is relatively insensitive, the increments of pain intensity are not numerically equal (e.g. the difference between mild and moderate pain is not necessarily equal to the difference between severe and very severe pain). This means that statistical analysis is more difficult and non-parametric testing must be used.

Instruction example

Circle the adjective best describing your pain: mild, moderate, severe, very severe, excruciating.

Numerical rating scales

Numerical rating scales offer numbers denoting increasing severity of pain, and are a compromise between VRS and visual analogue scales. The scale usually ranges from 1 to 10. Again, the scale is not even, i.e. 2 does not necessarily equal twice the pain of 1. Table 7.5 gives an example commonly used for endometriosis symptoms.

Instruction example

Circle the number from 1 to 10 which best describes your pain, 1 being mild pain and 10 being most severe pain.

Visual analogue scales

A visual analogue scale consists of a horizontal straight line, ideally 10 cm long (sometimes 15 cm or 20 cm), on which pain is represented as a continuum from no pain to worst possible pain. The patient marks a vertical stroke on the line where they judge their pain to lie between the two extremes. This method, when properly explained and understood, is thought to be more accurate, more sensitive and more reliable than the previous two methods. It also allows easier statistical analysis of pain symptoms.

Table 7.5 Pelvic pain scoring system

Deep dyspareunia	
None	0
Mild – present but tolerable	1
Moderate – severe enough to necessitate interruption of intercourse	2
Severe – severe enough to necessitate avoidance of intercourse	3
Dysmenorrhoea	
None	0
Mild – some loss of work efficiency	1
Moderate – in bed part of the day, occasional loss of work	2
Severe – in bed 1 or more days, in incapacitation	3
Pelvic pain	
None	0
Mild – occasional pelvic discomfort or premenstrual pain	1
Moderate – noticeable discomfort for most of cycle	2
Severe – requires strong analgesic, persistent during cycle other than with menses	3

Instruction example

Mark on the line where you judge your pain to lie between no pain and worst possible pain:

no pain ———————————————————— worst possible pain

These above methods of pain measurement, because they measure only one aspect of pain – its intensity – have been likened to giving a black-and-white picture of pain. Multidimensional methods are likened to giving a colour picture of pain.

McGill pain questionnaire

As previously stated, it is striking that, when patients presenting at an endometriosis clinic are asked to describe their pelvic pain in their own words, there is a remarkably high number of common descriptions: firstly, site – either one or both of the iliac fossae, or suprapubic pain or lower back pain – and then nature of the pain – dull, aching, dragging, burning, tiring, exhausting, depressing and draining. When asked to indicate the site, the patient will very often rub a general area and hardly ever point with a fingertip. This characteristic is shared with other visceral pain.

The McGill pain questionnaire was formulated by Melzack and Torgerson [30] and consists of groups of pain descriptors which describe the qualitative or sensory nature of the pain (e.g. pricking, burning) and its influence on the subject's emotions (e.g. frightening, vicious). The questionnaire records the site of the pain and there is also a small group of miscellaneous descriptors. Because it measures pain characteristics other than intensity, the McGill pain questionnaire is extremely useful as a diagnostic aid. Leavitt and Garron [31] used a modified form of the pain questionnaire to try to distinguish between organic and functional pain. They found an accuracy rate of 87% comparing questionnaire predictions with final diagnosis after exhaustive investigations. Different clinical syndromes, e.g. menstrual pain and cancer pain, can be distinguished with a high degree of accuracy using this questionnaire.

The questionnaire takes 5–10 min to administer. The patient is asked to respond only to the descriptions which describe her pain. Then, incorporated into the questionnaire are a visual analogue scale and a present pain intensity rating (a VRS). A shortened form of the McGill pain questionnaire [32] has been developed which correlates very highly with the long-form McGill pain questionnaire and is as useful for most purposes (see Fig. 7.5).

One criticism of the present pain index is that it uses two emotive words (distressing and horrible) with other words describing severity alone. This could be confounding as, for example to an infertile woman who wishes to conceive, any slight twinge of pain might be horrible as it might remind her of her unsatisfied fertility design, but the pain might not necessarily be severe.

Other multidimensional methods

Other multidimensional methods of pain measurement employ behavioural responses to pain as well as pain intensity as criteria. Analgesic use and incapacitation are two such examples. One such useful scoring system used specifically for women with pelvic pain and dysmenorrhoea has been developed by Andersch and Milsom [33] (Table 7.6).

Specific assessments for endometriosis

Other pain scoring systems for deep dyspareunia, dysmenorrhoea and pelvic pain have been used together to form a pelvic pain score (see Table 7.5). The scores are simply added together, with the ranges used to describe severity being 1–3 mild, 4–6 moderate and 7–9 severe.

RAFS pain assessment method

The latest multidimensional pain assessment instrument specifically tailored for patients with endometriosis was proposed by the American Fertility

Patient's name ____________________ Date __________ Time __________am/pm

PRI: S ________ (1–10) A ________ (11–15) E ________ (16) M ________ (17–20) PRI(T) ________ (1–20) PPI ________

1	Flickering Quivering Pulsing Throbbing Beating Pounding	11	Tiring Exhausting		
		12	Sickening Suffocating		
		13	Fearful Frightful Terrifying		
2	Jumping Flashing Shooting	14	Punishing Gruelling Cruel Vicious Killing		
3	Pricking Boring Drilling Stabbing Lancinating	15	Wretched Blinding		
4	Sharp Cutting Lacerating	16	Annoying Troublesome Miserable Intense Unbearable		
5	Pinching Pressing Gnawing Cramping Crushing	17	Spreading Radiating Penetrating Piercing		
6	Tugging Pulling Wrenching	18	Tight Numb Drawing Squeezing Tearing		
7	Hot Burning Scalding Searing	19	Cool Cold Freezing		
8	Tingling Itchy Smarting Stinging	20	Nagging Nauseating Agonizing Dreadful Torturing		
9	Dull Sore Hurting Aching Heavy	PPI			
10	Tender Taut Rasping Splitting	0 1 2 3 4 5	No pain Mild Discomforting Distressing Horrible Excruciating		

Brief Momentary Transient	Rhythmic Periodic Intermittent	Continuous Steady Constant

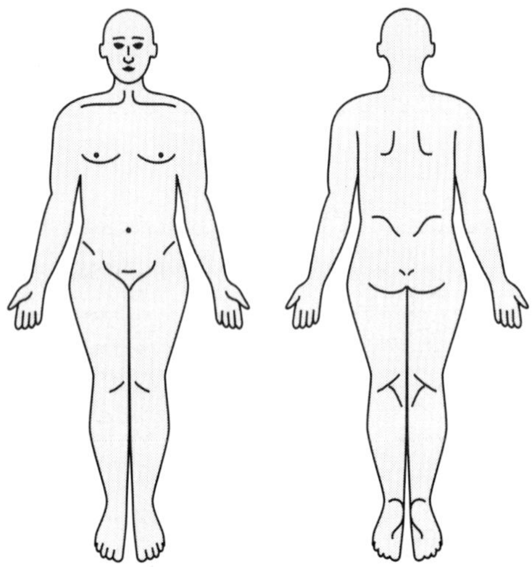

E = External
I = Internal

Comments:

(a)

Fig. 7.5 (a) The McGill pain questionnaire. Redrawn from [30] with permission.

Patient's name ______________________________ Date _______________

		None		Mild		Moderate		Severe
Throbbing	0		1		2		3	
Shooting	0		1		2		3	
Stabbing	0		1		2		3	
Sharp	0		1		2		3	
Cramping	0		1		2		3	
Gnawing	0		1		2		3	
Hot–Burning	0		1		2		3	
Aching	0		1		2		3	
Heavy	0		1		2		3	
Tender	0		1		2		3	
Splitting	0		1		2		3	
Tiring–Exhausting	0		1		2		3	
Sickening	0		1		2		3	
Fearful	0		1		2		3	
Punishing–Cruel	0		1		2		3	

No pain |―――――――――――――――――――――| Worst possible pain

PPI		
0	No pain	
1	Mild	
2	Discomforting	
3	Distressing	
4	Horrible	
5	Excruciating	

(b)

Fig. 7.5 (b) The short-form McGill pain questionnaire. Redrawn from [32] with permission.

Table 7.6 Andersch and Milsom's dysmenorrhoea scoring system: the verbal multidimensional scoring system for assessment of severity of dysmenorrhoea

Grade	Working ability	Systemic symptoms	Analgesics
Grade 0: Menstruation is not painful and daily activity is unaffected	Unaffected	None	Not required
Grade 1: Menstruation is painful but seldom inhibits the woman's normal activity. Analgesics are seldom required. Mild pain	Rarely affected	None	Rarely required
Grade 2: Daily activity affected. Analgesics required and give relief so that absence from work or school is unusual. Moderate pain	Moderately affected	Few	Required
Grade 3: Activity clearly inhibited. Poor effect of analgesics. Vegetative symptoms, e.g. headache, tiredness, nausea, vomiting and diarrhoea. Severe pain	Clearly inhibited	Apparent	Poor effect

Reproduced from [33] with permission.

Society in 1993 [34]. The site and quality of the pelvic pain are recorded, as well as incapacitation caused by pain. Quality and severity overlap on the five-point VRS used to judge quality – mild, discomforting, distressing, horrible, excruciating – the latter three descriptions indicating qualitative characteristics and the former two descriptions indicating severity. The site of the pain is documented in an anatomical diagram (Fig. 7.6).

The physical findings are recorded, including details of tenderness, nodularity and any immobility of pelvic organs on pelvic examination. At the time of laparoscopy or laparotomy, the presence and consistency of adhesions is noted, as well as their position. Individual endometriotic lesions are described according to their site, size and gross appearance (biopsies of suspected endometriotic areas are encouraged to confirm diagnosis). After treatment, new charts are used to document alteration in symptoms and the presence of disease at follow-up laparoscopy, if carried out.

Shortcomings of this proposed instrument could be, firstly, the snapshot picture of the pain when endometriosis pain is often cyclical, and secondly, that the VRS mixes descriptions which express emotive aspects of pain and pain severity. Pain need not be severe in order to be horrible. However, since it is now recognized that endometriosis has many guises at operation and the more recently recognized forms may be responsible for considerable amounts of pain, it is likely to prove a useful instrument to attempt to correlate site of endometriosis with site of pain – but we must await its further evaluation.

The multidimensional measurements of pain, which rely on pain behaviour to quantify the pain from none to severe, may be more reliable to compare pain severity between individuals, and may help to eliminate the discrepancy which would otherwise be observed if one asked a more stoical person and a more histrionic person to describe the same pain purely as they interpreted it, without having the anchors of different pain behaviours to modify or standardize the severity of the pain.

The level of pain at which an individual is incapacitated or at which an individual must seek relief in the form of analgesics is more useful when comparing pain between individuals, and it is probably more standard. If in the pain measurement score the level of pain at which an individual seeks analgesia is described as moderate, this would make the 'very severe' pain of the more histrionic person and the 'fairly mild' pain described by the more stoical person the same.

When studying pain in an individual over time or comparing pre-and post-treatment pain, visual analogue scales, VRS or numerical rating scales are more useful, but when comparing populations it is probably more useful to use pain scales which are graded from mild to severe according to the pain behaviour exhibited.

Clearly, it would be useful for meta-analysis of endometriosis if there could be a consensus of opinion on which pain scoring system should be used. At present, if two similar studies have been carried out for the evaluation of treatment of pelvic pain associated with endometriosis, comparison between one which has used, for example, a visual analogue scale for assessment of pain relief and another which has used a multidimensional method is impossible.

Personality, psychology and pelvic pain in endometriosis

Pain is both an emotional and a physical unpleasant sensation associated with actual or potential tissue damage. In the presence of chronic pain, however, there may no longer be an association with tissue damage, but the sensation and, usually, anxiety persist. It rarely or never occurs that pain is purely organic or purely psychogenic; there will almost always be at least a small/larger element of both making up the total experience. It is well known that emotional state influences pain perception, fear and depression tending to exacerbate pain experience. Conversely, chronic pain, especially, may cause anxiety and depression in an individual who did not previously have these personality traits.

Several studies have been carried out to investigate psychological characteristics associated with endometriosis. As the groups studied and questionnaires used differ slightly between the studies discussed below, it is not possible to compare directly the different results obtained.

MANAGEMENT OF ENDOMETRIOSIS IN THE PRESENCE OF PELVIC PAIN
A Clinical Instrument to Document the Extent of Endometriosis and Pelvic Pain[1]

Patient's Name ______________________ Age __________ Date __________

PRE-OPERATIVE ASSESSMENT OF PELVIC PAIN

Complaints ____

____

Describe the patient's symptoms of pain quality and position, and any limitation caused by these symptoms. Abbreviate quality of pain as **A = mild, B = discomforting, C = distressing, D = horrible, E = excruciating.** On the anatomic drawings below, draw a **SOLID LINE** around the area(s) of pain described by the patient, and mark the most intense area(s) with an **X.**

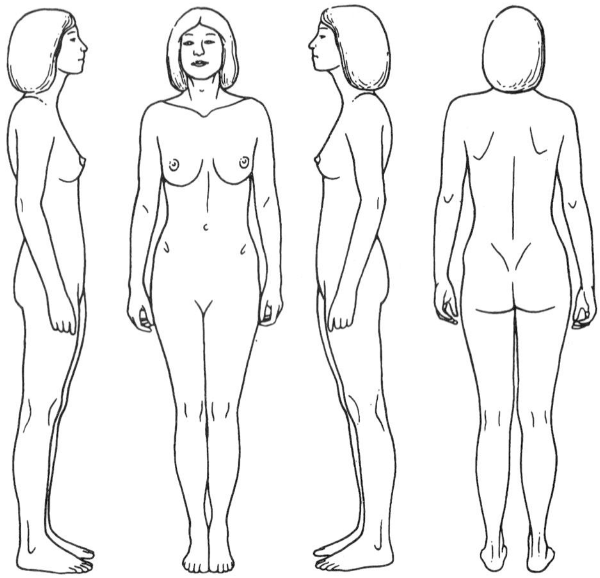

Physical findings ____

____

Identify the quality and site of tenderness caused by palpation, extent of nodularity, diffuse or focal distribution, and/or fixation of uterus/adnexa. On the anatomic drawings above, draw a **BROKEN LINE** around the area(s) of tenderness found on examination.

Adjuncts: [ ] IVP? [ ] BE? [ ] Sigmoidoscopy? [ ] Other? ______________________

____

[1] The association of pelvic pain and endometriosis remains enigmatic because the extent of disease by the previous AFS classifications does not dependably relate to the severity of pelvic pain or tenderness. This form was designed by the AFS Committee on Classification of Endometriosis to carefully document the location and intensity of pelvic pain and tenderness in addition to distribution of endometriosis and pelvic adhesions. Constant recording of this data will permit consistent management of the patient with endometriosis and pelvic pain, and facilitate clinical research.

(a)

Fig. 7.6 RAFS proposed pelvic pain assessment methods in endometriosis [34]. From The American Fertility Society. Management of endometriosis in the presence of pelvic pain. *Fertil Steril* 1993; **60**: 952–5. Reproduced with permission of the publisher, The American Fertility Society.

Procedure ____

____

OPERATIVE DESCRIPTION OF PELVIC ADHESIONS

Describe the location, points of attachment and characteristics of adhesions. Abbreviate characteristics as **A = avascular/thin, T = thick/dense, B = band/string-like, S = sheet-like.** Draw a picture of these adhesions at the appropriate location in each quadrant.

I (Anterior)

IIa (Left lateral)

IIb (Right lateral)

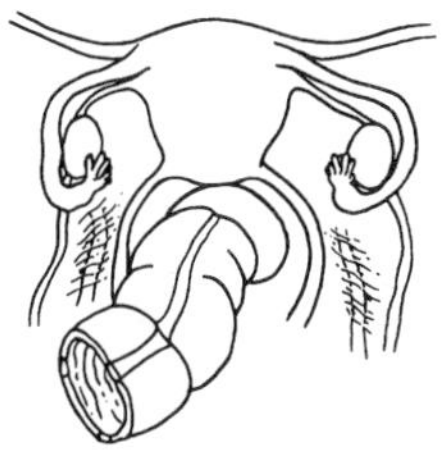

IV (Other sites)

III (Posterior)

OPERATIVE APPEARANCE OF THE DISTRIBUTION OF ENDOMETRIOSIS

After mobilizing the pelvic viscera, measure the size (mean diameter in millimeters) and depth of each visible lesion. Use a calibrated endoscopic probe, if necessary. Record the location, dimension, visual appearance and histologic confirmation of these lesions. Abbreviate the visual appearance as **C = clear, V = vesicles/blebs, P = pink, R = red/flame-like, B = black/blue, Y = yellow/brown, W = white, F = peritoneal fibrosis.** Document the site of each lesion by positioning the index number (No. on the table below) at the appropriate location in each quadrant.

I (Anterior)

IIa (Left lateral)

IIb (Right lateral)

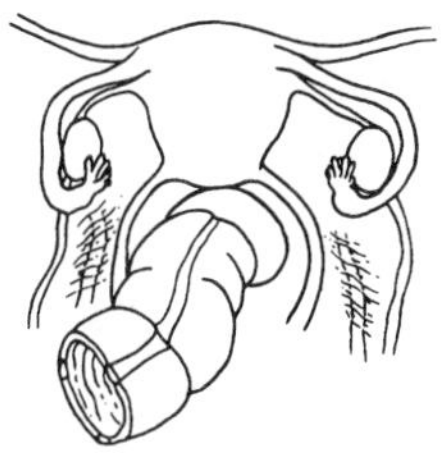

IVa (Other intra-abdominal sites)

IVb (Outside peritoneal cavity)

III (Posterior)

No.	Size in mm	Depth	Appearance	Histology	Location
i.e.	*8 m*	*2 mm*	*F*	*Glands & stroma*	*III*
1					
2					
3					
4					
5					
6					
7					
8					
9					
10					

No.	Size in mm	Depth	Appearance	Histology	Location
11					
12					
13					
14					
15					
16					
17					
18					
19					
20					

Histology ____

Results ____

(b)

Fig. 7.6 *Continued*

Beard *et al.* [35] conducted a prospective study into psychological characteristics of women complaining of pelvic pain prior to their diagnostic laparoscopy. They administered an Eysenck Personality Inventory, which screens for extroversion and neuroticism, and a Middlesex Hospital questionnaire, which measured free-floating and phobic anxiety, obsessional traits, depression and hysteria. They also included a control group who had no pelvic pain symptoms. They found that the group of women complaining of pelvic pain with a normal laparoscopy ($n = 18$) were psychologically significantly different from women without pelvic pain. They tended to be more neurotic and to have abnormal attitudes towards both their own and their partner's sexuality. There were no significant differences between the group with pain and a positive (abnormal) laparoscopy ($n = 17$) and the control group (women without pelvic pain, $n = 9$).

Beard *et al.* [35] postulated that these women with pelvic pain and a normal laparoscopy had consciously or unconsciously used this symptom to avoid close physical involvement with their partners. Their largely psychosomatic pain, they thought, was perceived to be pelvic in its localization as this corresponded to the physical forms of the psychological problem. A supporting observation for this hypothesis is that of women who have suffered from chronic pelvic pain in the absence of any abnormal pelvic pathology [36].

Waller and Shaw (unpublished data) compared psychological profiles of four different groups of women to investigate the evidence of psychological differences between women with symptomatic as opposed to asymptomatic mild endometriosis. The four different groups were:

1 A control group (admitted for laparoscopic sterilization with a normal pelvis).

2 Women with no pain but subsequently diagnosed as having mild or minimal endometriosis.

3 Women with pelvic pain and mild/minimal endometriosis.

4 Women with pelvic pain but a normal pelvis.

Waller and Shaw (unpublished data) found that depression scores and sexual dissatisfaction levels were significantly higher in women with pelvic pain symptoms, both with mild/minimal endometriosis and with a normal pelvis (groups **3** and **4**), compared with the control group and those women who were asymptomatic of their endometriosis. They concluded that pelvic pain symptoms in the presence of only mild or minimal endometriosis may not always be due to the disease.

Another study, conducted principally by psychologists [37] to investigate the possibility of a specific psychological profile associated with endometriosis, used the same questionnaires as Waller and Shaw (unpublished data) and also additional ones (the Eysenck Personality Questionnaire, the short-form McGill questionnaire and a general health questionnaire). They administered

Table 7.7 Study designs for investigation of specific psychological profiles with pelvic pain and/or endometriosis

Study	Questionnaires	Groups
[33]	(1) Eysenck Personality Inventory (EDI) [39] (2) Middlesex Hospital questionnaire [42] (3) Semantic differential scores (psychosexual profile)	(A) Pain and normal pelvis (B) Pain and abnormality in pelvis (C) Control
[35]	(1) Beck Depression Inventory (BDI) [43] (2) Spielberger State–Trait Analysis (SSTA) [41] (3) Golombok–Rust Inventory of Sexual Satisfaction (GRISS) [40]	(A) Control (B) No pain and endometriosis (C) Pain and endometriosis (D) Pain and a normal pelvis
[36]	(1) BDI (2) SSTA (3) GRISS (4) EPI (5) McGill short-form questionnaire [32] (6) General health questionnaire [44]	(A) Pain and endometriosis (B) Pain and other cause

the questionnaire to 40 women who were subsequently diagnosed as having endometriosis and 41 women in whom another diagnosis was made, such as pelvic inflammatory disease, cervicitis or pelvic adhesions. The results showed that endometriosis patients scored significantly higher for psychoticism, introversion and both state and trait anxiety in comparison with the other pain patients, although the two groups did not differ on pain rating scores.

Renaer *et al.* [38] also found higher scores for neuroticism, anxiety and introversion, as well as hypochondria and hysteria, using the Minnesota Multiphasic Personality Inventory (MMPI). They concluded, sensibly, that, as neuroticism is unlikely to cause endometriosis, pain itself is more likely to lead to neuroticism (Table 7.7) [32, 35, 37, 39–44] (KG Waller & RW Shaw; unpublished data).

Medical treatment

The main trophic hormone for the endometrium and for endometriotic deposits is oestrogen. The abolition of oestrogenic stimulation by bilateral oophorectomy, usually combined with hysterectomy, is the most effective method of treating endometriosis with the minimum risk of recurrence. Obviously this treatment option is tragic in nulliparous young women with pregnancy aspirations and highly undesirable even in those women without pregnancy expectations because of possible detrimental cardiovascular effects, decreasing bone density and atrophy of the genital tract, and other unpleasant concomitant menopausal symptoms (vasomotor, psychological and emotional).

Pregnancy has long been noticed to have a beneficial effect on the symptoms of endometriosis. The effect of high-dose oestrogens and progesterones brings about decidual changes in endometriotic deposits, which then undergo necrosis and atrophy following pregnancy [45].

Broadly, the main principles of hormonal medical therapy are to mimic the hormonal milieux of either the menopause or pregnancy, in order to produce disease regression. Alternatively, respite from symptoms for a period of time to allow pregnancy to occur or merely to delay surgical intervention for a period of time is a desirable aim. The hormonal medical treatment options shown to be effective in relief of pain in endometriosis are: danazol, combined oestrogens and progestogens, progestogens alone, gestrinone, and gonadotrophin-releasing hormone (GnRH) analogues.

Danazol

Danazol was introduced as a medical treatment option for endometriosis by Greenblatt *et al.* in 1971 [46] and has been the most commonly and widely used of all medical treatments for endometriosis to date. Its mode of action is dealt with in Chapter 10.

Danazol has proved itself effective in relieving symptoms of pelvic pain, dysmenorrhoea and dyspareunia in many studies (Table 7.8) [47–50]. Most earlier studies were conducted using a dose of danazol of 800 mg/day. The ideal or recommended dose of danazol is still a moot point. Two trials – double-blind and placebo-controlled – have been conducted to compare treatment with 100 mg, 200 mg, 400 mg or 600 mg of danazol [47, 49]. There was significant symptomatic improvement with all doses; however, recurrence rates were greater at the lower doses and pain relief tended to be better with higher doses (Table 7.8)

Ideally, amenorrhoea should be achieved as this abolishes the symptom of dysmenorrhoea and also ensures ovulation is not occurring, which is important not only to maintain a hypo-oestrogenic environment but also to ensure that conception does not occur, as danazol is potentially teratogenic. The minimum dose at which menstruation is suppressed is probably the ideal dose for satisfactory efficacy whilst minimizing the impact of side-effects.

Combined oestrogens and progestogens – pseudopregnancy

At high doses oestrogens and progestogens exert their therapeutic effect by bringing about pseudopregnancy with decidualization, followed by atrophy. The pseudopregnancy regime has been used since the late 1950s and, when

Table 7.8 Effect of danazol on pain

Reference	Dosage (mg)	Duration of treatment (months)	*n*	No. improved/no. with symptoms (%)			Recurrence rate (%)	Length of follow-up (months)
				Dysmenorrhea	Dyspareunia	Pelvic pain		
[47]	800	6	103	70/71 (99%)	—	54/56 (96%)	39	48
[48]	800	6	49	46/46 (100%)	28/28 (100%)	45/45 (100%)	33	36
[49]	100–600	6	32	20/27 (74%)	14/20 (70%)	15/26 (58%)	36	24
[50]	800	4–5	100	56/75 (75%)	26/42 (62%)	41/69 (59%)	33	60

followed, the regimen is efficacious in the relief of pain [51,52]. Success rates for improvement or pain relief are given from 75 to 89%.

The main problem with this regimen is that it is not well tolerated. In one study, the drop-out rate was 41% [53] due to unpleasant side-effects of nausea, acne, alopecia, decreased breast size and increased muscle mass. Generally, combined high-dose oestrogens and progestogens have fallen out of favour because of low patient acceptability and also because of the worries on the part of the physician regarding increased thrombotic tendencies.

An interesting paper by Vercellini *et al.* in 1993 [54] compared low-dose combined oral contraceptive administration with the GnRH analogue goserelin administration for 6 months in endometriosis-associated pelvic pain, dysmenorrhoea and dyspareunia. The dose of oestrogen was only 20 μg daily. They found that deep dyspareunia and non-menstrual pelvic pain symptoms were improved similarly in both groups. Dysmenorrhoea symptoms were not compared because the menses were suppressed with goserelin. Recurrence of symptoms was similarly high at follow-up at 6 months in both groups. The numbers of patients in this study were small, but, if repeated and the results confirmed, replacement of GnRH analogue treatment for endometriosis by the low-dose combined oral contraceptive/pill for longer-term suppression would be of tremendous economic advantage for health care expenditure.

Progestogens

Progestogens alone are better tolerated than pseudopregnancy regimens but without compromising efficacy. Oral and depot medroxyprogesterone acetate (MPA), lynoestrenol, dydrogesterone and norethisterone have all been used for the treatment of pain of endometriosis and have all been shown to be very effective. Moghissi and Boyce [55], using 30 mg oral MPA daily, claimed to have 100% pain relief in their study. Similarly impressive results for complete pain relief were obtained with 45 patients taking dydrogesterone 5 mg twice daily in Johnston's study [56]. Telimaa *et al.* [57] showed, in a prospective placebo-controlled trial comparing danazol with high-dose MPA at 100 mg/day, that pain relief with the progestogen was nearly as good as with danazol and both were significantly better than placebo.

Side-effects of progestogen therapy, in approximate order of decreasing frequency, are breakthrough bleeding, nausea, fluid retention and breast tenderness [58]. The serum lipid profile is adversely affected by progestogens, causing a rise in low-density lipoproteins (LDLs) and hence a more atherogenic lipid profile. With 19-nortestosterone-related progestogens, this effect is more significant (norethisterone, norgestrel and lynoestrenol) but the effect also exists with high doses of the 17-hydroxyprogesterone and MPA [59]. It is not known, nor can it be known for many years, what effect this treatment course may have on future mortality from ischaemic heart disease and arteriopathy, if any.

Gestrinone

Gestrinone is a synthetic trienic 19-norsteroid. It is predominantly antiprogestogenic but is also moderately antioestrogenic and it also displays low androgenic and oestrogenic activity. Sex-hormone-binding globulin (SHBG) levels fall, which leads to a rise in free testosterone levels [60] and hence its androgenic side-effects of seborrhoea, acne, hirsutism, alopecia and breast shrinkage. Muscle cramps and oedema are also relatively common side-effects.

One unusual and positive feature of the drug is that it need only be given twice weekly orally at a dose of 2.5 mg (total 5 mg/week) for 6 months.

Pain relief is usually achieved to a significant degree (> 90%) in reported studies [61, 62]. Recurrence of pain at 1 year following treatment was approximately 15–30%, depending on whether only partial or complete resolution of symptoms had been obtained at the end of the course, complete remission of pain was associated with a lower incidence of recurrence.

GnRH analogues

These are nona- or decapeptides which have a longer half-life and a greater affinity for GnRH pituitary receptors than native GnRH. Treatment with GnRH analogues effects a medical menopause, which is reversible on cessation of the treatment (see Chapter 11 for more details of mode of action).

The first report of GnRH analogue use in women with endometriosis was written by Meldrum *et al.* in 1982 on a series of five women [63]. The treatment was given for only 1 month but four out of the five women reported a disappearance of or an improvement in their symptoms. Since then, GnRH analogues have gained wide acceptance and have been shown to be effective in the treatment of pelvic pain [64], showing reductions in pelvic symptom scores by 93% at the end of 6 months' treatment, in a large group of women. Hardt *et al* in 1986 [65] showed 20 out of 26 women to be pain-free after 6 months' treatment with buserelin, and four of the remaining six had significant reduction in pain symptoms.

GnRH analogues have compared very favourably with the oldest-established medical treatment for endometriosis, danazol. The Naferelin European Endometriosis Trial Group [66] compared nafarelin with the standard regimen of 600 mg danazol daily and found that nafarelin was equally as effective as danazol in the relief of pain. This large study ($n = 307$) was unusual in having 10 patients on nafarelin ceasing to participate in the trial because of side-effects, compared with four danazol-treated patients. GnRH analogue vs. danazol studies in the main tend to have more drop-out patients in the danazol-treated group because of anabolic side-effects. During follow-up at 12 months in this study, 77% of nafarelin recipients had no symptoms or mild symptoms only, compared with 67% of danazol recipients.

The side-effects of GnRH analogues are those of the menopause: vasomotor symptoms of hot flushes, night sweats with insomnia at times, vaginal dryness, headache and emotional liability and depression are the most common but appear to be well tolerated. Bone changes are dealt with in detail elsewhere (Chapter 11).

Surgical treatment of endometriosis

The method of medical or surgical treatment chosen will be dictated by the extent and type of disease, the age of the patient, her desire for fertility and the severity of her symptoms. With the increasingly widespread availability of laparoscopic expertise, and experience with laser technology, minimally invasive surgery is becoming a more popular treatment option for endometriosis.

Surgical treatment may be conservative or radical. Usually, before reaching a management decision, a diagnostic laparoscopy will be performed to confirm the diagnosis of endometriosis and, if present, to ascertain its stage, the sites affected, the type (whether superficial or deeply infiltrating) and the extent and tenacity of the adhesions present.

Conservative surgery aims to eradicate as much of the endometriosis as possible whilst preserving ovarian and reproductive function. Laparoscopy is performed where possible but when disease and adhesions are more extensive, laparotomy is indicated. The operation may involve ablation of superficial deposits by diathermy or laser, adhesiolysis, endometrioma excision, enucleation of deeply infiltrating lesions, laparoscopic uterosacral nerve ablation or presacral neurectomy.

Radical surgery is not usually performed until other medical and surgical treatment options have been exhausted and is only employed in patients with severe persistent pelvic pain and recurrent disease resistant to treatment. It consists of total abdominal hysterectomy and bilateral salpingo-oophorectomy, as well as removal of all visible or accessible endometriotic deposits as far as possible. The women undergoing radical surgery are, sadly, often young and hormone replacement therapy (HRT) should be commenced after 6–9 months and then with symptomatic monitoring for recurrence. Progestogens may be used in this interim period, as they may minimize menopausal symptoms.

Conservative surgical techniques

Laser ablation

It is possible to destroy all visible endometriotic lesions by vaporizing and coagulating these discrete areas, using laser. There are various types of laser, all with their relative advantages and disadvantages, and these are discussed in Chapters 12–14.

Laser laparoscopy alone as a treatment for pelvic pain appears to be convincingly efficacious. Sutton [67] quotes rates of pain relief at 1 year as being 70%. However, few controlled studies have been carried out. A double-blind randomized prospective controlled study to investigate the effect of laser laparoscopy on pelvic pain has been conducted by Sutton [68]. The two treatment arms were a control group, who merely received hydrotubation and aspiration of peritoneal fluid but no laser therapy, and a definitive treatment arm, who underwent laser ablation of all endometriotic lesions, hydrotubation and aspiration of peritoneal fluid and, in addition, laparoscopic uterosacral nerve ablation (LUNA – see below). The results were unfortunately not conclusive, as the numbers enrolled did not allow statistical significance to be attained.

It would obviously be of value to receive further data from similar controlled studies to be convinced that laser laparoscopy is effective in the relief of pelvic pain due to endometriosis.

Laparoscopic uterosacral nerve ablation

The uterosacral ligaments are a commonly affected site in patients suffering from endometriosis. Infiltration of the uterosacral ligaments by endometriotic deposits results in invasion, inflammation and fibrosis of the inferior hypogastric and its anterior extension – the uterovaginal plexus (the Lee–Frankenhauser plexus). This manifests itself symptomatically with severe dysmenorrhoea, deep dyspareunia and pelvic pain, all referred to the midline. Ablation of the uterosacral ligaments can be performed at the time of laparoscopy, forming two small craters. The risks of the procedure are haemorrhage and ureteric damage (as they run parallel to the uterosacral ligament) at the point of insertion of the uterosacral ligaments into the cervix.

Studies performed demonstrating the efficacy of the procedure in abolishing midline dysmenorrhoea have ranged in their measurement of symptom relief from 70% [69] to 92% [70]. Few of these studies have managed to randomize significant numbers of patients into placebo-controlled treatment groups. One study, which is perhaps the best champion for the procedure, albeit small in numbers, was a randomized double-blind prospective controlled study on a group of women with severe midline dysmenorrhoea, conducted by Lichten and Bombard in 1987 [71]. They randomized 10 patients to a control (diagnostic laparoscopy) group and another 11 patients to a treatment (LUNA) group. All patients had completed an MMPI to screen for psychiatric illness. Those with an abnormal psychological profile had been excluded. Postoperatively none of the patients in the control group had relief of dysmenorrhoea, but nine of the 11 patients (81%) who had received LUNA treatment reported complete relief at 3 months post-surgery. Forty-five per cent of these women had persistent relief of dysmenorrhoea at 1 year follow-up. Unfortunately in this trial, endometriosis was an exclusion criterion. However, the study seems to suggest that the procedure is worth while carrying out when midline dysmenorrhoea is present in those receiving laser laparoscopic treatment for endometriosis.

Presacral neurectomy

Presacral neurectomy (PSN) was first described by Jaboulay [72] and Ruggi [73] in 1899. This operation was popular over 20 years ago but has generally fallen from popularity, possibly because of poor results due to poor patient selection and also because it was probably being superseded by the safer and arguably just as effective LUNA procedure. It should only be used for severe midline dysmenorrhoea or pelvic pain which is thought to be uterine in origin.

The operation is a major one, usually entails a laparotomy and excision of the meshwork of the inferior hypogastric plexus where it sits anterior to L5 and below the bifurcation of the aorta retroperitoneally. A 5 cm length of tissue is excised after the ureters have been identified and retracted. The hazards are quite considerable; the internal iliac artery may be divided, common iliac vein damage may be caused, the ureters are at risk and major pelvic haemorrhage is an intraoperative and postoperative complication [74].

In a large review or meta-analysis of pelvic denervation for chronic pelvic pain in endometriosis Vercellini *et al.* [75] lamented the absence of a large multicentre trial with precise baseline criteria and precise description of the surgical methods to be employed. They concluded that there are, to date, inadequate data to confirm or refute the effectiveness of PSN with uterosacral ligament amputation in the treatment of chronic pelvic pain associated with endometriosis. Individual studies vary widely in reports of results, from 100% success [76] to no difference between conservative surgery alone and the addition of PSN to conservative surgery [77]. Tjaden *et al.*'s study in 1990 [76] involved only four patients in each treatment group, who were actually randomized, whereas in Candiani *et al.*'s study [77], 40 were randomly assigned to conservative surgery alone and 38 to conservative surgery with additive PSN. Candiani's study was more powerful and showed no benefit with the addition of PSN. They concluded that PSN should only be considered in selected patients with mainly midline pain.

Conclusion

Endometriosis without doubt is associated with and produces a variety of pain symptoms. The mechanisms of pain induction in endometriosis are likely to be multiple and perhaps variable as the disease deposits themselves progress from the fresh red haemorrhagic lesions, through to their final white scarified 'invasive' implants. The failure of a correlation between site or number of implants and type or severity of pain is an area which requires further investigations, as indeed does the development of appropriate assessment schemes for pain type and severity.

References

1 Shaw RW. *An Atlas of Endometriosis*, 1993, p. 19, Table 4. Carnforth, Parthenon Publishing Group.

2 Buttram VC. Conservative surgery for endometriosis in the infertile female: a study of 206 patients with implications for both medical and surgical therapy. *Fertil Steril* 1979 **31**: 117.

3 Bayer SR, Seibel MM. Endometriosis: clinical symptoms and infertility. In: Rolland R, Chanda Dev R, Willemsen W (eds). *Gonadotrophin Down-regulation in Gynaecological Practice*, 1988, p. 103. New York, Alan R. Liss.

4 Greenblatt RB, Dmowski WP, Mahesh VB, Scholer HFL. Clinical studies with an anti-gonadotrophin – danazol. *Fertil Steril* 1971 **22**: 102.

5 O'Connor DT. Clinical features in diagnosis. In: Jordan A, Singer A (eds). *Endometriosis* 1987, vol. 5, pp. 68–78. Edinburgh, Churchill Livingstone.

6 McMinn RH (ed.) *Last's Anatomy*, 8th edn, 1990, pp. 398–400. London, Churchill Livingstone.

7 Tindall VR (ed.). *Jeffcoate's Principles of Gynaecology*, 5th edn, 1987, pp. 49–52. London, Butterworths.

8 Moore KL. *Clinically Orientated Anatomy*, 3rd edn, 1992, pp. 281–289. London, Williams and Wilkins.

9 De Swiet M, Chamberlain G (eds). *Basic Sciences in Obstetrics and Gynaecology*, 2nd edn, 1992, p. 79. London, Churchill Livingstone.

10 Zimmerman M. Peripheral and central nervous mechanisms of nociception. Pain and pain therapy: facts and hypotheses. In: Bonica JJ, Liebeskind JC, Albe-Fessard DG (eds). *Advances in Pain Research and Therapy*, 1979, vol 3, pp. 3–32. New York, Raven Press.

11 Iggo, A. Mechanisms of nociception in persistent pain. In: Lipton S, Miles J (eds). *Persistent Pain: Modern Methods of Treatment*, 1983, vol. 3, pp. 1–16. London, Academic Press.

12 Cervero F. Mechanisms of visceral pain. In: Lipton S (ed.). *Persistent Pain: Modern Methods of Treatment*, 1983 vol. 4, pp. 1–19. London, Academic Press.

13 Wellstood-Eason MJH. Relief of chronic pain. In: Smith G, Aikenhead AR (eds). *Textbook of Anaesthesia*, 1985, pp. 529–538, London, Churchill Livingstone.

14 Barlow DH, Glynn CJ. Endometriosis and pelvic pain. In: Brosens I (ed.). *Endometriosis*, 1993. Clinical Obstetrics and Gynaecology Series. London, Ballière & Tindall.

15 Head H. On disturbances of sensation with special reference to the pain of visceral disease. *Brain* 1893 **16**: 1–133.
16 Ruch TC. Visceral sensation and referred pain. In: Fulton JF (ed.). *Howell's Textbook of Physiology*, 15th edn, 1946, pp. 385–401. Philadelphia, W.B. Saunders.
17 Shaw RW. *An Atlas of Endometriosis*, 1993, p. 18. Carnforth, Parthenon Publishing Group.
18 Acosta AA, Butram VC Jr, Besch PK *et al.* A proposed classification of pelvic endometriosis. *Obstet Gynecol* 1973 **42**: 19.
19 Fedele L, Parazzini F, Bianchi S, Arcaini L, Candiani GB. Stage and localization of pelvic endometriosis and pain. *Fertil Steril* 1990 **53**: 155–173.
20 Mahmood TA, Templeton A. The impact of treatment on the natural history of endometriosis. *Human Reprod* 1990 **5**: 965–970.
21 American Fertility Society. Revised American Fertility Society classification of endometriosis. *Fertil Steril* 1985 **43**: 351.
22 Koninckx PR, Meuleman C, Demeyere S, Lesaffre E, Cornillie F. Suggestive evidence that pelvic endometriosis is a progressive disease whereas deeply infiltrating endometriosis is associated with pelvic pain. *Fertil Steril* 1991 **55**: 759–765.
23 Cornillie FJ, Oosterlynck D, Lauwergus JM, Koninckx PR. Deeply infiltrating pelvic endometriosis histology and significance. *Fertil Steril* 1990 **53**: 978–983.
24 Martin DC (ed.). *Atlas of Endometriosis*, 1993, p. 9.5. London, Gower Medical Publishing.
25 Vernon M, Beard J, Graves K, Wilson EA. Classification of endometriotic implants in morphologic appearance and capacity to synthesise prostaglandin F. *Fertil Steril* 1986 **46**: 801–805.
26 Jansen RPS, Russell P. Non pigmented endometriosis: clinical laparoscopic and pathological definition. *Am J Obstet Gynecol* 1986 **155**: 1154–1159.
27 Redwine DB. Age-related evolution in colour appearance of endometriosis. *Fertil Steril* 1987 **48**: 1062–1063.
28 Mersky H. Taxonomy of pain. *Pain* 1987 **6**: 249–252.
29 Huskisson EC. Measurement of pain. *Lancet* 1974 **ii**: 1127.
30 Melzack R. The McGill pain questionnaire: major properties and scoring methods. *Pain* 1975 **1**: 275–299.
31 Leavitt F, Garron DC. Validity of a back pain classification scale for detecting psychological disturbance as measured by MMPI. *J Clin Psych* 1980 **36**: 186–189.
32 Melzack R. The short-form McGill pain questionnaire. *Pain* 1987 **30**: 191–197.
33 Andersch B, Milsom I. An epidemiologic study of young women with dysmenorrhoea. *Am J Obstet Gynecol* 1982 **144**: 656–660.
34 American Fertility Society. Management of endometriosis in the presence of pelvic pain. *Fertil Steril* 1993 **60**: 952–955.
35 Beard RW, Belsey EH, Lieberman MB, Wilkinson JCM. Pelvic pain in women. *Am J Obstet Gynecol* 1977 **128**: 566–570.
36 Reiter RC, Gambone JC. Demographic and historic variables in women with idiopathic chronic pelvic pain. *Obstet Gynecol* 1990 **75**: 428–432.
37 Low WY, Edelmann RJ, Sutton C. A psychological profile of endometriosis patients in comparison to patients with pelvic pain of other origins. *J Psychosomatic Res* 1993 **37**: 111–116.
38 Renaer M, Vertanmen H, Nijs P, Wagemans L, Van Hemelrijk T. Psychological aspects of chronic pelvic pain in women. *Am J Obstet Gynecol* 1979 **134**: 75–80.
39 Eysenck HJ, Eysenck SBG. *Manual of the Eysenck Personality Questionnaire*, 1975. London, Hodder and Stoughton.
40 Rust J, Bennum I, Crowe M, Golombok S. *Manual of the Golombok Rust Inventory of Marital State*, 1986. Windsor, NFER-Nelson.
41 Spielberger CD, Gorsuch RL, Lushene R. *Manual of the State–Trait Anxiety Inventory*,

1979. Palo Alto, CA, Consulting Psychologists Press.
42 Crown S, Crisp AH. A short clinical diagnostic self-rating scale for psychoneurotic patients: the Middlesex Hospital questionnaire. *Br J Psychiatry* 1966 **112**: 917.
43 Beck AT. *Depression: Causes and Treatment*, 1972. Philadelphia, University of Philadelphia.
44 Goldberg DP, Williams PA. *A User's Guide to the General Health Questionnaire*, 1988. Windsor, NFER-Nelson.
45 Kistner RW. The treatment of endometriosis by inducing pseudopregnancy with ovarian hormones: a report of fifty-eight cases. *Fertil Steril* 1959 **10**: 539.
46 Greenblatt RB, Dimowski WP, Mahesh VB, Scholer HFL. Clinical studies with an antigonadotrophin danazol. *Fertil. Steril.* 1971 **22**: 102.
47 Dmowski WD & Cohen MR. Treatment of endometriosis with an antigonadotrophin, danazol: a laparoscopic and histological education. *Obstet Gynecol* 1975 **46**: 147.
48 Greenblatt RB, Tzigownis V. Danazol treatment of endometriosis: long-term follow-up. *Fertil Steril* 1979 **32**: 518.
49 Biberoglu KO, Behrman SJ. Dosage aspects of danazol therapy in endometriosis: short term and long term effectiveness. *Am J Obstet Gynecol* 1981 **139**: 645.
50 Barbieri RL, Cauich JA, Mahris A *et al.* Danazol inhibits steroidogenesis. *Fertil Steril* 1977 **28**: 809.
51 Andrews MC, Andrews WC, Strauss AF. Effects of progestin-induced pregnancy on endometriosis: clinical and microscopic studies. *Am J Obstet Gynecol* 1959 **78**: 776.
52 Kourides PR, Kistner RW. Three new synthetic progestins in the treatment of endometriosis. *Obstet Gynecol* 1968 **31**: 821.
53 Noble AD, Letchworth AT. Medical treatment of endometriosis: a comparative trial. *Postgrad Med J* 1979 **55** (Suppl. 5): 37.
54 Vercellini P, Trespidi L, Colombo A *et al.* A gonadotropin-releasing hormone agonist versus a low-dose oral contraceptive for pelvic pain associated with endometriosis. *Fertil Steril* 1993 **60**: 75–79.
55 Moghissi KS, Boyce CRK. Management of endometriosis with oral medroxyprogesterone acetate. *Obstet Gynecol* 1976 **47**: 265.
56 Johnston WI. Dydrogesterone and endometriosis. *Br J Obstet Gynaecol* 1976 **83**: 77.
57 Telimaa S, Puolakka J, Ronuberg L, Kauppila A. Placebo controlled comparison of danazol and high dose medroxyprogesterone acetate in the treatment of endometriosis. *Gynaecol Endocrinol* 1987 **1**: 13–23.
58 Luciano AA, Turksoy RN, Carleo JL. Clinical and endocrine evaluation in the treatment of endometriosis (Abstract). Presented at 41st Annual Meeting of the American Fertility Society, 27 Sept. – 2 Oct. 1985, p. 134.
59 Telimaa S, Penttila L, Puolakka J, Ronnberg L, Kauppila A. Circulating lipid and lipoprotein concentration during danazol and high-dose medroxyprogesterone acetate therapy of endometriosis. *Fertil Steril* 1989 **52**: 31–35.
60 Venturini PL, Bertolini S, Bruneghi MCM *et al.* Endocrine metabolic and clinical effects of gestrinone in women with endometriosis. *Fertil Steril* 1989 **52**: 589–595.
61 Azadien-Boulanger G, Secchi J, Tournemine C *et al.* Hormonal activity profiles of drugs for endometriosis therapy. In: Raynoud JP, Ojassoo T, Martini L (eds). *Medical Management of Endometriosis*, 1984, p. 125. New York, Raven Press.
62 Couthinho EM, Husson JM, Azadieu-Boulanger G. Treatment of endometriosis with gestrinone – five years' experience. In: Raynoud JP, Ojassoo T, Martini L (eds). *Medical Management of Endometriosis*, 1984, p. 249. New York, Raven Press.
63 Meldrum DR, Chang RJ, Lu J *et al.* Medical oophorectomy using a long-acting GnRH agonsit: a possible new approach for the treatment of endometriosis. *J Clin Endocrinol Metab* 1982 **54**: 1081–1083.
64 Reichel RP, Schweppe KW, Zoladex Endometriosis Study Group. Goserelin (Zoladex)

depot in the treatment of endometriosis. *Fertil Steril* 1992 **57**: 1197–1202.

65 Hardt W, Schmidt-Gollwitzer M, Schmidt-Gollwitzer K *et al.* Erste Ergebnisse bei der Behandlung der Endometriose mit dem LH-RH Analogen Buserelin. *Geburtshilfe Frauenheilkunde* 1986 **46**: 483.

66 Nafarelin European Endometriosis Trial Group (NEET). Nafarelin for endometriosis: a large-scale, danazol-controlled trial of efficacy and safety, with 1 year follow-up. *Fertil Steril* 1992 **57**: 514–522.

67 Sutton CJG. Laparoscopic treatment of endometriosis. In: Sutton CJG (ed.). *New Surgical Techniques in Gynaecology*, 1991, pp. 107–119. Carnforth, Parthenon Publishing Group.

68 Sutton CJG. Laser laparoscopy in the treatment of endometriosis. In: Thomas EJ, Rock JA (eds). *Modern Approaches to Endometriosis*, 1991, pp. 199–220. Academic Publishers.

69 Sutton C, Hill D. Laser laparoscopy in the treatment of endometriosis. *Br J Obstet Gynaecol* 1990 **97**: 181–185.

70 Davies GD. Management of endometriosis and its associated adhesions with the CO_2 laparoscope. *Obstet Gynaecol* 1985 **68**: 422–425.

71 Lichten EM, Bombard J. Surgical treatment of primary dysmenorrhoea with laparoscopic uterosacral nerve ablation. *J Reprod Med* 1987 **32**: 37–41.

72 Jaboulay M. Le traitement de la névralgie pelvienne par la paralysie du sympathique sacré. *Lyon Med* 1899 **90**: 102–108.

73 Ruggi C. La simpaticectania addominale utro-ovaria come mezzo di cura di alcuhe lesion interne degli orgain genitali della donna. *Bologna Zanichelli* 1899.

74 Howkins J, Stallworthy J (eds). *Bonney's Gynaecological Surgery: Pre-sacral Neurectomy*, 1974, pp. 488–491. London, Baillière & Tindall.

75 Vercellini P, Fedele L, Bianchi S *et al.* Pelvic denervation for chronic pain associated with endometriosis: fact or fancy? *Am J Obstet Gynecol* 1991 **165**: 745–749.

76 Tjaden B, Schlaff WS, Kinball A *et al.* The efficacy of presacral neurectomy for the relief of midline dysmenorrhoea. *Obstet Gynecol* 1990 **76**: 89–91.

77 Candiani GB, Fedele L, Vercellini P *et al.* Presacral neurectomy for the treatment of pelvic pain associated with endometriosis: a controlled study. *Am J Obstet Gynecol* 1992 **167**: 100–103.

Chapter 8
Infertility and Endometriosis

S. INGAMELLS AND E.J. THOMAS

Introduction

There can be little doubt that the relationship between endometriosis and infertility continues to excite considerable debate. One camp would argue that there is little place for a chapter addressing this relationship in a modern textbook on endometriosis, whilst the opposing camp would say that the relationship is so obvious that the facts do not bear repetition. Certainly research into it continues. We found 728 articles in the last 10 years up to 1 January 1994. The pace of publication is also accelerating, with 30 papers in 1984 and 90 in 1993. In spite of this, there is still doubt whether there is a causal relationship between endometriosis and infertility that is not associated with tubal or ovarian damage. Previous reviews addressing this issue have been unable to make definitive conclusions because of the lack of randomized controlled prospective studies and the inadequate sample numbers involved for meaningful statistical analysis [1–3]. In recent years, both scientific and clinical research into this enigmatic disease has been prolific and has produced many advances in our understanding of it. In view of that, we wish to explore whether we are better able to form definitive conclusions now or whether the available literature is still as confusing.

We are assuming that it is evident that endometriosis that structurally damages the tubes and ovaries causes infertility. Therefore, this chapter will mainly concentrate on the association of endometriosis with infertility when no structural damage is present. We will call such disease mild endometriosis. In order to prove a causal association between mild endometriosis and infertility, a number of specific criteria must be fulfilled. Firstly, the disease must be shown to be more prevalent in women with infertility. Secondly, an aetiological basis must be shown. Thirdly, the presence of the disease must adversely affect fertility and, lastly, successful treatment must restore fertility to normal. The aim of this chapter is to review the available evidence that any or all of these criteria are met.

The prevalence of endometriosis in women with infertility

Laparoscopic confirmation

The possibility of a causal link between endometriosis and infertility first arose when it was noted that infertility was seen in patients with endometriosis twice as frequently as in the general population. Laparoscopic studies in infertile women confirmed the finding that endometriosis was more common in infertile women than fertile women [4]. Subsequent retrospective studies reported the prevalence of endometriosis in infertile women as 20–40% [2]. A recent prospective study compared the prevalence of endometriosis in infertile women with women undergoing laparoscopic sterilization, abdominal hysterectomy and laparoscopy for abdominal pain [5]. This confirmed the findings of the retrospective studies and showed that endometriosis was present in 21% of infertile women. This study reported that only 6.2% of women undergoing laparoscopic sterilization had endometriosis [5]. Similar figures, ranging from 1 to 7%, have been obtained for the general population by these means [6]. In all these studies it was assumed that women undergoing laparoscopic sterilization were representative of the general population, which is not necessarily correct.

As direct visualization of the endometriosis at laparoscopy or laparotomy is considered essential to the diagnosis, the precise prevalence of the disease in the general population may be impossible to determine accurately. A recent prospective study has suggested that the prevalence of endometriosis in a group of randomly selected normal women is much higher than this. The prevalence of endometriosis was investigated in the partners of infertile men and it was assumed that the partners of azoospermic men are normal women who are not becoming pregnant because of male-factor infertility. In these women, the prevalence of endometriosis was 20.7% [7].

Subtle lesions

The problem is further complicated by the changes in our understanding of the presentations of endometriosis. Jansen and Russell [8] reported that the disease was not only present in blue-black lesions but also in vesicular, petechial and haemorrhagic lesions, as well as peritoneal defects and fibrous scars. It is believed that powderburn lesions may represent burnt-out disease and that the vesicular and haemorrhagic lesions represent active disease. Redwine [9] has described an age-related evolution from active to inactive disease that follows this postulated model. Furthermore, microscopic endometriosis has been reported in up to 15% of normal peritoneal biopsies at laparoscopy [10]. These changes mean that the denominator used to define the disease in infertile women is constantly changing and makes comparisons between studies very difficult.

Epidemiological studies

While most epidemiological studies have shown an increased prevalence of endometriosis in infertile patients, they have not indicated whether the infertility predisposed women to endometriosis or vice versa. A case–control study investigating the factors predisposing women to endometriosis found prolonged nulliparity was a significant risk factor for the development of endometriosis [11]. These data were further supported by Vessey *et al.* [12], who showed that pregnancy had a protective effect on endometriosis. Clearly, infertile women are less likely to experience pregnancy. In addition, prolonged and uninterrupted exposure to menstruation has been reported as a risk factor for endometriosis, and infertile women will be more likely to experience this than fertile women. Finally, repeat laparoscopies in women with prolonged unexplained infertility and previously normal laparoscopies with no evidence of endometriosis have demonstrated endometriosis in 12–20% of women [2, 13]. As the infertility existed before the endometriosis, it is unlikely that endometriosis caused infertility in these women.

In conclusion, the evidence supports an increased prevalence of endometriosis in infertile women. However, there is no epidemiological evidence to support a causal relationship, nor is there evidence to support the hypothesis that infertility causes endometriosis or that some common factor causes both. Until there is a robust consensus over what constitutes active endometriosis and what represents inactive disease, good epidemiological studies addressing this problem will be impossible to perform.

The aetiology of infertility in women with endometriosis

The next section will discuss the factors thought to be involved in causing infertility in women with endometriosis. The first part of this section will be devoted to a brief discussion of the aetiology of infertility in severe endometriosis. The second part will concentrate on the aetiology of infertility in mild endometriosis when no structural damage is apparent.

Severe endometriosis

An obvious causal relationship exists between severe endometriosis and infertility when structural damage is apparent. The distortion of the pelvic anatomy by adhesions and scarring leads to a mechanical disturbance in fertility. The presence of periovarian adhesions restricts the available surface for oocyte release, while fimbrial and tubal adhesions prevent successful ovum retrieval and transport to the uterine cavity.

Mild endometriosis

The relationship between mild endometriosis and infertility is less obvious. The frequent finding of mild endometriosis in women undergoing infertility investigations has led to the assumption that an association exists [2]. Numerous hypotheses have been proposed to explain how mild endometriosis could affect fertility. Putative abnormalities at each stage in the female reproductive cycle have been investigated, including genetic predisposition, the development of an autoimmune response, endocrinological and immunological abnormalities and an increased incidence of spontaneous abortion. These factors and the evidence for their involvement in associating infertility with mild endometriosis will be discussed next.

Genetic predisposition

In recent years, many common disorders have been shown to have strong genetic components, with conditions such as heart disease, diabetes and cancer showing a familial tendency. Twin studies and studies of the families of affected individuals have shown that many of these disorders are caused by the interaction of environmental factors with several genes at different loci [14]. The individual genes and their interaction in these polygenic diseases are now being identified by recombinant deoxyribonucleic acid (DNA) technology. Identification of these genes is leading to advances in understanding the mechanisms involved in the diseases and to new treatments.

The study of individuals and families affected by endometriosis has revealed that there is a genetic component in endometriosis [15, 16]. Genetic studies in patients with histologically proved endometriosis have suggested a polygenic or multifactorial mode of inheritance for the disease [16, 17]. A sevenfold increased risk of endometriosis has been found in first-degree relatives [16, 18, 19] and patients with an affected first-degree relative were found to be more likely to have severe endometriosis [16, 20]. Twin studies have confirmed that endometriosis has a genetic trait [21].

It is tempting to conclude from these data that there is a clear case for a genetic predisposition to endometriosis. However, caution must be exercised, as there are a number of confounding variables. It may be that the diagnosis in one first-degree relative is educational for the rest of the family, resulting in earlier recourse to medical consultation and diagnostic techniques. Another explanation may be that there are genetic and social influences on pain tolerance that will affect the use of medical resources. To date, there have been no gene-mapping studies or attempts to identify the genes involved, although studies are currently being undertaken. Efforts must be directed towards identifying the genes involved in endometriosis in these twin and familial cases. With more genetic information available, elucidation of the molecular basis of endometriosis may be achieved and further advances made in understanding the disease. Linkage studies can then be carried out to determine if there is a link between genes controlling endometriosis and fertility. However, these studies are impossible to perform without a well-defined denominator and, as in epidemiological research, the absence of such a clear definition is very disabling.

Autoimmune response

It has been postulated that the presence of ectopic endometrial implants in women with endometriosis leads to an autoimmune response [22], resulting in implantation failure and subsequent infertility. The evidence in the literature to support the hypothesis is conflicting. Autoantibodies to endometrial tissue have been identified in the serum and peritoneal fluid of women with endometriosis [22, 23], although other studies have failed to confirm these findings [24, 25]. Antiendometrial antibodies have been found more frequently in infertile women than fertile women [26] but the significance of antiendometrial antibodies is unclear as they have also been noted in several other gynaecological conditions [27]. Furthermore no correlation has been found between the severity of endometriosis and the level of the antibody detected in the serum and peritoneal fluid [23]. Treatment for endometriosis has not been found to alter antiendometrial antibody levels [26] but the effect of this treatment on subsequent fertility was not reported. The hypothesis that endometriosis and infertility are causally related by an autoimmune mechanism is also not supported by the clinical results from *in vitro* fertilization programmes, which show no difference in implantation between women with endometriosis and women with tubal infertility [3]. With the current evidence available, it must be concluded that there is no evidence to support the causal relationship between endometriosis and autoimmunity.

Endocrine abnormalities

The concomitant occurrence of mild endometriosis and abnormalities of pituitary ovarian function in infertility has led to the assumption that an association exists between these two factors. However, identical abnormalities have been described in the infertile population in the absence of endometriosis, and proof that the abnormalities actually cause infertility *in vivo* is conflicting [13]. Proof of a causal association between these abnormalities and endometriosis relies on demonstrating the abnormalities in consecutive menstrual cycles and in patients with endometriosis more commonly than in other infertile groups [1].

The abnormalities of pituitary ovarian function that have been identified in mild endometriosis include defective folliculogenesis, anovulation, luteinized unruptured follicle syndrome (LUF) and luteal phase defects. These different endocrine factors will be discussed in turn.

Folliculogenesis

A variety of follicular phase defects have been observed in women with mild endometriosis. These have included abnormal hormone levels [28], abnormal follicular growth [29], decreased follicular size [30] and a shortened follicular phase [30]. More recent studies have failed to confirm that any of these abnormalities exist in women with mild endometriosis. One controlled study, which used a combination of ovarian ultrasound and hormone radioimmunoassay, compared women with mild endometriosis and otherwise unexplained infertility and in a healthy control group. In only two of the 22 cycles studied were abnormalities of follicular development detected [31]. Unfortunately, consecutive cycles were not studied so it is not known whether these phenomena occurred consistently in each menstrual cycle in these individuals. In agreement with Bancroft *et al.* [31], a study by Mahmood and Templeton [32] has found that follicular development in infertile women with laparoscopically documented mild endometriosis was normal in the majority of patients. Only one patient had abnormal endocrinology, with evidence of premature ovulation over two cycles.

Ovulation defects

The frequency of anovulation among infertile women with endometriosis has been reported at levels up to 10% [2]. The significance of ovulatory dysfunction in association with endometriosis is difficult to assess, as similar levels have been observed among infertile women in general [33]. In addition, in a recent study in infertile women whose only demonstrable abnormality was a finding of mild endometriosis at laparoscopy, ovulation was found to be normal [32].

In endometriosis, it has been suggested that ovulatory dysfunction may be primarily related to the presence of adhesions and not to other endocrine abnormalities. In rabbits, studies controlling for adhesions in minimal ovarian endometriosis indicated that impaired ovulation was primarily related to the presence of periovarian adhesions [34]. This finding has been supported by studies in an adhesion-free rabbit model, where the isolated influence of peritoneal endometrial implants on fertility could be examined [35]. In this study, ovulation was not impaired by the presence of the endometrial implants. Further support for the association of impaired ovulation only in the presence of adhesions has been obtained by Chillik *et al.* [36] in women with endometriosis undergoing *in vitro* fertilization. Oocyte recovery in this study was only reduced in the presence of endometriosis associated with adhesions [36].

Luteinized unruptured follicle syndrome

LUF has been considered as a putative endocrine mechanism linking endometriosis and infertility. In this syndrome, the dominant follicle fails to rupture after the occurrence of the luteinizing hormone (LH) surge and this persists for extended periods. Diagnosis is made when an ovulatory stigma is absent at laparoscopy or when changes indicating follicular rupture cannot be demonstrated by serial ultrasound scans. Initial reports demonstrated the presence of LUF in a high proportion of patients with mild endometriosis [37]. However, when comparable figures were found in control populations [38] and among normal fertile women [39], the significance of LUF in infertility was questioned. LUF has been demonstrated as a rare occurrence in women with mild endometriosis [31, 32, 40].

Animal evidence has further questioned the LUF as an aetiological mechanism linking endometriosis and infertility. Although LUF was a more frequent finding in monkeys with endometriosis, the finding was inconsistent between consecutive cycles in individual animals [41]. Unfortunately, the incidence of LUF in consecutive menstrual cycles in infertile women with and without endometriosis is unknown. At the present time, it must be concluded that LUF is unlikely to be an important contributing factor to either infertility or endometriosis.

Luteal phase defects

The criteria for the diagnosis of luteal phase deficiency have been defined and include shortened duration to less than 11 days, aberrant basal body temperature chart, histologically delayed endometrial maturation and lower progesterone production. Abnormalities in all these factors have been reported in both endometriosis and infertility, although evidence remains conflicting as to the contribution luteal phase defects have in infertility.

Luteal function has been studied in 24 infertile patients who had endometriosis and compared with the luteal function of 20 patients who had unexplained infertility [42]. Peak and late luteal progesterone levels were found to be similar in both the groups, while early luteal progesterone levels were lower on the 2 days after the LH surge. Endometrial biopsy specimens obtained in eight of the patients with endometriosis showed luteal phase patterns in all except one patient. Thus, in this controlled study no evidence was obtained to substantiate the hypothesis that luteal phase defects are seen in association with endometriosis in infertile patients. Other studies have confirmed the normal progesterone profiles during the luteal phase in infertile patients with endometriosis [43] but, in contrast, found a significantly higher prevalence of retarded endometrium in women with endometriosis and unexplained infertility. As 13 of the 15 cases of retarded endometrial development were associated with normal progesterone levels, Li *et al.* [43] suggest that the response of the endometrium to progesterone is abnormal. Morphological studies may help to elucidate these abnormalities.

Hyperprolactinaemia

Women with endometriosis have been shown to have higher plasma prolactin levels [44, 45] than both normal and infertile controls. However, the levels are only significantly different between normal controls and women with moderate or severe endometriosis [45]. Although it has been suggested that prolactin hypersecretion has a role in infertility in conjunction with luteal phase defects, there is no evidence to support this hypothesis in mild endometriosis.

The peritoneal environment

Alterations in the peritoneal environment that may interfere with fertility have been demonstrated in women with endometriosis [46]. The presence of ectopic endometrium in the pelvis is thought to provide an antigenic stimulus that induces inflammatory changes in the peritoneal fluid. The inflammatory changes observed include increased peritoneal fluid volumes and elevated macrophage numbers and activity, as well as higher levels of cytokines and prostanoids [2].

The peritoneal fluid of women with mild endometriosis [47] and infertility [48] has been shown to have a higher total macrophage content and a higher percentage of activated macrophages when compared with fertile women [49, 50]. These activated macrophages are thought to affect fertility by their cytotoxic effect on the oocyte, spermatozoa and embryo. When peritoneal fluid from women with and without endometriosis was analysed in an assay investigating sperm–egg interaction, a significant decrease in the number of ova penetrated was observed with the peritoneal fluid from women with endometriosis [49]. In addition, peritoneal fluid from women with mild or minimal endometriosis adversely affects sperm movement [51] and decreases sperm motility and velocity [52]. Peritoneal macrophages have also been shown to increase sperm phagocytosis in women with endometriosis [53]. Mouse embryo development has been shown to be adversely affected by the peritoneal fluid from women with mild endometriosis [54, 55]. Furthermore, treatment for endometriosis has been found to alter the peritoneal fluid. In experiments investigating the cytotoxicity of peritoneal fluid, the peritoneal fluid from women who had undergone medical treatment for endometriosis ceased to be embryo-toxic [55].

High levels of interleukin 1 were demonstrated in the peritoneal fluid of women with endometriosis [54]. Interleukin 1 is primarily thought to stimulate the synthesis of a variety of active substances from macrophages, endometriotic deposits and inflammatory cells present in the peritoneum [56]. However, elevated prostanoid concentrations in peritoneal fluid of women with endometriosis are not found consistently [2, 49, 57, 58]. This makes the significance of elevated prostaglandin levels in altering fertility difficult to interpret.

Prostaglandins are thought to affect fertility by altering tubal motility and by interfering with ovulatory and luteal function. Tubal motility has been reported to be stimulated by prostaglandins [59] and could theoretically result in the more rapid transport of the gamete along the tube so that the embryo arrives in the uterine cavity at an inappropriate time for implantation. There is no direct evidence to support this hypothesis.

Most studies agree that alterations in the immunological activity of peritoneal fluid can affect fertility. The inhibition of macrophage activity in animals with endometriotic implants has been shown to restore fertility [60, 61] but no improvement in fecundability is seen in humans following treatment of endometriosis [2]. The reason for this apparent discrepancy may have been identified in a recent study which analysed the cytotoxicity of peritoneal macrophages in women with endometriosis [62]. This study suggests that the immunological reactions seen in mild endometriosis may actually be essential to the process of eliminating ectopic endometrium. Lack of macrophage cytotoxicity in this study was associated with more advanced disease and it was suggested that the increased macrophage cytotoxicity seen in mild endometriosis may limit the growth of ectopic endometrial cells [62]. Confirmation of these observations has been provided by Haney *et al.* [63], who found a negative correlation between the peritoneal leucocyte count and the extent of endometriosis. Further studies on this complex subject are essential to clarify the importance of these observations.

Spontaneous abortion rate

The relationship of endometriosis to spontaneous abortion was suggested following reports documenting higher abortion rates in women with endometriosis than in normal populations [64, 65]. Further evidence for this relationship was obtained following observations that treatment of endometriosis significantly reduced the spontaneous abortion rate [66]. More recent controlled prospective [67] and retrospective studies [68] have failed to confirm these earlier findings. Metzger *et al.* [67] found dramatic reductions in the spontaneous abortion rate in patients with endometriosis after surgical treatment for endometriosis. However, similar reductions were also found in the untreated group and spontaneous abortion rates comparable with the general population were recorded [67]. When pregnancy outcomes were retrospectively analysed in women with endometriosis and women with tubal disease, no significant differences could be found between the two groups [68]. These two controlled studies concluded that the high spontaneous abortion rates observed are characteristic of other subgroups of women with secondary infertility and no causal relationship exists between endometriosis and spontaneous abortion.

In conclusion, although a variety of causal mechanisms have been postulated for infertility in mild endometriosis, none has been shown to occur consistently and there is as much evidence to disprove such a relationship in each case as there is to support one. At present, no causal mechanism has been shown to exist between mild endometriosis and infertility.

The effect of treatment on fertility in women with endometriosis

The natural history of endometriosis must be fully understood before an assessment of the effects of treatment for endometriosis on fertility can be made. The first part of this section will outline our current knowledge about the natural history of the disease. This will be followed by a review of the evidence that endometriosis adversely affects fertility. The impact the different surgical techniques have made on restoring fertility in women whose endometriosis has caused obvious structural damage will then be discussed. The impact that treatment of mild endometriosis has on fertility will then be addressed. Finally, the place techniques of assisted conception have in the treatment of infertility in women with both mild and severe endometriosis will be discussed.

The natural history of endometriosis

Our knowledge about the natural history of endometriosis is limited. Assumptions regarding the natural progression of the disease from mild to severe forms have been questioned and it is now thought that mild endometriosis could be an entirely different disease entity from severe endometriosis [69, 70]. It appears that the presence of ectopic endometrium within the peritoneum may be a normal physiological phenomenon [69, 71]. Histological studies of normal peritoneum and biopsied peritoneal lesions suggest that endometriosis is a common, and possibly a ubiquitous, finding in normally menstruating women [8, 10, 72]. Epidemiological studies reporting the high prevalence of mild endometriosis in normal [7] and multiparous women [73] would support this suggestion.

It appears that it is the activity and not merely the presence of the endometriotic implants within the peritoneum that is of importance. In normal individuals it is postulated that ectopic endometrial cells present within the peritoneum are routinely eliminated by a cell-mediated immune response. The endometriotic deposits visualized in these women are assumed to reflect cytolysis of recently implanted endometrium [62]. Certainly laparoscopically, there is evidence that the disease progresses with time from an active stage, characterized by vesicular and nodular lesions, to an inactive stage, characterized by powderburn spots [9]. Further evidence that the activity of endometriotic implants does change with time has been provided by Evers [74] who conducted review laparoscopies in patients with endometriosis. Using a revised American Fertility Society classification score, this team found that the lesions seen at the first laparoscopy showed a changing pattern of disappearance and appearance. A number of other prospective studies have confirmed that mild endometriosis can spontaneously regress without treatment [5, 75, 76]. Similarly, mild forms of endometriosis have been found to progress to more severe forms. In these same studies, endometriosis worsened in 23–79% [5, 75, 76]. It has been postulated that progression of the disease occurs in women with defective immunological responses to the ectopic endometrium. The implants could then progress to the infiltrating lesions seen in florid endometriosis [71]. Only when the natural history of the disease in the absence of treatment is known can the results of studies assessing the effect of treatment on infertility in patients with endometriosis be assessed.

Evidence that endometriosis adversely affects fertility

The evidence in the literature that mild or minimal endometriosis has an adverse effect on fertility is conflicting. In animals, the creation of experimental endometriosis has been reported to influence future fertility in a number of studies. However, only primates have spontaneous endometriosis and a recent study reported no difference in fertility in monkeys with spontaneous disease compared with normal controls [77].

In humans, there is one controlled prospective study investigating patients undergoing artificial insemination by donor (AID) for azoospermia or severe oligospermia. All women underwent diagnostic laparoscopy prior to commencing AID. Seven women were found to have mild endometriosis and their fecundability (a mean monthly probability of pregnancy) was significantly lower (0.036) than patients without endometriosis (0.12) [78]. This is an important and frequently quoted study but there are limitations to the interpretation of the data. There were only seven patients in the endometriosis group and, if the results are compared using 95% confidence limits, there is considerable overlap. Secondly, it was assumed that endometriosis would have a deleterious effect and therefore a one-tailed analysis was performed. If a two-tailed analysis is performed, then the statistical difference disappears. Finally, men with both oligo- and azoospermia were included, meaning that it cannot be concluded that the degree of male infertility did not act as an independent variable, which would have been especially strong in a group which only contained seven individuals.

A much larger retrospective study of infertile women examined whether the presence and severity of endometriosis affected the reproductive outcome of infertile patients. Conception rates were found to be comparable in women with mild endometriosis (30.7%) and without endometriosis (30.0%). This study concluded that endometriosis had no impact on the reproductive outcome of infertile patients unless distortion of the pelvic anatomy occurred [79]. Current data, therefore, do not consistently support the hypothesis that endometriosis adversely affects fertility.

The impact of treatment on fertility where structural damage is present

For infertile patients with severe pelvic endometriosis and structural damage, the best pregnancy rates are achieved with surgical treatment. Treatment of both the endometriosis and the adhesions present in these women can be achieved by conservative surgery at laparotomy or by laparoscopy coupled with cautery or laser treatment. The effectiveness of these treatments has been analysed in a number of studies, but differences in treatment regimes, disease severity, duration of follow-up and study design make comparison of the findings impossible [80–82].

Laparotomy with conservative surgery has for many years been the treatment of choice for women with severe endometriosis and dense adhesions [83]. Pregnancy rates of approximately 50% have been obtained when the normal pelvic anatomy is restored at laparotomy by dividing adhesions and mobilizing the Fallopian tubes and ovaries [84, 85]. Similar results have also been obtained after treating severe endometriosis laparoscopically [86].

The high costs of in-patient care and loss of work time after laparotomy have encouraged the development and use of laparoscopic methods to restore pelvic anatomy to normal in women with severe endometriosis [81,87]. However, few well-designed studies have been conducted to identify the optimal mode of surgical treatment. The effect of surgical treatment on pregnancy rates in infertile women with endometriosis has been analysed in one prospective controlled clinical trial [88]. Sixty-three women with moderate/severe endometriosis were treated surgically by either laparotomy or laparoscopy. Laparoscopic treatment resulted in statistically better pregnancy rates than treatment by laparotomy. A further study has compared the use of the CO_2 laser at laparoscopy or laparotomy in women with severe endometriosis [85]. The CO_2 laser was used to treat 13 patients at laparotomy and 11 patients at laparoscopy. Comparable pregnancy rates of 53.8% and 54.5%, respectively, were found.

As experience with the laser at laparoscopy increases, many gynaecologists are finding that advanced endometriosis can be treated more effectively laparoscopically than by laparotomy. The laser allows very effective adhesiolysis and restores the pelvic anatomy to normal with minimal damage to adjacent tissues [89]. At the same time as adhesiolysis, the laser can be used to destroy disease by excising endometriomas and vaporizing endometrial deposits. In addition, after treatment laparoscopically the adhesions appear less likely to recur than after laparotomy [86]. In surgically experienced hands, laser laparoscopic treatment of severe endometriosis can yield pregnancy rates as high as 68.6% [90]. Further controlled studies must be carried out to substantiate these claims so that the treatment of endometriosis where structural damage is present can be optimized. While it is preferable for financial and economic reasons to treat severe endometriosis laparoscopically, good controlled prospective studies must be conducted to ensure that the high financial outlay for lasers is justified in the treatment of infertile women with severe endometriosis.

The impact of treatment on fertility where no structural damage is present

If endometriosis is causally associated with infertility, then treatment resulting in the elimination of the endometriotic lesions should restore fertility to normal. Significant improvements in endometriosis can be found at second-look laparoscopies carried out 9–18 months after completion of treatment for endometriosis [5]. However, unless studies also report the effect treatment has on fertility, they are of little use in determining the management of women with infertility and endometriosis.

Four randomized controlled prospective studies, with pregnancy rates as the end-point, have been conducted in infertile women with endometriosis [91–94]. Collectively, these studies compared the fertility rates in infertile women after treatment with drugs (danazol, medroxyprogesterone acetate and gestrinone) known to be efficacious in the treatment of endometriosis with those after placebo or no treatment. The women studied all had unexplained infertility and minimal endometriosis. In the two studies investigating the efficacy of danazol treatment in infertile women with mild endometriosis, the treatment and non-treatment groups had similar pregnancy rates [92,93]. The 12-month cumulative pregnancy rates in the group treated with gestrinone were 25%, which was not statistically different from the rate of 24% seen in women receiving placebo [94]. In the final study, women were treated surgically before being randomly allocated to receive danazol, medroxyprogesterone acetate or placebo. The 30-month pregnancy rate in patients receiving placebo was 46%, which was not statistically different from the treated groups [91]. Thus, randomized controlled clinical trials do not demonstrate any benefit from the present treatment modalities to the fertility of women with endometriosis [74,79].

Assisted conception in women with endometriosis

The outcome of *in vitro* fertilization, donor insemination and other assisted conception methods in women with endometriosis is controversial. Some studies have found that endometriosis reduces fecundity in women undergoing assisted conception regimes [77,95–97], while others found that endometriosis had no effect on the outcome [78,98,99].

Two studies have reported reduced fecundability in women with endometriosis undergoing donor insemination [77,95]. However, both studies involved very small numbers of women with endometriosis ($n = 7$ and $n = 8$, respectively). A further study, in a larger group of women with minimal endometriosis, compared the monthly fecundity rate in women undergoing donor insemination with women whose partners had normal semen analysis [99]. No differences were seen in the fecundity rates between the two groups. An improvement in fecundity rates is seen in women with mild endometriosis undergoing donor insemination in combination with ovulation induction regimes [100,101]. However, no improvements are seen in the cumulative pregnancy rates in these women.

A large retrospective study has assessed the conception rate in women with mild endometriosis undergoing *in vitro* fertilization. A total of 309 patients with endometriosis and 392 without endometriosis and otherwise unexplained infertility were studied. The presence of endometriosis had no effect on the pregnancy rates per embryo transfer. In addition, the severity of the disease did not affect the pregnancy rates either per patient or per embryo transfer [78]. This finding is in contrast to studies on the role of *in vitro* fertilization in infertile women which showed reduced pregnancy rates in women with endometriosis [36, 97]. However, when donor eggs from women without endometriosis were used for *in vitro* fertilization in women with endometriosis, pregnancy rates were not reduced. Pregnancy rates were only reduced when oocytes were derived from women with endometriosis. These women had significantly reduced implantation rates compared with women whose oocytes were derived from non-endometriotic ovaries [97].

As with all the other major areas addressed in this review, there is no consistent evidence to support the hypothesis that treatment of endometriosis improves fertility. In fact, the balance of evidence would support the absence of any effect.

Conclusion

The extensive research conducted into endometriosis in recent years has added further evidence to refute the hypothesis that mild endometriosis is causally associated with infertility. Many of the aetiological theories that have been postulated have no supporting evidence now that good randomized controlled studies have been conducted. Certainly there is no evidence to support the theory that endometriosis causes infertility either through auto-immune mechanisms or by altering the spontaneous abortion rate. There are so many different endocrine abnormalities that can lead to infertility that investigating the association between them all and endometriosis is an extremely complicated task. Good animal studies have helped to clarify some of the endocrine aspects involved in endometriosis, but direct extrapolation from animal models of endometriosis to the human is fraught with hazards. Only when more is understood about the endocrine control of the disease will it be possible to separate out and logically investigate any causal relationship to infertility. Our understanding of the effect endometriosis may have on the peritoneal environment has increased dramatically recently. However, research seems to be posing more questions than it is answering, at the moment. We need to know why mild endometriotic implants should spontaneously regress in some women and yet show rapid progression to advanced disease in others.

It bears repetition that no large review of the relationship between mild endometriosis and infertility has concluded either that it is causal or that treatment benefits the patient. At the beginning of this chapter, we defined four specific criteria that needed to be fulfilled if mild endometriosis was to be considered relevant in infertility, namely: an increased prevalence of the disease in infertile women, a clear aetiological basis, that the presence of the disease must decrease fertility and that treatment of it should increase fertility.

We have only been able to show that the first criterion is fulfilled and that the other three are not.

We conclude that it is the correct time for the paradigm of mild endometriosis causing infertility to be rejected. Neither surgical nor medical treatment should be initiated in these patients. The majority of evidence would support the paradigm that these patients have unexplained infertility, with mild endometriosis being either a coincidental factor or caused by childlessness. Until there is any significant body of evidence to reject the new paradigm, patients should be recommended to pursue infertility investigations and treatment appropriate to a couple with unexplained infertility. Active treatment of endometriosis should only be instigated in patients with symptoms or in whom there is documented evidence of deterioration of the disease which compromises fertility.

Finally, for the future, it should be stressed that all studies of treatments of endometriosis in infertile women should be constructed so as to demonstrate a clinically significant benefit. It is clearly inadequate for treatment to be comparable to non-intervention. Medical therapy is contraceptive, laparoscopic equipment is expensive and the procedure carries a small hazard to the patient. We would consider that, to justify these two negative factors, cumulative conception rates after 1 year should be improved by a minimum of 20%, although we appreciate that such an opinion is subjective. It does, however, provide a basis for designing meaningful, prospective studies.

References

1 Thomas EJ. Endometriosis and infertility. In: Thomas E, Rock J (ed.). *Modern Approaches to Endometriosis*, 1991, pp. 113–128. Dordrecht, Kluwer Academic Publishers.

2 Mahmood TA, Templeton A. Pathophysiology of mild endometriosis: review of literature. *Hum Reprod* 1990 **5**: 765–784.

3 Brosens I. Endometriosis related to infertility. *Curr Opin Obstet Gynaecol* 1991 **3**: 205–210.

4 Strathy JH, Molgaard CA, Coulam CB, Melton LJ. Endometriosis and infertility: a laparoscopic study of endometriosis among fertile and infertile women. *Fertil Steril* 1982 **38**: 667–672.

5 Mahmood TA, Templeton A. The impact of treatment on the natural history of endometriosis. *Hum Reprod* 1990 **5**: 965–970.

6 Barbieri RL. Etiology and epidemiology of endometriosis. *Am J Obstet Gynecol* 1990 **162**: 565–567.

7 Waller KG, Lindsay P, Curtis P, Shaw RW. The prevalence of endometriosis in women with infertile partners. *Eur J Obstet Gynaecol Reprod Biol* 1993 **48**: 135–139.

8 Jansen RP, Russell P. Non-pigmented endometriosis: clinical, laparoscopic and pathologic definition. *Am J Obstet Gynecol* 1986 **155**: 1154–1159.

9 Redwine DB. Age-related evolution in color appearance of endometriosis. *Fertil Steril* 1987 **48**: 1062–1063.

10 Nisolle M, Paindaveine B, Bourdon A *et al.* Histologic study of peritoneal endometriosis in infertile women. *Fertil Steril* 1990 **53**: 984–988.

11 Candiani GB, Danesino V, Gastaldi A, Parazzini F, Ferraroni M. Reproductive and menstrual factors and risk of peritoneal and ovarian endometriosis. *Fertil Steril* 1991 **56**: 230–234.
12 Vessey MP, Villard-Mackintosh L, Painter R. Epidemiology of endometriosis in women attending family planning clinics. *Br Med J* 1993 **306**: 182–184.
13 Pepperell RJ, McBain JC. Unexplained infertility: a review. *Br J Obstet Gynaecol* 1985 **92**: 569–580.
14 Weatherall DJ. *The New Genetics and Clinical Practice*, 3rd edn, 1991. Oxford, Oxford University Press.
15 Ranney B. Endometriosis. IV. Hereditary tendency. *Obstet Gynecol* 1971 **37**: 734–737.
16 Simpson JL, Elias S, Malinak LR, Buttram VC. Heritable aspects of endometriosis. 1. Genetic studies. *Am J Obstet Gynecol* 1980 **137**: 327–331.
17 Lamb K, Hoffmann RG, Nichols TR. Family trait analysis: a case–control study of 43 women with endometriosis and their best friends. *Am J Obstet Gynecol* 1986 **154**: 596–601.
18 Moen MH, Magnus P. The familial risk of endometriosis. *Acta Obstet Gynecol Scand* 1993 **72**: 560–564.
19 Coxhead D, Thomas EJ. The familial inheritance of endometriosis in a British population: a case–control study. *J Obstet Gynaecol* 1993 **13**: 42–44.
20 Malinak LR, Buttram VC, Elias S, Simpson JL. Heritable aspects of endometriosis. II. Clinical aspects of familial endometriosis. *Am J Obstet Gynecol* 1980 **137**: 332–336.
21 Moen MH. Endometriosis in monozygotic twins. *Act Obstet Gynaecol Scand* 1994 **73**: 59–62.
22 Weed JC, Arquembourg PC. Endometriosis: can it produce an autoimmune response resulting in infertility? *Clin Obstet Gynecol* 1980 **23**; 885–893.
23 Badawy SZA, Cuenca V, Freliech H, Stefanu C. Endometrial antibodies in serum and peritoneal fluid of infertile patients with and without endometriosis. *Fertil Steril* 1990 **53**: 930–932.
24 Joshi SG, Zamah NM, Raikar RS *et al.* Serum and peritoneal fluid proteins in women with and without endometriosis. *Fertil Steril* 1986 **46**: 1077–1082.
25 Switchenko AC, Kauffman RS, Becker M. Are there endometrial antibodies in sera of women with endometriosis? *Fertil Steril* 1991 **56**: 235–241.
26 Fernandez-Shaw S, Hicks BR, Yudkin PL *et al.* Anti-endometrial and anti-endothelial auto-antibodies in women with endometriosis. *Hum Reprod* 1993 **8**: 310–315.
27 Kennedy SH, Starkey PM, Sargent IL, Hicks BR, Barlow DH. Antiendometrial antibodies in endometriosis measured by an enzyme-linked immunosorbent assay before and after treatment with danazol and nafarelin. *Obstet Gynecol* 1990 **75**: 914–918.
28 Ayers JWT, Birenbaum DL, Menon KML. Luteal phase dysfunction in endometriosis; elevated progesterone levels in peripheral and ovarian veins during follicular phase. *Fertil Steril* 1987 **47**: 925–929.
29 Doody MC, Gibbons WE, Buttram VC. Linear regression analysis of ultrasound follicular growth series: evidence for an abnormality of follicular growth in endometriosis patients. *Fertil Steril* 1988 **49**: 47–51.
30 Tummon IS, Maclin VM, Radwanska E, Binor Z, Dmowski WP. Occult ovulatory dysfunction in women with minimal endometriosis or unexplained infertility. *Fertil Steril* 1988 **50**: 716–720.
31 Bancroft K, Vaughan Williams CA, Elstein M. Pituitary–ovarian function in women with minimal or mild endometriosis and otherwise unexplained infertility. *Clin Endocrinol* 1992 **36**: 177–181.
32 Mahmood TA, Templeton A. Folliculogenesis and ovulation in infertile women with mild endometriosis. *Hum Reprod* 1991 **6**: 227–231.

33 Soules MR, Malinak LR, Bury R, Poindexter A. Endometriosis and anovulation: a co-existing problem in the infertile female. *Am J Obstet Gynecol* 1976 **125**: 412–417.

34 Kaplan CF, Eddy CA, Olive DL, Schenken RS. Effect of ovarian endometriosis on ovulation in rabbits. *Am J Obstet Gynecol* 1989 **160**: 40–44.

35 Dunselman GAJ, Dumoulin JCM, Land JA, Evers JLH. Lack of effect of peritoneal endometriosis on fertility in the rabbit model. *Fertil Steril* 1991 **56**: 340–342.

36 Chillik CF, Acosta AA, Garcia JE *et al.* The role of *in vitro* fertilisation in infertile patients with endometriosis. *Fertil Steril* 1985 **44**: 56–61.

37 Brosens IA, Koninckx PR, Corveleyn PA. A study of plasma progesterone, oestradiol 17β, prolactin and LH levels and of the luteal phase appearance of the ovaries in patients with endometriosis and infertility. *Br J Obstet Gynaecol* 1978 **85**: 246–250.

38 Dmowski WP, Rao R, Scommegna A. The luteinized unruptured follicle syndrome and endometriosis. *Fertil Steril* 1980 **33**: 30–34.

39 Vanrell JA, Balasch J, Fuster JS, Fuster R. Ovulation stigma in fertile women. *Fertil Steril* 1982 **37**: 712–713.

40 Thomas EJ, Lenton EA, Cooke ID. Follicle growth patterns and endocrinological abnormalities in infertile women with minor degrees of endometriosis. *Br J Obstet Gynaecol* 1986 **93**: 852–858.

41 Schenken RS, Asch RH, Williams RF, Hodgen GD. Etiology of infertility in monkeys with endometriosis: luteinized unruptured follicles, luteal phase defects, pelvic adhesions and spontaneous abortions. *Fertil Steril* 1984 **41**: 122–130.

42 Kusuhara K. Luteal function in infertile patients with endometriosis. *Am J Obstet Gynecol* 1992 **167**: 274–277.

43 Li T-C, Dockery P, Cooke ID. Endometrial development in the luteal phase of women with various types of infertility: comparison with women of normal fertility: *Hum Reprod* 1991 **6**: 325–330.

44 Muse K, Wilson EA, Jawad MJ. Prolactin hyperstimulation in response to thyrotropin-releasing hormone in patients with endometriosis. *Fertil Steril* 1982 **38**: 419–422.

45 Acien P, Lloret M, Graells M. Prolactin and its response to the luteinizing hormone-releasing hormone thyrotropin-releasing hormone test in patients with endometriosis before, during, and after treatment with danazol. *Fertil Steril* 1989 **51**: 774–780.

46 Halme J. Role of peritoneal inflammation in endometriosis-associated infertility. *Ann N Y Acad Sci* 1991 **622**: 266–274.

47 Haney AF, Muscato JJ, Weinberg JB. Peritoneal fluid cell populations in infertility patients. *Fertil Steril* 1981 **35**: 696–698.

48 Olive DL, Weinberg JB, Haney AF. Peritoneal macrophages and infertility: the association between cell number and pelvic pathology. *Fertil Steril* 1985 **44**: 772–777.

49 Chacho KJ, Chacho MS, Andreson BS, Scommegna A. Peritoneal fluid in patients with and without endometriosis: prostanoids and macrophages and their effect on the spermatozoa penetration assay. *Am J Obstet Gynecol* 1986 **154**: 1290–1299.

50 Halme J, Becker S, Haskill S. Altered maturation and function of peritoneal macrophages: possible role in pathogenesis of endometriosis. *Am J Obstet Gynecol* 1987 **156**: 783–789.

51 Curtis P, Lindsay P, Jackson AE, Shaw RW. Adverse effects on sperm movement characteristics in women with minimal and mild endometriosis. *Br J Obstet Gynaecol* 1993 **100**: 165–169.

52 Oak MK, Chantler EN, Williams CA, Elstein M. Sperm survival studies in peritoneal fluid from infertile women with endometriosis and unexplained infertility. *Clin Reprod Fertil* 1985 **3**: 297–303.

53 Muscato JJ, Haney AF, Weinberg JB. Sperm phagocytosis by human peritoneal macrophages: a possible cause of infertility in endometriosis. *Am J Obstet Gynecol* 1982 **144**: 503–510.

54 Fakih H, Baggett B, Holtz G *et al.* Interleukin-1: a possible role in the infertility associated with endometriosis. *Fertil Steril* 1987 **47**: 213–217.

55 Taketani Y, Kuo T-M, Mizuno M. Comparison of cytokine levels and embryo toxicity in peritoneal fluid in infertile women with untreated or treated endometriosis. *Am J Obstet Gynecol* 1992 **167**: 265–270.

56 Bancroft K, Vaughan Williams CA, Elstein M. Minimal/mild endometriosis and infertility: a review. *Br J Obstet Gynaecol* 1989 **96**: 454–460.

57 Dawood MY, Khan-Dawood FS, Wilson L. Peritoneal fluid prostaglandins and prostanoids in women with endometriosis, chronic pelvic inflammatory disease and pelvic pain. *Am J Obstet Gynecol* 1984 **148**: 391–395.

58 De Leon FD, Vijayakumar R, Brown M *et al.* Peritoneal fluid volume, estrogen, progesterone, prostaglandin and epidermal growth factor concentrations in patients with and without endometriosis. *Obstet Gynecol* 1986 **68**: 189–194.

59 Wilhelmsson L, Lindblom B, Wiqvist N. The human uterotubal junction: contractile patterns of different smooth muscle layers and the influence of prostaglandin E2, prostaglandin F2a and prostaglandin I2 *in vitro. Fertil Steril* 1979 **32**: 303–307.

60 Steinleitner A, Lambert H, Roy S. Immunomodulation with pentoxifylline abrogates macrophage-mediated infertility in an *in vivo* model: a paradigm for a novel approach to the treatment of endometriosis-associated subfertility. *Fertil Steril* 1991 **55**: 26–31.

61 Steinleitner A, Lambert H, Suarez M *et al.* Periovulatory calcium channel blockade enhances reproductive performance in an animal model for endometriosis-associated subfertility. *Am J Obstet Gynecol* 1991 **164**: 949–952.

62 Braun DP, Gebel H, Rotman C, Rana N, Dmowski WP. The development of cytotoxicity in peritoneal macrophages from women with endometriosis. *Fertil Steril* 1992 **57**: 1203–1210.

63 Haney AF, Jenkins S, Weinberg JB. The stimulus responsible for the peritoneal fluid inflammation observed in infertile women with endometriosis. *Fertil Steril* 1991 **56**: 408–413.

64 Naples JD, Batt RE, Sadigh H. Spontaneous abortion rate in patients with endometriosis. *Obstet Gynecol* 1981 **57**: 509–512.

65 Jansen RPS. Spontaneous abortion incidence in the treatment of infertility. *Am J Obstet Gynecol* 1982 **143**: 451–473.

66 Wheeler JM, Johnston BM, Malinak LR. The relationship of endometriosis to spontaneous abortion. *Fertil Steril* 1983 **39**: 656–660.

67 Metzger DA, Olive DL, Stohs GF, Franklin RR. Association of endometriosis and spontaneous abortion: effect of control group selection. *Fertil Steril* 1986 **45**: 18–23.

68 Pittaway DE, Vernon C, Fayez JA. Spontaneous abortions in women with endometriosis. *Fertil Steril* 1988 **50**: 711–715.

69 Audebert A, Backstrom T, Barlow DH *et al.* Endometriosis 1991: a discussion document. *Hum Reprod* 1992 7: 432–435.

70 Candiani GB, Vercellini P, Fedele L, Colombo A, Candiani M. Mild endometriosis and infertility: a critical review of epidemiologic data, diagnostic pitfalls, and classification limits. *Obstet Gynecol Surv* 1991 **46**: 374–382.

71 Vercellini P, Bocciolone L, Crosignani PG. Opinion – is mild endometriosis always a disease? *Hum Reprod* 1992 7: 627–629.

72 Murphy AA, Green WR, Bobbie D, dela Cruz ZC, Rock JA. Unsuspected endometriosis documented by scanning electron microscopy in visually normal peritoneum. *Fertil Steril* 1986 **46**: 522–524.

73 Kirshon B, Poindexter AN, Fast J. Endometriosis in multiparous women. *J Reprod Med* 1989 **34**: 215–217.

74 Evers JLH. The pregnancy rate of the no-treatment group in randomized clinical trials of endometriosis therapy. *Fertil Steril* 1989 **52**: 906–907.

75 Thomas EJ, Cooke ID. Impact of gestrinone on the course of asymptomatic endometriosis. *Br Med J* 1987 **294**: 272–274.
76 Telimaa S, Ronnberg L, Kauppila A. Placebo-controlled comparison of danazol and high-dose medroxyprogesterone acetate in treatment of endometriosis after conservative surgery. *Gynecol Endocrinol* 1987 **1**: 363–371.
77 D'Hooghe TM, Bambra CS, Koninckx PR. Cycle fecundity in baboons of proven fertility with minimal endometriosis. *Gynecol Obstet Investig* 1994 **37**: 63–65.
78 Jansen RPS. Minimal endometriosis and reduced fecundability: prospective evidence from an artificial insemination by donor program. *Fertil Steril* 1986 **46**: 141–143.
79 Inoue M, Kobayashi Y, Honda I, Awaji H, Fujii A. The impact of endometriosis on the reproductive outcome of infertile patients. *Am J Obstet Gynecol* 1992 **167**: 278–282.
80 Hughes EG, Fedorkow DM, Collins JA. A quantitative overview of controlled trials in endometriosis-associated infertility. *Fertil Steril* 1993 **59**: 963–970.
81 Gant NF. Infertility and endometriosis: comparison of pregnancy outcomes with laparotomy versus laparoscopic techniques. *Am J Obstet Gynecol* 1992 **166**: 1072–1081.
82 Olive DL, Haney AF. Endometriosis-associated infertility: a critical review of therapeutic approaches. *Obstet Gynecol Surv* 1986 **41**: 538–555.
83 Candiani GB, Fedele L, Vercellini P. Laparotomy versus laparoscopy in the surgical treatment of endometriosis: the end of an era? *Acta Eur Fertil* 1989 **20**: 163–166.
84 Rock JA, Guziak DS, Sengos C *et al.* The conservative surgical treatment of endometriosis: evaluation of pregnancy success with respect to the extent of disease as categorized using contemporary classification systems. *Fertil Steril* 1981 **35**: 131–137.
85 Chong AP, Luciano A, O'Shaughnessy AM. Laser laparoscopy versus laparotomy in the treatment of infertility patients with severe endometriosis. *J Gynecol Surg* 1990 **6**: 179–183.
86 Sutton C. Lasers in infertility. *Hum Reprod* 1993 **8**: 133–146.
87 Luciano AA, Lowney J, Jacobs SL. Endoscopic treatment of endometriosis associated infertility – therapeutic, economic and social benefits. *J Reprod Med Obstet Gynecol* 1992 **37**: 573–576.
88 Adamson GD, Hurd SJ, Pasta DJ, Rodriguez BD. Laparoscopic endometriosis treatment: is it better? *Fertil Steril* 1993 **59**: 35–44.
89 Kurtz BR, Daniel JF. The role of lasers in the laparoscopic treatment of infertility and endometriosis. *Reprod Med Rev* 1993 **2**: 85–94.
90 Nezhat C, Crowgey S, Nezhat F. Videolaseroscopy for the treatment of endometriosis associated with infertility. *Fertil Steril* 1989 **51**: 237–240.
91 Telimaa S. Danazol and medroxyprogesterone acetate inefficacious in the treatment of infertility in endometriosis. *Fertil Steril* 1988 **50**: 872–875.
92 Seibel MM, Berger MJ, Weinstein FG, Taymor ML. The effectiveness of danazol on subsequent fertility in minimal endometriosis. *Fertil Steril* 1982 **38**: 534–537.
93 Bayer SR, Seibel MM, Saffan DS, Berger MJ, Taymor ML. Efficacy of danazol treatment for minimal endometriosis in infertile women – a prospective randomized study. *J Reprod Med* 1988 **33**: 179–183.
94 Thomas EJ, Cooke ID. Successful treatment of asymptomatic endometriosis: does it benefit infertile women? *Br Med J* 1987 **294**: 1117–1119.
95 Yeh J, Seibel M. Artificial insemination with donor sperm: a review of 108 patients. *Obstet Gynecol* 1987 **70**: 313–316.
96 Matson PL, Yovich JL. The treatment of infertility associated with endometriosis by *in vitro* fertilization. *Fertil Steril* 1986 **46**: 432–434.
97 Simon C, Gutierrez A, Vidal A *et al.* Outcome of patients with endometriosis in assisted reproduction: results from *in-vitro* fertilization and oocyte donation. *Hum Reprod* 1994 **9**: 725–729.

98 Jones HW, Acosta AA, Andrews MC *et al.* Three years of *in vitro* fertilisation at Norfolk. *Fertil Steril* 1984 **42**: 826–834.

99 Rodriguez-Escudero FJ, Neyro JL, Corcostegui B, Benito JA. Does minimal endometriosis reduce fecundity? *Fertil Steril* 1988 **50**: 522–524.

100 Fedele L, Bianchi S, Marchini M *et al.* Superovulation with human menopausal gonadotropins in the treatment of infertility associated with minimal or mild endometriosis: a controlled randomized study. *Fertil Steril* 1992 **58**: 28–31.

101 Deaton JL, Gibson M, Blackmer KM *et al.* A randomised controlled trial of clomiphene citrate and intrauterine insemination in couples with unexplained infertility or surgically corrected endometriosis. *Fertil Steril* 1990 **54**: 1083–1088.

Chapter 9
Classification of Endometriosis

M.J. CANIS, F.H. LOH, A. WATTIEZ, J.L. POULY, E. GLOWACZOVER AND J. RAIGA

Introduction

As there is no correlation between the anatomical lesions and the clinical findings in patients with endometriosis, the term pelvic endometriosis has to be illustrated using an adjective and/or a score to provide some information about the extent of the disease. Because it included a complete and simple description of surgical findings and easily comprehensible adjectives to describe each stage, the American Fertility Society (AFS) endometriosis classification system became the international language of endometriosis [1]. However, endometriosis is still an 'enigmatic' disease and we have yet to find the perfect system which would provide a correct prognosis for post-treatment fertility, relief of pelvic pain and the risk of recurrence.

This major difficulty should be kept in mind when proposing new systems or changes to the current classification. A change in the language can only be introduced prospectively, implying that within a few years part of the results provided by clinical studies is lost, as comparison with previous reports becomes difficult or impossible. Therefore, although our current language, the revised American Fertility Society (RAFS) classification [2] needs to be improved and adapted to new treatments, the changes should be prospectively evaluated by some groups particularly interested in endometriosis, so as to avoid unnecessary and/or detrimental modifications.

Historical review

In 1949 Wicks and Larson [3] stated: 'It is left to the individual surgeon to practice what he thinks best, without a road being opened to correct his decision for future reference. They proposed the first classification of endometriosis, which included histologic criteria. Cyst walls lined by phagocytic cells containing blood pigments and cellular debris were classified as grade I, whereas lesions with endometrium resembling normal endometrium and supported by an abundant endometrial stroma were described as grade IV. Sixty-one per cent of their patients were found to have grade I or II disease, which can be described as non- or low-'active'. Making a plea for more conservative surgical treatment of endometriosis, they proposed a conservative treatment for patients with low-active disease. As the grading can be accomplished accurately from frozen section, the surgical management may be decided intraoperatively. This approach still appears interesting when so few scientific data are available to help the intraoperative decisions. Histologic grading was established from a peritoneal implant in only one case, probably suggesting that most of their patients would be included in stage IV of the RAFS classification, and that the percentage of patients with low-active endometriosis would be very different when studying patients with minimal or mild disease. Consequently, their treatment guidelines cannot be applied in current clinical practice. In contrast, their histologic criteria may need to be reconsidered to improve the intraoperative indications of the medical treatment.

In 1951, Huffman [4] first emphasized the need for a common language. He proposed a surgical system similar to that used when staging cervical cancer [4]. Adhesions were not staged, but mild disease was included. A similar surgical classification was designed in 1974 by Mitchell and Farber [5] who proposed a stage V for malignant transformation of ovarian endometriomas.

In 1962, Riva *et al.* [6] tried to classify their patients according to the number of pelvic areas involved. They concluded 'that the objective categorizing of patients according to the severity of the disease has defied us'. In their opinion the number of areas involved is not sufficient to adequately stage a patient. The volume of the lesions as well as the surrounding adhesions should be included.

In 1966, Beecham [7] proposed a classification which included surgical and clinical data, making it well suited to record responses to medical treatments.

The pregnancy rates reported before 1973 ranged between 13 and 94% [8] suggesting that the populations studied were dissimilar. Because of this problem, a classification scheme was designed by several investigators on a flight returning from a medical conference [9]. It included the size of the lesions and scarring and retraction around the implants, as well as adnexal adhesions. In a retrospective study, Acosta *et al.* [10] reported a direct relationship between the initial extent of the disease and the postoperative pregnancy rates. This relationship was confirmed in other studies [6, 11, 12] and this system became widely accepted. Essential data, such as ovarian endometrioma diameter, were included and staged, accounting for the high incidence of adnexal adhesions after ovarian surgery. However, this classification had several disadvantages:

1 It did not distinguish between unilateral and bilateral adnexal disease.

2 Some lesions were insufficiently described, resulting in doubts when staging.

3 This first international classification appeared too inflexible when classifying patients with minimal unilateral periadnexal adhesions as moderate, or patients with endometriomas of less than 2 cm as moderate and patients with endometriomas of more than 2 cm as severe [8].

In 1977, the Kistner *et al.* [13] classification emphasized the importance of tubo-ovarian adhesions and classified them according to their amenability to laparoscopic adhesiolysis. This system was more complex than the Acosta *et al.* [10] classification, and did not allow the distinction between unilateral and bilateral adnexal involvement. In order to allow the distinction between unilateral and bilateral disease, Buttram [14] proposed an 'expanded classification of endometriosis', which was no better than the Acosta *et al.* [10] classification in predicting postoperative fertility [15].

In 1978 the American Fertility Society appointed a committee, who published the first AFS classification [1], which became widely accepted. Each location was scored using a weighted point system to distinguish endometriotic lesions of different size. The patients were then classified in four stages: mild, moderate, severe and extensive. This first AFS classification and the subsequent schemes have several advantages:

1 The scoring system is flexible enough to describe each case, including those which do not follow the usual progression of the disease. This is a major improvement as compared with previous systems which tried to follow the natural history of the disease.

2 When filling out the form, the physician has to describe all the pelvic areas, thus avoiding incomplete or vague operative reports.

3 A scoring system is suitable for computerized analysis of data.

Unfortunately, the scores and cut-off points are chosen arbitrarily.

As expected, numerous criticisms have been published. The 1979 AFS classification [1] was reliable for postoperative fertility only if comparing combined stages (stages I and II versus stages III and IV) [15]. W.C. Andrews [16] suggested that more points should be given to bilaterality. Hasson [17] emphasized that uterosacral ligament endometriotic implants should be differentiated from other peritoneal lesions in patients with chronic pelvic pain and that a three-dimensional assessment would allow an easier differentiation of superficial and deep lesions than a two-dimensional description. Too much importance was given to tubal lesions, which are rare [8]. The scores attributed to 3 cm endometriomas or to complete cul-de-sac obliteration were too low [18]. Guzick *et al.* [19], studying 214 patients treated surgically, found no significant relation between the stages and subsequent fertility.

Following all these comments, the committee was convened again and elaborated in the RAFS 1985 endometriosis classification system [2], which is still used for infertile patients. The committee decided to separate patients with minimal and mild disease, whose fertility prognosis is similar, and to group patients with severe and extensive disease. Consequently, patients with bilateral and unilateral severe adnexal involvement were included in the same stage [20]. However, this new scheme includes major improvements: tubal endometriosis is excluded from the score and described under additional endometriosis; peritoneal implants are described using a two- and a three-dimensional assessment; patients with complete posterior cul-de-sac obliteration are classified as severe; 16 points are attributed to dense adhesions enclosing the fimbria; high scores are attributed to dense adnexal adhesions; points attributed to solitary adnexa are multiplied by two. This scheme is presented in Fig. 9.1.

Rationale for a classification

A classification should be a common language, allowing us to communicate easily [18], and an expert system, in order to provide guidelines for the treatment and prognosis for post-treatment fertility, relief of pelvic pain and recurrences.

A language

The extent of the disease is essential when discussing a patient's files or treatments. To avoid a time-consuming description, the lesions should be summarized using one word or a score, thus providing a much better description than the word endometriosis alone. These words are essential when there is no correlation between the clinical symptoms and the anatomical lesions. Operative reports are improved when using the RAFS classification [2], since a complete description of the pelvis is required. As improved operative reports are written with the same words all around the world, a valuable comparison of the results obtained with various treatments becomes possible.

This language should satisfy some requirements. The translation from anatomical lesions to 'words' should be simple, fast, easy and clear, thus minimizing the surgeon's interpretation. The language should be flexible enough to allow an easy description of any case. This language needs a glossary including an accurate and simple description of each word. This glossary, which is not yet available, is essential, as, when discussing issues with foreign colleagues, we have often noticed that words very commonly used in clinical practice do not have the same meaning in different countries. For instance, deep peritoneal implants are not clearly described in the current system. Should we consider all the typical black puckered lesions as deep lesions, or should this term be reserved for deeply infiltrating implants (more than 3 mm) [21, 22]? Similarly, the term complete cul-de-sac obliteration

Patient's name ____________________ Date ____________

Stage I (Minimal) 1–5
Stage II (Mild) 6–15
Stage III (Moderate) 16–40
Stage IV (Severe) >40
Total ____________

Laparoscopy ________ Laparotomy ________ Photography ________
Recommended treatment ____________________
____
Prognosis ____________________

		Endometriosis	< 1 cm	1–3 cm	> 3 cm
Peritoneum		Superficial	1	2	4
		Deep	2	4	6
Ovary	R	Superficial	1	2	4
		Deep	4	16	20
	L	Superficial	1	2	4
		Deep	4	16	20

Posterior cul-de-sac obliteration	Partial	Complete
	4	40

		Adhesions	<1/3 enclosure	1/3–2/3 enclosure	>2/3 enclosure
Ovary	R	Filmy	1	2	4
		Dense	4	8	16
	L	Filmy	1	2	4
		Dense	4	8	16
Tube	R	Filmy	1	2	4
		Dense	4*	8*	16
	L	Filmy	1	2	4
		Dense	4*	8*	16

*If the fimbriated end of the Fallopian tube is completely enclosed, change the point assignment to 16.

Additional endometriosis ____________________
____
____
____

Associated pathology ____________________
____
____
____

To be used with normal tubes and ovaries

To be used with abnormal tubes and ovaries

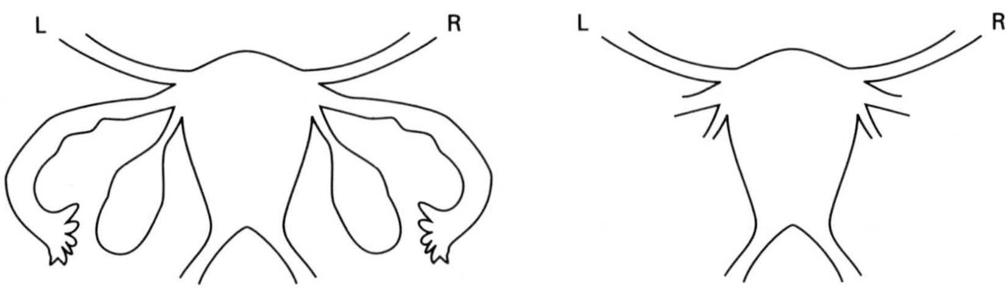

Fig. 9.1 Revised American Fertility Society classification of endometriosis (1985) [2]. From The American Fertility Society. Revised American Fertility Society classification of endometriosis. *Fertil Steril* 1985 **43**: 351. Reproduced with permission of the publisher, The American Fertility Society.

may be confusing for those who do not know the initial description from Sampson.

An expert system

A perfect classification should allow an accurate prognosis for post-treatment fertility and relief of pelvic pain and should indicate the risk of recurrence [18]. Such an expert system is much more difficult to define. It is obtained by attributing a score to each lesion and deciding the cut-off points between the stages. Until now, these scores and breakpoints have been empirically decided. The present classification is not an expert system.

When attributing a score to a lesion, one is trying to assess the effect of this lesion on postoperative outcome. This depends on several factors:

1 The effect of the lesion itself on the outcome, something that is rarely known, as demonstrated by numerous studies on the treatment of minimal disease.

2 The usefulness, effectiveness, difficulties, failures and complications of the treatment.

3 The various treatments which may be proposed, according to the patient's age and previous medical history.

4 The delay necessary to obtain the desired outcome.

5 The frequency and the consequences of the lesions often associated with the considered lesion.

Except for patients with mechanical infertility, our understanding of the disease is too poor to design a true expert system, which will probably not be established solely using data obtained at laparoscopy or laparotomy. As lesions found at surgery represent only one day in the spontaneous evolution of the disease, a marker for the disease 'activity' would be essential to decide the management.

Staging technique

Although surgical staging is now considered the gold standard, no statement has been made concerning the best surgical approach, laparoscopy or laparotomy, and what surgical procedures are required to accurately stage a patient. When evaluating patients retrospectively from videotapes, we found that a patient with severe endometriosis cannot be staged only from laparoscopic inspection. For example, a complete examination of the pelvic peritoneum and of the posterior cul-de-sac is impossible unless large endometriomas have been punctured and emptied.

Operative laparoscopy is the best surgical staging technique. However, guidelines for laparoscopic staging are required and it is necessary to report on the form whether or not a complete pelvic examination has been achieved and which parts of the pelvis have not been fully inspected.

As ovarian punctures and adhesiolysis are often required, prerequisites for laparoscopic staging are very similar to those for laparoscopic treatment of endometriosis [23]. The following conditions are required: (i) patients informed of a possible laparotomy; (ii) a bowel preparation administered on the day before surgery; and (iii) adequate laparoscopic retractors available (10–15° Trendelenburg position, efficient uterine cannulation, a good pneumoperitoneum, two or three ancillary trocars inserted in the suprapubic area). The laparoscopic staging includes the following steps:

1 By means of the Trendelenburg position and atraumatic forceps, the bowel and the omentum are pushed over the superior pelvic brim.

2 The magnification provided by the laparoscope is used to inspect the anterior and posterior cul-de-sac, looking for small and atypical peritoneal implants.

3 Peritoneal cytology and/or peritoneal washing are sampled, as in any patient with an ovarian cystic mass.

4 The tubes and the ovaries are mobilized, looking for tubal and ovarian adhesions.

5 To diagnose ovarian endometriomas a complete ovariolysis is required.

6 The broad ligaments and the anterior ovarian surface are inspected.

7 Enlarged ovarian and/or star-like ovarian scars are routinely punctured, looking for small endometriomas [24].

8 The posterior cul-de-sac and the rectum are assessed, using vaginal examination and/or vaginal and rectal probes [25].

9 If an ovarian endometrioma has been opened, the pelvis is copiously irrigated; the internal cyst wall is inspected and biopsied in order to rule out malignancy and to differentiate endometriomas from functional chocolate cysts [26, 27].

10 The upper part of the abdomen is carefully inspected, looking for bowel or appendicular endometriosis.

Expertise in operative laparoscopy is a prerequisite to accurate staging of patients with severe disease. Similarly, awareness of the various visual appearances of peritoneal and ovarian endometriotic implants is required [22]. Moreover, a recommended cycle day for diagnostic laparoscopy would be invaluable to obtain consistent descriptions of atypical implants.

As the laparoscope is a lens, subjective assessment of the size is obviously unreliable. The size of an implant on the video screen depends on the distance between the lens and the lesion. Therefore, the diameter of the lesions should be measured by comparing it with laparoscopic instruments of known dimensions.

Approaching the 'activity' of endometriosis

Endometriosis 'activity' has not yet been clearly defined. However, this term is often used in comments and discussions, as most authors agree to say that the clinical consequences of endometriosis are more related to the 'activity' than to the extent of the disease. The implants and the peritoneal environment have been proposed to evaluate endometriosis activity.

The implants have been studied using *in vitro* prostaglandin synthesis [28] and pathological examination [29–31]. Vernon *et al.* [28] demonstrated that *in vitro* reddish implants produced twice the amount of prostaglandin F (PGF) compared with brown implants, whereas black implants did not have the *in vitro* capacity to produce PGF. More recently, Nisolle *et al.* [30, 31] and Donnez *et al.* [29] confirmed, using a usual and a three-dimensional pathologic examination, that red implants are more active than black puckered lesions and have a higher vascularization and increased mitotic activity.

The peritoneal environment has been studied using peritoneal fluid volume, peritoneal cell number, concentration, activation or production of cytokine or growth factors and aminoterminal propeptide of type III procollagen and endometrial stromal cell proliferation [32–36]. Syrop and Halme [36] demonstrated that postoperative fertility was related to peritoneal fluid volume. Spuijbroek *et al.* [34] correlated for the first time the results obtained studying the peritoneal fluid and the laparoscopic appearance of peritoneal implants. They suggested that early peritoneal endometriosis is an invasive disease since the peritoneal fluid concentration of aminoterminal propeptide type III collagen was significantly increased in patients with subtle lesions [34], whereas it was not different from controls in patients without early implants.

As already suggested by Weitzman and Buttram [9], physiologic parameters will have to be incorporated into new classification systems. In our opinion, after a careful scientific evaluation, the good marker for endometriosis 'activity' will have to be cost-effective, simple and easy to assess during or just before the surgical diagnosis in every hospital. Before it can be proposed for clinical practice, the marker will have to be carefully related to anatomical data and postoperative results, using prospective clinical studies. Surprisingly, the peritoneal fluid volume on a recommended cycle day, which appeared very attractive, has never been re-evaluated.

Description of peritoneal endometriosis

Since 1986, several authors have emphasized the importance of atypical and subtle peritoneal implants [5, 29, 36–38]. These descriptions are essential when the study of the implants is the main approach of the 'activity' of endometriosis. The relationships between laparoscopic appearances and clinical data are unclear since atypical and typical lesions are often associated in the same patient. To perform prospective studies of this essential problem, a classification of implant appearances is required. This classification of atypical lesions should include simple descriptions and carefully selected colour pictures [23]. This description of peritoneal implants is now included in the management of endometriosis in the presence of pelvic pain [39, 40]. The words used to describe the implants are similar to those used in the reports about subtle and atypical lesions. However, these words may not have the same meaning for all these experts. Unfortunately, colour pictures to document each appearance have not been published with this form. These pictures, which are being prepared by the AFS committee, are urgently required, as the distinction between clear implants and vesicles or between white lesions and peritoneal fibrosis may not appear obvious and easy to everyone. Similarly, a simple description and examples of what should be considered as superficial and deep peritoneal endometriosis and how to assess the depth of an implant are necessary.

Comments on the RAFS classification system for infertile patients

A simplified RAFS classification

Based on the unexplained strong association of endometriomas and adhesions, Koninckx *et al.* [21] proposed an attractive simplified classification. They suggested that, by increasing the points for endometriomas, adhesions could be omitted, whereas >95% of the patients would be staged identically. However, the following arguments should be considered:

1 Adhesions need to be fully described in infertile patients.

2 The association between endometriomas and adhesions may be absent in patients who have undergone previous treatment; the main advantage of the AFS classification is to be flexible enough to describe lesions which do not follow the usual progression of the disease.

3 The adhesion scoring system is easy to use, and the simplification would be more apparent than real.

4 A complete description is essential in clinical and research studies.

Should a stage V be included?

We recently proposed that a stage V needs to be considered in the next AFS classification scheme [20]. This modification is supported by the following arguments:

1 When studying fertility after laparoscopic treatment of endometriosis, we found an intrauterine pregnancy rate of 37.5% [41]; however, we obtained no pregnancy when the AFS score was > 70, whereas 52.9% of the patients who had a score of 70 or less conceived.

2 As shown in Table 9.1, this significant difference was explained by the difficulties encountered when treating patients with extensive dense adhesions; complete treatment of ovarian endometriomas was achieved significantly less often when the adhesions score, including posterior cul-de-sac obliteration, was > 50.

3 As presented in Table 9.2, we also found that the incidence of bilateral endometriomas and bilateral severe adhesions was significantly more common in patients with a score > 70 [20].

Table 9.1 Immediate anatomical results of laparoscopic treatment (79 patients)

	Adh. score > 50		Adh. score ⩽ 50		Total	
	n	%	*n*	%	*n*	%
Adhesiolysis	33		46		79	
Complete	11*	33.3	33*	71.7	44	55.6
Partial	22	66.6	13	28.3	35	44.3
Treatment of ovarian endometriomas	40		53		93	
Complete	31†	77.5	51†	96.2	82	88.2
Drainage	9	22.5	2	3.8	11	11.8

* $P < 0.001$.
† $P < 0.01$.

Table 9.2 Incidence of bilateral lesions according to the AFS score

	Group 1 (AFS ⩽ 70) $N = 46$		Group 2 (AFS > 70) $N = 43$	
Bilateral lesions	*n*	%	*n*	%
Adnexal score ⩾ 16	23*	50.0	39*	90.7
Adnexal score ⩾ 20	16*	34.8	35*	81.4
Adhesions score ⩾ 16	9*	19.6	28*	65.1
Ovarian score ⩾ 16	13†	28.3	24†	55.8
Ovarian score ⩾ 20	11†	23.9	22†	51.2

N = Total number of patients in the group studied; n = number of patients who had the considered anatomical lesion on both adnexa.
* $P < 0.001$.
† P0.02.

4 The prognosis is better in patients with normal adnexa [8].
5 We and others recently demonstrated that adhesion reformation is an all too frequent occurrence after laparoscopic treatment of dense adhesions [42,43]. Therefore, in patients with bilateral dense adhesions, conservative surgery is not an efficient treatment of infertility. This conclusion is confirmed by the results obtained at routine second-look laparoscopy performed in 53 patients with RAFS stage IV endometriosis. At second-look laparoscopy, the AFS score of patients who had an initial score >70 was 56.6 ± 33.6, still very high (Table 9.3). This poor result is mainly explained by adhesion re-formation, since the adhesion score (cul-de-sac obliteration excluded) is not improved by the laparoscopic procedure ($P > 0.2$).

Table 9.3 Comparison of AFS and of adhesion score at laparoscopic treatment and at second-look laparoscopy

	Laparoscopic treatment	Second-look laparoscopy	P
AFS score ≤ 70; $n = 53$			
AFS score	55.3 ± 7.8	21.6 ± 18.4	< 0.001
Implants score	27.2 ± 14.7	5.4 ± 6.3	< 0.001
Adhesions score	16.1 ± 11.4	12.2 ± 12.6	< 0.04
AFS score > 70; $n = 22$			
AFS score	96.8 ± 14.1	56.6 ± 33.6	< 0.001
Implants score	34.1 ± 13.4	8.9 ± 13.1	< 0.001
Adhesions score	39.6 ± 15.4	33.4 ± 16.8	> 0.2

6 Studying the adnexal adhesion score at laparoscopic treatment and at second-look laparoscopy in 180 adnexa, we confirmed that adhesion re-formation is an essential problem and that, in contrast, postoperative adhesion formation is uncommon after laparoscopic treatment (Table 9.4).
7 Endometriosis appears to be a good indication for *in vitro* fertilization (IVF) and embryo transfer; IVF is probably the best treatment for infertile patients with extensive adhesions.
8 An extensive stage was included in the 1979 AFS classification scheme [1].
9 This stage is not uncommon; as can be seen from Fig. 9.2, in our current experience, stage V endometriosis is as common as stage IV or stage II, and represents about 14% of our patients.

As the surgeon's interpretation is important when assessing the extent of the disease, breakpoints should be established from multicentre prospective studies, using carefully recorded videotapes so that the lesions could be staged by several investigators. A score of 70 is probably not a correct breakpoint,

Table 9.4 Comparison of adnexal adhesion scores at laparoscopic treatment and at second-look laparoscopy

Group	*n*	Laparoscopic treatment	Second-look laparoscopy	*P*
All adnexa	180	9.7 ± 9.8	7.9 ± 9.8	> 0.05
Severe	106	12.9 ± 10.5	10.5 ± 10.9	< 0.05
Moderate	74	4.0 ± 5.5	4.2 ± 6.3	> 0.6
40 < AFS < 71	62	8.0 ± 8.1	6.1 ± 8.1	< 0.02
AFS > 70	44	19.8 ± 9.6	16.7 ± 11.6	> 0.2
Cyst > 3 cm	72	12.6 ± 10.6	11.1 ± 11.3	> 0.3
Cyst none	108	7.1 ± 9.3	5.9 ± 8.7	> 0.05
Adh. ⩽ 4	50	1.1 ± 1.6	3.3 ± 5.9	< 0.01
Adh. ⩾ 16	45	23.4 ± 6.3	16.8 ± 11.2	< 0.01
AFS < 71	14	21.0 ± 5.6	13.4 ± 9.5	< 0.02
AFS > 70	31	24.9 ± 6.1	19.5 ± 11.6	> 0.05

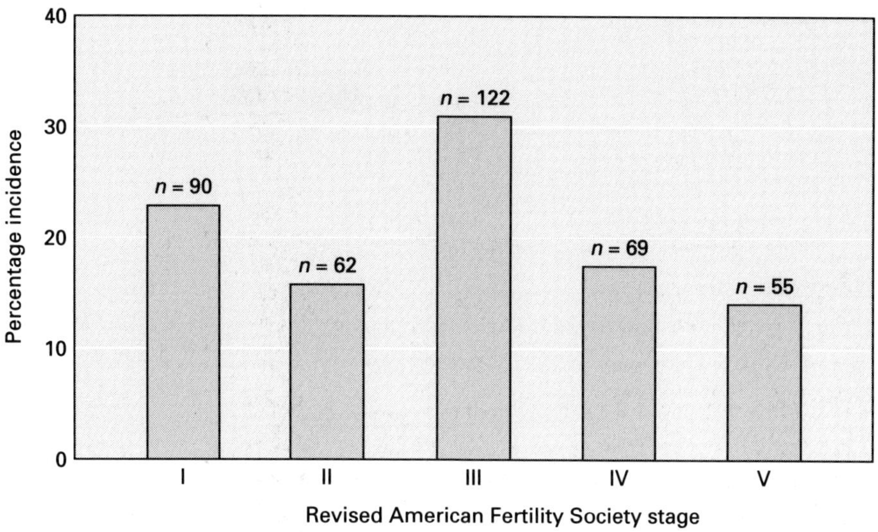

Fig. 9.2 Incidence of each American Fertility Society stage among 398 patients treated by laparoscopy.

since a patient with this score and a complete cul-de-sac obliteration may have normal adnexa.

Chronic pelvic pain (Fig. 9.3)

The AFS committee was convened again in October 1992. As the current AFS classification was designed for women with infertility and the incidence of deep infiltrating disease and pelvic adhesions is different in chronic pelvic pain

MANAGEMENT OF ENDOMETRIOSIS IN THE PRESENCE OF PELVIC PAIN
A Clinical Instrument to Document the Extent of Endometriosis and Pelvic Pain[1]

Patient's Name ____________________ Age __________ Date __________

PRE-OPERATIVE ASSESSMENT OF PELVIC PAIN

Complaints ____________________

Describe the patient's symptoms of pain quality and position, and any limitation caused by these symptoms. Abbreviate quality of pain as **A = mild, B = discomforting, C = distressing, D = horrible, E = excruciating.** On the anatomic drawings below, draw a **SOLID LINE** around the area(s) of pain described by the patient, and mark the most intense area(s) with an **X.**

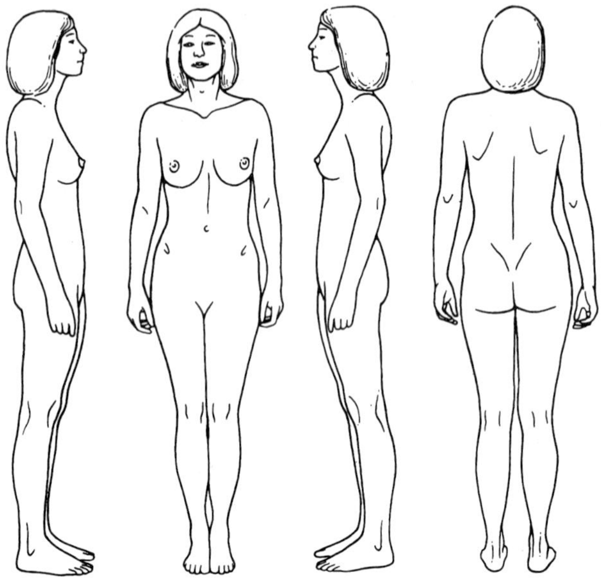

Physical findings ____________________

Identify the quality and site of tenderness caused by palpation, extent of nodularity, diffuse or focal distribution, and/or fixation of uterus/adnexa. On the anatomic drawings above, draw a **BROKEN LINE** around the area(s) of tenderness found on examination.

Adjuncts: [ ] IVP? [ ] BE? [ ] Sigmoidoscopy? [ ] Other? ____________________

[1] The association of pelvic pain and endometriosis remains enigmatic because the extent of disease by the previous AFS classifications does not dependably relate to the severity of pelvic pain or tenderness. This form was designed by the AFS Committee on Classification of Endometriosis to carefully document the location and intensity of pelvic pain and tenderness in addition to distribution of endometriosis and pelvic adhesions. Constant recording of this data will permit consistent management of the patient with endometriosis and pelvic pain, and facilitate clinical research.

Fig. 9.3 RAFS proposed pelvic pain assessment methods in endometriosis (1993) [40]. From The American Fertility Society. Management of endometriosis in the presence of pelvic pain. *Fertil Steril* 1993; **60**: 952–5. Reproduced with permission of the publisher, The American Fertility Society.

patients, it was decided to propose a new system for the management of chronic pelvic pain [44]. The system proposed in December 1993 [40] is not a classification but a form designed to standardize data collection. It includes clinical and surgical data, so as to study the relationship between endometriotic lesions and clinical signs and to permit the construction of a true classification for chronic pelvic pain patients.

This approach is reasonable, as our knowledge of endometriosis is too poor to propose a true classification. This first and preliminary step will soon appear as an essential progress in the difficult management of chronic pain associated with pelvic endometriosis. To fill this form the surgeon has to document the appearances of peritoneal endometriotic implants. Unfortunately, the system used to describe pelvic adhesion is slightly different from that used in infertile patients. This difference may appear confusing for most gynaecologists used to staging their patients with the 1985 RAFS classification [2]. The previous adhesion scoring system was easy to use and more precise. The advantages and potential disadvantages of this new adhesion scoring system have to be carefully evaluated. In our clinic we use both systems in pain patients so as to have all the information about the extent of adnexal adhesions and to know which system is the best one in our hands.

Conclusion

A scientifically based score for each lesion would be necessary to establish a perfect expert system. We have to accept that our current knowledge is not good enough to propose such a perfect system, and that long and difficult work will be required to improve our understanding, our management and our classification of endometriosis.

References

1 American Fertility Society. Classification of endometriosis. *Fertil Steril* 1979 **32**: 633.

2 American Fertility Society. Revised American Fertility Society classification of endometriosis. *Fertil Steril* 1985 **43**: 351.

3 Wicks MJ, Larson CP. Histologic criteria for evaluating endometriosis. *Northwest Med J* 1949 **48**: 611–613.

4 Huffman JW. External endometriosis. *Am J Obstet Gynecol* 1951 **62**: 1243–1250.

5 Mitchell GW, Farber M. Medical versus surgical management of endometriosis. In: Reed D, Christian D (eds). *Controversies in Obstetrics and Gynecology*, vol. 2, 1974, pp. 631–636. Philadelphia, WB Saunders.

6 Riva HL, Kawasaki DM, Messinger AJ. Further experience with norethynodrel in treatment of endometriosis. *Obstet Gynecol* 1962 **19**: 111–117.

7 Beecham CT. Classification of endometriosis. *Obstet Gynecol* 1966 **28**: 437.

8 Buttram VC. Evolution of the revised American Fertility Society classification of endometriosis. *Fertil Steril* 1985 **43**: 347–350.

9 Weitzman GA, Buttram VC. Classification of endometriosis. *Obstet Gynecol Clin North Am* 1989 **16**: 61–77.

10 Acosta AA, Buttram VC, Besch PK *et al.* A proposed classification of pelvic endometriosis. *Obstet Gynecol* 1973 **42**: 19–23.

11 Buttram VC, Reiter RC, Ward S. Treatment of endometriosis with danazol: report of a 6-year prospective study. *Fertil Steril* 1985 **43**: 353–360.

12 Schenken RS, Malinak LR. Reoperation after initial treatment of endometriosis with conservative surgery. *Am J Obstet Gynecol* 1978 **131**: 416–421.
13 Kistner RW, Siegler AM, Berhman SJ. Suggested classification for endometriosis relationship to infertility. *Fertil Steril* 1977 **28**: 1008–1010.
14 Buttram VC. An expanded classification of endometriosis. *Fertil Steril* 1978 **9**: 240–242.
15 Rock JA, Guzick, DS, Sengos C *et al.* The conservative surgical treatment of endometriosis: evaluation of pregnancy success with respect to the extent of the disease as categorized using contemporary classification systems. *Fertil Steril* 1981 **35**: 131–137.
16 Andrews WC. Classification of endometriosis. *Fertil Steril* 1981 **35**: 124–125.
17 Hasson HM. Classification for endometriosis (Letter). *Fertil Steril* 1981 **35**: 368–369.
18 Candiani GB. The classification of endometriosis: historical evolution, critical review and present state of the art. *Acta Eur Fertil* 1986 **17**: 85–92.
19 Guzick DS, Bros DS, Rock JA, Assessing the efficacy of the American Fertility Society's classification of endometriosis: application of a dose–response methodology. *Fertil Steril* 1982 **38**: 171–176.
20 Canis M, Pouly JL, Wattiez A *et al.* Incidence of bilateral adnexal disease in severe endometriosis (revised-American Fertility Society, stage IV). Should a stage V be included in the American Fertility Society classification? *Fertil Steril* 1992 **57**: 691–692.
21 Koninckx PR, Meuleman C, Demeyere S, Lesaffre E, Cornillie F. Suggestive evidence that pelvic endometriosis is a progressive disease, whereas deeply infiltrating endometriosis is associated with pelvic pain. *Fertil Steril* 1991 **55**: 759–765.
22 Martin DC, Hubert G, Levy B. Depth of infiltration of endometriosis. *J Gynecol Surg* 1989 **5**: 55–59.
23 Canis M, Bouquet de Jolinières J, Wattiez A *et al.* Classification of endometriosis. *Baillère's Clin Obstet Gynecol* 1993 **7**: 759–774.
24 Candiani GB, Vercellini P, Fedele L. Laparoscopic ovarian puncture for correct staging of endometriosis. *Fertil Steril* 1990 **53**: 994–997.
25 Reich H, McGlynn F, Salvat J. Laparoscopic treatment of cul de sac obliteration secondary to retrocervical deep endometriosis. *J Reprod Med* 1991 **36**: 516–522.
26 Mage G, Canis M, Manhes H *et al.* Laparoscopic management of adnexal cystic masses. *J Gynecol Surg* 1990 **6**: 71–79.
27 Martin DC, Demos Berry J. Histology of chocolate cysts. *J Gynecol Surg* 1990 **6**: 43–46.
28 Vernon MW, Beard JS, Graves K, Wilson EA. Classification of endometriotic implants by morphologic appearance and capacity to synthesize prostaglandin F. *Fertil Steril* 1986 **46**: 801–806.
29 Donnex J, Nisolle M, Casanas-Roux F. Three dimensional architectures of peritoneal endometriosis. *Fertil Steril* 1992 **57**: 980–983.
30 Nisolle M, Paindaveine B, Bourdon A *et al.* Histologic study of peritoneal endometriosis. *Fertil Steril* 1990 **53**: 984–988.
31 Nisolle M, Casanas-Roux F, Anaf V, Mine JM, Donnez J. Morphometric study of the stromal vascularization in peritoneal endometriosis. *Fertil Steril* 1993 **59**: 681–684.
32 Halme J, Becker S, Haskill S. Altered maturation and function of peritoneal macrophages: a possible role in pathogenesis of endometriosis. *Am J Obstet Gynecol* 1986 **157**: 783–789.
33 Olive DL, Montoya I, Riehl RM, Schenken RS, Macrophage-conditioned media enhance endometrial stromal cell proliferation *in vitro*. *Am J Obstet Gynecol* 1991 **164**: 953–958.
34 Spuijbroek MDEH, Dunselman GAJ, Menheere PPCA, Evers JLH. Early endometriosis invades the extracellular matrix. *Fertil Steril* 1992 **58**: 929–933.
35 Surey ES, Halme J. Effect of platelet-dervied growth factor on endometrial stromal cell proliferation *in vitro*: a model for endometriosis? *Fertil Steril* 1991 **56**: 672–679.
36 Syrop CH, Halme J. A comparison of peritoneal fluid parameters of infertile patients and the subsequent occurrence of pregnancy. *Fertil Steril* 1986 **46**: 631–635.

37 Jansen RPS, Russell P. Non pigmented endometriosis: clinical laparoscopic and pathologic definition. *Am J Obstet Gynecol* 1986 **155**: 1154–1158.
38 Martin DC, Hubert GD, Vander Zwaag R, El-Zeky F. Laparoscopic appearances of peritoneal endometriosis. *Fertil Steril* 1989 **51**: 63–67.
39 American Fertility Society. Classification. Plenary Session VII, Third World Congress on Endometriosis, Brussels, 1–3 June 1992.
40 American Fertility Society. Management of endometriosis in the presence of pelvic pain. *Fertil Steril* 1993 **60**: 952–955.
41 Canis M, Mage G, Manhes H *et al.* Laparoscopic treatment of endometriosis. *Acta Obstet Gynecol Scand* 1989 **150** (Suppl.): 15–20.
42 Canis M, Mage G, Wattiez A *et al.* Second-look laparoscopy after laparoscopic cystectomy of large ovarian endometriomas. *Fertil Steril* 1992 **58**: 617–619.
43 Operative Laparoscopy Study Group. Postoperative adhesion development after operative laparoscopy: evaluation at early second-look procedures. *Fertil Steril* 1991 **55**: 700–704.
44 Rock JA. Endometriosis and pelvic pain. *Fertil Steril* 1993 **60**: 950–951.

Part 3
Medical Treatments

Chapter 10
Medical and Endocrine Modulatory Treatments

P.C. LINDSAY

Introduction

Endometriosis is diagnosed in women from a wide range of presentations. The most common presenting symptoms are pelvic pain, dysmenorrhoea, dyspareunia and infertility. It may also be diagnosed in asymptomatic women undergoing elective procedures, such as laparoscopic sterilization, or it may be diagnosed following the detection of an adnexal mass during well-woman screening. The wide range of presentations is matched by an ever-widening range of medical and surgical treatment options, which allows treatment to be tailored to the individual, taking into account factors such as age, symptoms, reproductive status and fertility demands.

An understanding of the benefits, side-effects, risks and limitations of different treatments is essential to make the most appropriate choice of treatment for an individual. In this chapter, general aspects of medical treatment of endometriosis will be discussed, including a critical review of the types of study used to look at the efficacy of medical treatment. This will be followed by a review of different types of medical treatments. Gondatrophin-releasing hormone (GnRH) analogues, which have become an established treatment for endometriosis during the last decade, will be discussed in greater depth in Chapter 11, p. 206.

Background considerations

Before discussing the efficacy of treatments for endometriosis, it is important to review the natural history of endometriosis. Most endometriosis is intra-abdominal, and conventionally a laparoscopy or laparotomy is essential to make the diagnosis and establish the extent of the disease. The diagnosis is usually made on visual inspection and therefore depends on how thorough the inspection is. While many pigmented endometriotic lesions are characteristic, some lesions are more subtle and may be missed by the less than astute observer. There is a wide range of appearances for peritoneal endometriosis and there is evidence that non-pigmented endometriosis is the most common variety [1]. This is the type that is more likely to be overlooked and may thus lead to bias in our interpretation of results from studies using visual diagnosis to assess the disease or its treatment. Murphy *et al.* [2] suggested that some endometriosis is microscopic, having found endometriosis using scanning electron microscopy in 25% of peritoneal biopsies taken from normal-looking peritoneum during laparotomies in women with stage III or IV endometriosis. The concept of microscopic disease has not been backed up by other studies in which the diagnosis of normal peritoneum is made by close laparoscopic inspection prior to biopsy [3].

It is difficult to establish the true prevalence and natural progression of the condition. It is not ethical to perform repeated laparoscopies on patients with untreated endometriosis just to observe any changes that might be occurring. Although there have been many studies of endometriosis over the past 30 years, there are relatively few controlled studies where placebo groups have been laparoscoped before and after treatment with a placebo. In these studies, progression of disease was noted during intervals ranging from 6 months to 1 year in 23–47% of patients on placebo [4, 5]. However, regression or resolution of the disease was noted in 18–53% of patients on placebo. These studies were performed on patients whose primary complaint was infertility. To date, there is one placebo-controlled study on patients whose primary complaint is pain. Dlugi *et al.* [6] compared depot leuprolide acetate with placebo, looking specifically at pain symptoms. While it was shown that leuprolide acetate was more effective in the first 3 months of treatment, the study design allowed non-responders to drop out at this stage. In the placebo group, 27 out of 31 patients dropped out, making it impossible to assess the placebo group. Fedele *et al.* [7] have, however, compared expectant management of pelvic pain associated with minimal–mild endometriosis with buserelin treatment. In the group managed expectantly, spontaneous remission of pain symptoms occurred in three of 16 cases. It is difficult to extrapolate this data and ascertain its significance, given the small numbers. The above data and assumptions must, however, be borne in mind when looking at the results of trials of treatment for endometriosis, since it would seem that both appearances and symptoms may improve on no treatment at all.

When judging the merits of clinical trials studying endometriosis treatment, the variables being assessed should be considered. Assessment of symptoms is mainly subjective and therefore prone to imprecision but is probably the most important assessment. Objective assessments, such as laparoscopic scoring systems, used before and after treatment, also have limitations. Severity of symptoms may not correlate with the extent of the disease seen laparoscopically. The widely used scoring system of the American Fertility Society (AFS) [8] is good at assessing disease at first laparoscopy but it was not designed to assess the impact of treatment on endometriosis. Medical treatments may cause involution and regression of endometrial implants but they do not lyse adhesions or ablate large endometriomata. Scoring systems that are heavily weighted towards adhesions and endometriomata will thus not show what may be quite effective reductions in the number and/or size of deposits and symptom relief from medical treatment.

If laparoscopic assessment is the means by which the efficacy of a treatment is judged, it is important to consider the timing of the second laparoscopy, i.e. whether it was performed during treatment or after finishing treatment. Evers [9] demonstrated the importance of this in a study he performed treating patients with danazol. Follow-up laparoscopy was performed either at the end of a 6-month course of danazol or 2 months after the end of treatment. In those patients who underwent laparoscopy whilst on danazol, there was a significant reduction in the size and number of implants, as would have been expected from the results of previous studies. In those patients who had their laparoscopy 2 months after treatment finished, when ovarian function had returned, there was no significant reduction in implant size or number of implants. From this study, it was concluded that the 'cure rate' of endometriosis therapy depended on when the second-look laparoscopy was performed.

This study also reinforces the point that medical treatment for endometriosis does not eradicate the disease. It shows that endometriosis is more difficult to identify when suppressed and, with the return of cyclical ovarian activity, it becomes evident again. This finding concurs with most studies of medical treatment for endometriosis in which there has been a follow-up phase. The follow-up in these studies generally measures symptom recurrence and there appears to be a recurrence rate of 30–53% within 1–5 years [10, 11].

If it is accepted that endometriosis is not eradicated by medical treatment but only suppressed, the next question should be: 'How long should it be treated for?' To date, most papers report treatment regimens lasting from 3 to 6 months. There are few papers directly comparing different durations of treatment. Doberl *et al.* [12] showed that 6 months' treatment with danazol was more effective in terms of implant regression than 4 months' treatment. The duration of treatment is relatively arbitrary. Factors such as symptomatic and metabolic side-effects, cost and a desire to give as few drugs as possible tend to limit the duration for which treatment is given. There is little work in the literature on more prolonged treatment of endometriosis or on the prevention of recurrence of symptoms in treated patients.

Medical treatment of endometriosis varies from regimens designed to give symptom relief primarily to regimens which through endocrine modulation aim to suppress and 'cure' endometriosis. The rest of this chapter will look at specific medical treatments for endometriosis.

Analgesics and prostaglandin synthetase inhibitors

Dysmenorrhoea is a very common symptom and how much of it is due to endometriosis is unknown. Retrospective studies of patients with symptomatic endometriosis have shown that symptoms are present for many years before the diagnosis is confirmed laparoscopically. Most of these patients have used proprietary analgesics purchased at their local pharmacy before presenting to the medical profession for help. How many women with dysmenorrhoea and possibly endometriosis use regular analgesics is not known but the number is likely to be substantial.

The association between prostaglandins and dysmenorrhoea is long established, although its nature is less than clear. It has been shown that women with endometriosis have increased levels of prostaglandin $F_{2\alpha}$ ($PGF_{2\alpha}$) and PGE_2 in their endometrium [13]. It has also been shown that endometriotic ovarian tissue produces greater levels of PGF than healthy ovarian tissue [14]. One might therefore expect that prostaglandin synthetase inhibitors (PGSIs) might have a beneficial effect on endometriosis.

PGSIs are a heterogeneous group of non-steroidal anti-inflammatory agents that act mainly by inhibiting the production of prostaglandins though some (fenamates) also antagonize prostaglandins at the target level. There are a limited number of studies looking specifically at their use in endometriosis. Kauppila *et al.* [15] compared acetylsalicylic acid, indomethacin and tolfenamic acid with placebo. There was no difference in premenstrual complaints between the groups. During menstruation tolfenamic acid relieved endometriotic symptoms more effectively than placebo, while acetylsalicylic acid and indomethacin did not differ from placebo. In a later crossover study [16], they showed that naproxen sodium produced significantly more pain relief than placebo in patients with endometriosis.

There are no studies of the effect of PGSIs on fertility rates in humans with endometriosis. It would appear from the limited evidence available that some but not all PGSIs are effective in treating dysmenorrhoea associated with endometriosis.

It is likely that there are women with endometriosis who manage their symptoms successfully with self-administered PGSIs and do not present to their general practitioners or to gynaecologists. If patients whose symptoms do not respond to these simple treatments are those that present to gynaecologists, they are, perhaps, a selected group of poor responders and therefore it is not surprising that clinical trials with PGSIs do not show more positive results in these patients.

Endocrine modulation in endometriosis

Endometriosis is a hormone-dependent condition requiring ovarian steroids for its continued presence. It is not seen before menarche, is rare after the menopause and tends to regress during pregnancy. Endometriotic tissue can possess oestrogen, progestogen and androgen receptors, although these are in a lower concentration than seen in eutopic endometrium. The presence of receptors in endometriotic tissue, however, allows us to treat endometriosis by altering the sex steroid environment and it is this manipulation that has been the basis of medical management of the condition over the past 50 years.

Oestrogens and androgens

The first attempts to treat endometriosis by endocrine modulation involved the use of either oestrogens or androgens. Stilboestrol was the form of oestrogen used in the 1940s and effective pain relief was reported using high doses [17]. It was reputed to cause softening and atrophy of the lesions. Side-effects of thromboembolic disorders, hypertension, severe nausea and vomiting, however, make solitary oestrogen therapy unacceptable today. Methyltestosterone was another agent used in early attempts to treat endometriosis [18]. Again, claims were made for good pain relief, but virilizing side-effects, such as acne, deepening of the voice and hirsutism, make it currently unacceptable.

Oestrogens and progestogens

The beneficial effects of pregnancy on endometriosis was the basis of the 'pseudopregnancy' regimen advocated by Kistner [19]. He used varied oestrogen/progestogen combinations to mimic the hormonal effects of a normal pregnancy. Efficacy of treatment was assessed in terms of symptom relief and pelvic examination, and 'satisfactory' results were noted in 50 out of 58 patients. In the same paper, he also summarized other investigators' experience with pseudopregnancy regimens, finding a 'satisfactory' result in 98 out of 116 patients treated.

A more objective study of combined oestrogen/progesterone therapy randomized patients to treatment with enavid (mestranol 75 μg and norethynodrel 5 mg) or danazol for 6 months [20]. Twenty out of 23 patients treated with enavid experienced side-effects and seven patients failed to complete treatment because of serious side-effects. Only one patient in the danazol group stopped treatment. Danazol completely relieved or improved symptoms of pain in 20 out of 23 patients, while enavid only helped in five of 14 patients. Laparoscopy was performed in all patients 6 months after starting treatment. Twenty-three of the 27 patients treated with danazol were either cured or improved, while only six of 23 patients treated with enavid had any objective improvement. Overall, this high-dose combined therapy compared poorly with danazol.

Oestrogen/progesterone combinations are, of course, most commonly used in combined oral contraceptives (COCs). COCs are well known to reduce dysmenorrhoea in young women, but whether any of this effect is due to treatment of endometriosis is unknown. The effect of COCs on the presentation of endometriosis has been studied. Buttram [21] noted a trend in patients with endometriosis suggesting that, the longer the duration of COC use, the greater the chance of mild rather than severe endometriosis. Mahmood and Templeton [22], in a prospective study investigating the prevalence of endometriosis, noted that the total duration of COC use was significantly higher in subjects with a normal pelvis than in those with endometriosis. A recent review of the literature concluded that there was no consensus on a link between COC use and the risk of endometriosis [23].

There are few data on the use of modern low-dose COCs for treating endometriosis. Vercellini *et al.* [24] have recently reported on a randomized trial comparing goserelin, a GnRH agonist, with a cyclical low-dose COC in the treatment of pelvic pain associated with endometriosis. After 6 months' treatment, there was a significant reduction in dyspareunia in both groups, with goserelin being superior. Non-menstrual pain was diminished in both groups and women taking the COC experienced a significant reduction in dysmenorrhoea. There was a return of symptoms in the 6 months following treatment in most patients.

One area of COC use, which is often mentioned but rarely (if ever) objectively studied, is the use of COCs to prevent recurrence of endometriosis following treatment with danazol or a GnRH agonist. Given that the present generation of COCs are progestogen-dominant and appear safe for long-term use, many gynaecologists advocate their use for patients who have been treated for endometriosis who do not wish to conceive. COCs may be given either on the usual monthly cyclical basis or without a pill-free period for 2 or 3 months at a time. By reducing the number of menses per year, the rate of recurrence may be reduced and less frequent menstrual symptoms may be acceptable. Experience from contraceptive studies shows that, while there is an increasing incidence of breakthrough bleeding (BTB) with prolonged periods of COC use [25], this is generally acceptable to patients on a 49-day cycle but less so with a 91-day cycle [26–28]. It may be more acceptable to patients with endometriosis, though, who are spared monthly menstrual symptoms.

Preventing recurrence of endometriosis symptoms is an area of increasing importance and further studies are required in this field to assess the value of COCs as long-term therapy.

Progestogens

A range of progestogens have been used to treat endometriosis over the past 30 years. They have been given continuously, in periods ranging from 3 months to 2 years, or in cyclical regimens. The types used vary from progesterone derivatives, such as medroxyprogesterone acetate (MPA), to 19-nortestosterone derivatives, such as norethisterone or dienogest, or retroprogesterones, such as dydrogesterone.

Progestogens, regardless of their type, act in two ways. They have a direct effect on the implants. *In vitro* studies have shown that MPA exerts a significant antiproliferative effect on stromal cell preparations [29]. They also act by suppressing ovarian function. Telimaa *et al.* [30] studied the endocrine effect of a high dose of MPA – 100 mg daily – compared with placebo. They found normal gonadotrophin levels and low oestradiol and progesterone levels. They also found that this dose suppressed levels of sex-hormone-binding globulin (SHBG) and the free androgen index. The direct effect and the endocrine changes cause decidualization, initially followed by atrophy of the ectopic implants [31]. Cornillie *et al.* [32] looked at the histological and ultrastructural changes of ectopic endometrium during treatment with dydrogesterone. They found in four of 18 patients focal secretory transformation with decidualization, which they described as no response. In the remaining patients, the endometriotic implants were either undifferentiated or revealed features of involution. Total eradication of implants was never observed. Interestingly, a marked improvement in endometriosis symptoms and signs was found by Johnston [33], who treated 49 patients with low-dose dydrogesterone, 5 mg twice daily. On this dose, patients continued to have a regular cycle. Endocrine parameters were not measured and it was proposed that low-dose progestogens may act preferentially on ectopic endometrium, as at that dose no decidualization was noted in eutopic endometrium.

Treatment with progestogens is effective in relieving pain symptoms. In studies using MPA, 30 mg/day, symptomatic improvement was noted in all patients [31, 34]. In another study, Luciano *et al.* [35] using a higher dose of MPA – 50 mg/day – found improvement in 80% of patients who had mainly moderate to severe disease. In a placebo-controlled trial, Telimaa *et al.* [4] found that MPA 100 mg/day was as effective as danazol in reducing symptoms and was significantly better than placebo. Kohler *et al.* [36], using dienogest 2 mg/day, noted an 83% global improvement in all subjective symptoms. Schlaff *et al.* [37] found that 86% of patients treated with an adequate course of megestrol acetate noted an improvement in their symptoms.

Second-look laparoscopies have been used to assess response to treatment in several studies. Complete healing was noted in 15 of 22 patients treated with MPA, 30 mg/day for 90 days, with the remaining seven showing improvement [34]. In patients treated with dienogest, 2 mg/day for 6 months, 80% of patients showed a marked improvement, with complete resolution seen in 62% [36].

There are few controlled studies looking at the effect of progestogens on endometriosis-associated infertility. Hull *et al.* [38] reported a comparative controlled trial with expectant management, danazol and MPA 30 mg/day. Pregnancy rates after 30 months were 55%, 46% and 71%, respectively, a non-significant difference. Telimaa [39] in a similar study compared a placebo with danazol or MPA 100 mg/day and found no difference in the pregnancy rates – 46%, 33% and 42%, respectively. These studies show that medical treatment of endometriosis is not effective in treating infertility.

The main side-effect noted with continuous progestogens is irregular spotting or BTB. The incidence of BTB or spotting in patients treated with MPA in one study was 12% [34] but most studies show a higher incidence, ranging from 25% [35] to 67% [4]. Changing the dose of MPA does not seem to influence this. Schlaff *et al.* [37] found BTB in 12 of 29 patients treated with megestrol acetate. Other side-effects noted by patients included decreased libido [36], weight gain, oedema and bloating [4].

One concern with long-term use of progestogens is associated with changes in the lipid profile. The magnitude of these changes depends on the dose and type of progestogen used. Telimaa *et al.* [40] showed a 26% reduction in high-density lipoprotein cholesterol (HDL-C) in patients treated with 100 mg/day MPA. This compared with a 53% reduction in HDL-C in patients treated with danazol 600 mg/day. There was no change in low-density lipoprotein cholesterol (LDL-C), but a rise in lipoprotein A was noted. While theoretically increasing the risk of atheroma formation and cardiovascular disease, the clinical significance of these changes for periods of up to 1 year is unclear. Newer progestogens have fewer metabolic effects. Dienogest, whilst a 19-nortestosterone derivative, causes fewer changes in the lipid profile [36]. When used in a relatively low but effective dose, a small decrease in HDL-C and triglycerides was observed, along with a small rise in LDL-C. None of these changes were significant. No effect on carbohydrate metabolism has been noted with dienogest [41].

Progestogens have been used for many years now and still have an important role to play in the medical management of endometriosis in the 1990s. They are effective in reducing pain symptoms, they are relatively cheap, their metabolic side-effects are not profound, especially in low-dose regimens, and their side-effects, whilst common, are acceptable to many patients. The new generation of progestogens, currently to be found in the newer contraceptive pills, have potential as agents for long-term treatment of endometriosis as they have fewer metabolic side-effects. Their formal assessment in the treatment of endometriosis is awaited.

Danazol

Danazol was synthesized in the early 1960s and the first report of its use in endometriosis was in 1971 by Greenblatt *et al.* [42]. It was subsequently approved for use in 1976 and has become the most commonly prescribed drug for endometriosis worldwide. It is an isoxazol derivative of the synthetic steroid 17α-ethinyltestosterone. It is absorbed well by the gastrointestinal tract. An oral dose of 400 mg gives peak levels at 2 hours and is undetectable at 8 hours. The serum half-life is 4–5 hours and ideally it should be given at least three times a day. It is metabolized by the liver and over 60 metabolites have been identified by thin-layer chromatography [43]. Most of the metabolites are thought to be inactive, although the principal metabolite, 2-hydroxymethylethisterone, exhibited mild progestogenic and androgenic activities. Once metabolized, danazol is excreted equally in urine and faeces.

Mode of action

Danazol acts by a variety of mechanisms. It interacts with intracellular steroid receptors, enzymes of steroidogenesis and circulating steroid-binding hormones.

1 Danazol acts directly on intracellular steroid receptors. Steroid hormones bind to intranuclear steroid receptors and alter the rate of transcription of tissue-specific genes. Natural steroids tend to be very specific as to which type of receptor they bind to, whilst synthetic steroids such as danazol are less specific and can bind to different types of receptor. When a synthetic steroid binds to a receptor, it may act as an agonist, an antagonist or a mixed agonist–antagonist. Danazol has a high affinity for testosterone receptors and has an agonistic action there. It has a moderate affinity for progesterone and glucocorticoid receptors and has agonist–antagonist and agonist effects on them, respectively [44].

2 Danazol has a direct effect on steroidogenesis by competitively inhibiting multiple steroidogenic enzymes, including 20–22-desmolase, 3β-hydroxysteroid dehydrogenase, 17β-hydroxysteroid dehydrogenase, 17α-hydroxylase, 17–20-hydroxylase, 11-hydroxylase and 21-hydroxylase. Steingold *et al.* [45] demonstrated this effect *in vivo*. Women were given either human menopausal gonadotrophins (HMG) or HMG and danazol. Danazol produced a 50% decrease in the oestradiol response to HMG, demonstrating that it blocks the effects of gonadotrophins on the ovary by a direct action on the ovary.

3 Danazol binds to circulating steroid-binding proteins, causing displacement of testosterone from SHBG and cortisol from cortisol-binding globulin (CBG). The displacement of testosterone leads to an increase in the total amount of free testosterone in the circulation [46]. This effect is further compounded by danazol, as it reduces the production of SHBG by the liver, which in turn increases the amount of free testosterone in the circulation.

The overall effect of these various mechanisms is to create a hypo-oestrogenic, hyperandrogenic environment. It reduces ovarian production of oestrogen by inhibiting ovarian steroidogenesis. Danazol does not reduce the basal levels of the gonadotrophins in premenopausal women but does diminish the mid-cycle surge [47]. The combination of suppressed gonadotrophins and direct inhibition of ovarian steroidogenesis creates a relatively hypo-oestrogenic state, which inhibits the growth of endometriosis. The direct androgenic effect of danazol plus the increased levels of free testosterone cause atrophy of endometriotic implants.

A further mechanism of action for danazol has been suggested. The immune system plays a role in the pathophysiology of endometriosis, although the exact nature of this role is not clear. Danazol is known to cause clinical improvement in autoimmune conditions, such as idiopathic thrombocytopenic purpura [48] and systemic lupus erythematosus [49], associated with a fall in the levels of the appropriate autoantibodies. *In vitro*, danazol displays an immunosuppressive effect on macrophage-dependent T cell proliferation, similar to the effect of glucocorticoids. In one study where autoantibody levels were measured during treatment with danazol or GnRH agonists, there was a significant reduction in the total levels of immunoglobulin G (IgG), IgM and IgA in the danazol group [50]. This group also had a reduction in the number of autoantibodies at the end of treatment. The effect of danazol on immunoregulation has not been fully established, nor has the importance of this aspect of danazol's activity in the treatment of endometriosis.

Side-effects

The symptomatic side-effects of danazol are mainly related to the hyperandrogenic state that it creates. The incidence of side-effects is dose-dependent and they include weight gain, muscle cramps, oily skin, acne and hirsutism [51]. Deepening of the voice is an uncommon side-effect but of importance as it appears to be irreversible [52]. Other side-effects are hypo-oestrogenic, such as decreased libido, decreased breast size and hot flushes.

Danazol has several metabolic side-effects. It alters the levels of blood lipoproteins, decreasing high-density lipoproteins (HDL) and increasing low-density lipoproteins (LDL) [40, 53]. These changes are reversible on stopping danazol. However, they are potentially atherogenic and theoretically increase the risk of heart disease. The risk is thought to be minimal with 6 months' treatment but may be significant with longer courses of treatment. Danazol should not be used in patients with hyperlipidaemia. Danazol also effects carbohydrate metabolism, causing a rise in insulin and glucagon levels [54]. It also causes a rise in lean tissue mass independent of the rise in free testosterone [55].

Clinical effect

The effect of danazol therapy on endometriotic implants, pain and endometriosis-related infertility has been studied.

The effect of treatment on implants can be assessed by means of second-look laparoscopy, although, as has been pointed out in the introduction to this chapter, the timing of the second-look laparoscopy is critical to the apparent results [9]. The visual appearance of treated endometriosis depends on whether laparoscopy is performed during ovarian suppression with danazol or after the resumption of cyclical menses. In the majority of studies of danazol, second-look laparoscopy has been performed during ovarian suppression.

The clinical effect of danazol is dose-dependent. Dose-finding studies suggest that at least 400 mg/day is needed [56] and that higher doses are needed in severe disease [57]. Dmowski and Cohen [58] found complete resolution of disease in patients with mild endometriosis after treatment with 800 mg danazol daily for 6 months. There was no effect on adhesions.

Danazol is very effective at relieving endometriosis-related pain symptoms. A recent review of the effect of danazol on pain has shown that it is most effective in the treatment of dysmenorrhoea, with over 90% of patients noting complete resolution or improvement of their symptoms [11]. It is less effective in the treatment of dyspareunia and pelvic pain, possibly reflecting that these symptoms more commonly result from adhesions and scarring.

Symptom recurrence after stopping treatment with danazol occurs in up to 51% of patients, depending on the dose used, lower doses being associated with higher recurrence rates [11, 57].

Many early studies reported respectable pregnancy rates following danazol treatment of endometriosis-related infertility. However, when prospective, randomized, placebo-controlled studies were performed, the results showed no beneficial effect for danazol. Siebel *et al.* [59] reported on patients who were randomized to receive either danazol for 6 months or no treatment. Thirty per cent of the danazol-treated patients conceived after treatment, compared with 50% of the untreated group, within 6 months of observation. Telimaa [39] found similar results in his study, confirming the view that medical treatment on its own is inappropriate treatment for endometriosis-related infertility.

Gestrinone

Gestrinone is a steroid derived from 19-nortestosterone. It was initially developed as an oral contraceptive; however, its interactions with various steroid receptors suggested a possible use in the treatment of endometriosis. In the human, gestrinone acts as an androgen, a progestogen and an anti-progestogen. It reduces the plasma concentration of SHBG, which causes a lowering of total plasma testosterone concentration but an increase in free plasma testosterone [60]. A similar effect occurs with danazol. There is no consistent lowering of luteinizing hormone (LH) concentration but the mid-cycle surge of LH is obliterated. In a placebo-controlled study, plasma oestradiol concentration was significantly lower in patients treated with gestrinone 2.5 mg twice weekly, compared with the placebo group, the levels in the treated group being comparable to those seen in the early follicular stage of the menstrual cycle [5].

The effect of gestrinone on eutopic and ectopic endometrium has been studied. In one study, endometrial samples were obtained before and after 3 and 6 months of treatment with either gestrinone 5.0 mg/week or danazol 600 mg/day [61]. At 3 months the endometria of the women treated with danazol were more atrophic than those of the women who received gestrinone. At 6 months marked endometrial atrophy was observed in all samples. Another study looked at the histological appearance of endometriotic tissue before and after treatment with gestrinone 1.25 mg/day for 2 months [62]. Cornillie *et al.* [62] found differentiated lesions in only one of 13 women following treatment and implant involution could be seen in 11 of 13 biopsies. The American Fertility Society (AFS) staging score was not significantly reduced following treatment but this might have been different had a longer course of treatment been used.

Gestrinone is administered orally in doses of 2.5–10 mg weekly on a daily, twice weekly or three times weekly schedule. The clinical effect is to suppress ovulation, which results in amenorrhoea or oligomenorrhoea. The side-effects of gestrinone are androgenic and antioestrogenic in nature, the most common being seborrhoea, acne, weight gain and breast hypotrophy. One study, which looked at vaginal administration of gestrinone, showed fewer androgenic side-effects but no difference in the efficacy of treatment [63].

Gestrinone has been found to be significantly better than placebo in terms of reducing implant size, as scored by the AFS system [5]. Two studies have compared dose regimens of 1.25 mg twice weekly with 2.5 mg twice weekly [64, 65]. Both studies assessed the effect of treatment by laparoscopy before and at the end of treatment, and found that both doses were equally effective in reducing the AFS score.

Gestrinone 2.5–5 mg twice a week orally for 6 months, in uncontrolled trials gave excellent resolution of endometriosis-related pain symptoms. In a comparative study of gestrinone 5–7.5 mg/week with danazol 600 mg/day for 6 months, there was no difference between the two groups with regard to improvement in pain scores while on treatment [66]. There was a similar reduction in endometriosis scores in the subgroup who had second laparoscopies. Pain symptoms recurred during the 18-month follow-up period in 57% of the patients treated with gestrinone and 53% of the patients treated with danazol. The cumulative pregnancy rate was 33% in the patients treated with gestrinone and 40% in those treated with danazol. Side-effects were more frequent and severe with the danazol group. This study concluded that gestrinone was as effective as danazol but was better tolerated.

There is only one placebo-controlled study assessing the value of gestrinone in the management of endometriosis-associated infertility. Patients were treated with either placebo or gestrinone 2.5 mg orally twice weekly for 24 weeks [67]. Cumulative pregnancy rates 12 months after the end of treatment were 25% for the gestrinone group and 24% for the placebo group. Furthermore, there was no difference in the pregnancy rates between patients in either arm of the study who had complete remission of their disease at the second laparoscopy and those who had residual disease.

Gestrinone would appear to be an effective treatment for endometriosis when given for 6 months. The symptom recurrence rate of 57% after 12 months of treatment [66] is in keeping with other medical treatments, again emphasizing the fact that medical treatment results in regression but not disappearance of endometriotic foci. Treatment is limited to 6 months because of asymptomatic side-effects. The principal concern with long-term use of gestrinone is the atherogenic effect on the lipid profile. One study has looked at the effect of 1.25 mg or 2.5 mg twice weekly on both the lipid profile and bone density [65]. No significant difference was noted between the different dose regimens. In both groups, the plasma concentrations of LDL rose by 13% and those of HDL fell by 40%, both changes being potentially adverse in terms of cardiovascular risk. These changes are similar to those seen with danazol. There was no significant change in bone density in either the lumbar spine or the proximal femur with treatment. Another study showed similar changes in the lipid profile but noted a dose-dependent effect when higher doses of gestrinone (5 and 10 mg/week) were given [68].

RU486 (mifepristone)

RU486 (mifepristone) is a steroidal antiprogesterone with antiglucocorticoid and antioestrogenic properties. It has a fourfold higher affinity for progesterone receptors than progesterone itself and has a much longer half-life than progesterone. These characteristics make it a potential treatment for endometriosis. One prospective study has looked at the effect of RU486 in patients with pelvic endometriosis [69]. Six patients with cyclical pelvic pain due to endometriosis were treated with RU486 100 mg/day for 3 months. All women became amenorrhoeic. LH levels increased on treatment but there was no change in follicle-stimulating hormone (FSH). Ovarian steroid levels did not change during treatment, oestradiol levels remaining in the follicular range. An increase in serum cortisol and adrenocorticotrophic hormone (ACTH) was noted, reflecting the antiglucocorticoid effect of RU486. Treatment resulted in an improvement in pelvic pain in all subjects. Follow-up laparoscopy was performed in five of the six patients. Endometriotic implants had resolved in one subject and persisted in all others. Side-effects reported included anorexia, nausea and fatigue in one patient. Three patients reported hot flushes during the first 8 weeks of treatment. In another study, the effect of a higher dose of RU486 on experimentally induced endometriosis implants in rats was observed [70]. No difference in implant size was noted between treated groups and control groups with up to 8 weeks' treatment. Both of these studies showed no effect of RU486 on size of implant; however, despite this, symptom relief was good in the human study. The mechanism of the pain relief in this situation is not clear but is probably not due to a direct effect on the endometriosis. Further studies are required to establish whether RU486 has a role in the treatment of endometriosis. Lower doses may avoid the antiglucocorticoid effect of RU486, whilst longer courses of treatment may result in regression of the implants.

Tamoxifen

Tamoxifen is a non-steroidal antioestrogen capable of antagonizing many of the actions of oestrogen. There is long-term nuclear retention of the tamoxifen–receptor complex, which, by suppressing oestrogen receptor production, causes oestrogen antagonism after an initial oestrogen-like response [71]. Tamoxifen is commonly used in the treatment of hormone-dependent breast cancer. Premenopausal women, who are given tamoxifen long-term, do not have suppression of their menstrual cycle and their mean mid-cycle oestradiol levels are higher than in non-treatment cycles [72]. They have mid-luteal progesterone levels suggestive of ovulation.

A single report has looked at the effect of tamoxifen on two patients with recurrent endometriosis after treatment with danazol [73]. Both were given tamoxifen 10 mg twice daily for 6 months. Both reported improvement in their symptoms, and laparoscopic assessment at the end of treatment showed 'an occasional trace of inactive endometriosis' only. Both patients complained of hot flushes in the early part of treatment. Other side-effects were fatigue, constipation and acne. Both noted their side-effects to be less pronounced than during their treatment with danazol. Neither patient became pregnant.

It would therefore appear that tamoxifen can cause regression of endometriosis without affecting ovulation. Theoretically, it should be possible to use tamoxifen for treatment of endometriosis in women with pain and infertility. This potential to conceive whilst on treatment raises the problem of the teratogenicity of tamoxifen. Animal data suggest that reproductive tract anomalies might occur but the human data are too limited at present to assess its teratogenic potential [74]. Further studies are required to establish whether tamoxifen has a role in the treatment of endometriosis.

Conclusion

Medical treatment has an important role to play in the management of endometriosis. Progestogens, danazol and gestrinone are all established treatments and effective in the management of endometriosis-related dysmenorrhoea, dyspareunia and pelvic pain. As there is little to choose between them in terms of efficacy, the choice between them should be based on the side-effect profile, patient choice and cost. Placebo-controlled trials have shown no benefit from their use in treating infertility.

It should be emphasized that medical treatment leads to regression rather than elimination. Pain symptoms recur in a large proportion of patients after stopping all forms of medical therapy. At present, treatment is given for a finite period because of the potential harm from metabolic side-effects. Future research needs to address long-term medical treatment with a view to finding therapies which are both effective at controlling symptoms and acceptable in terms of symptomatic and metabolic side-effects.

References

1 Redwine DB. The distribution of endometriosis in the pelvis by age groups and fertility. *Fertil Steril* 1987 **47**: 173–175.

2 Murphy AA, Green WR, Bobby D, de la Cruz ZC, Rock JA. Unsuspected endometriosis documented by scanning electron microscopy in visually normal peritoneum. *Fertil Steril* 1986 **46**: 522–524.

3 Redwine RB. Is 'microscopic' peritoneal endometriosis invisible? *Fertil Steril* 1988 **50**: 665–666.

4 Telimaa S, Puolakka J, Ronnberg L, Kauppila A. Placebo-controlled comparison of danazol and high-dose medroxyprogesterone acetate in the treatment of endometriosis. *Gynecol Endocrinol* 1987 **1**: 13–23.

5 Thomas EJ, Cooke ID. Impact of gestrinone on the course of asymptomatic endometriosis. *Br Med J* 1987 **294**: 272–274.

6 Dlugi AM, Miller JD, Knittle J, Lupron Study Group. Lupron depot (leuprolide acetate for depot suspension) in the treatment of endometriosis: a randomised, placebo-controlled, double blind study. *Fertil Steril* 1990 **54**: 419–427.
7 Fedele L, Bianchi S, Bocciolone L, Di Nola G, Franchi D. Buserelin acetate in the treatment of pelvic pain associated with minimal and mild endometriosis: a controlled study. *Fertil Steril* 1993 **59**: 516–521.
8 American Fertility Society. Revised American Fertility Society classification of endometriosis: 1985. *Fertil Steril* 1985 **43**: 351–352.
9 Evers JLH. The second-look laparoscopy for evaluation of the result of medical treatment of endometriosis should not be performed during ovarian suppression. *Fertil Steril* 1987 **47**: 502–504.
10 Waller KG, Shaw RW. Gonadotropin-releasing hormone analogues for the treatment of endometriosis: long-term follow-up. *Fertil Steril* 1993 **59**: 511–515.
11 Bayer SR, Seibel MM. Medical treatment: danazol. In: Schenken RS (ed.). *Endometriosis: Contemporary Concepts in Clinical Management*, 1989, p. 179. Philadelphia, JB Lippincott.
12 Dorberl A, Bergqvist A, Jeppsson S. *et al.* Regression of endometriosis following shorter treatment with, or lower dose of danazol. *Act Obstet Gynecol Scand Suppl* 1984 **123**: 51–58.
13 Williams EA, Collins VP, Clayton SG. Studies in the involvement of prostaglandins in uterine symptomatology and pathology. *Br J Obstet Gynaecol* 1976 **83**: 337–341.
14 Pickles WR, Hall WJ, Best FA, Smith GN. Prostaglandins in endometrium and menstrual fluid from normal and dysmenorrheic subjects. *J Obstet Gynaecol Br Commonwealth* 1965 **72**: 185–192.
15 Kauppila A, Poulakka J, Ylikorkala O. Prostaglandin biosynthesis inhibitors and endometriosis. *Prostaglandins* 1979 **18**: 655–661.
16 Kauppila A, Rönnberg L. Naproxen sodium in dysmenorrhoea secondary to endometriosis. *Obstet Gynecol* 1985 **65**: 379–383.
17 Karnaky KJ. The use of stilbestrol for endometriosis. *South Med J* 1948 **41**: 1109– 1111.
18 Hamblen EC. Androgen treatment of women. *South Med J* 1957 **50**: 743–745.
19 Kistner RW. The treatment of endometriosis by inducing pseudopregnancy with ovarian hormones. *Fertil Steril* 1959 **10**: 539–556.
20 Noble AD, Letchworth AT. Treatment of endometriosis: a study of medical management. *Br J Obstet Gynaecol* 1980 **87**: 726–728.
21 Buttram VC. Cyclic use of combination oral contraceptives and the severity of endometriosis. *Fertil Steril* 1979 **31**: 347–348.
22 Mahmood TA, Templeton A. Prevalence and genesis of endometriosis. *Hum Reprod* 1991 **6**: 544–549.
23 Vercellini P, Ragni G, Trespid L, Oldani S, Crosignani PG. Does contraception modify the risk of endometriosis? *Human Reprod* 1993 **8**: 547–551.
24 Vercellini P, Trespidi L, Colombo A *et al.* A gonadotropin-releasing hormone agonist versus a low-dose oral contraceptive for pelvic pain associated with endometriosis. *Fertil Steril* 1993 **60**: 75–79.
25 Loudon NB, Foxwell M, Potts DM, Guild AL, Short RV. Acceptability of an oral contraceptive that reduces the frequency of menstruation: the tri-cycle pill regimen. *Br Med J* 1977 **2**: 487–490.
26 Kornaat H, Geerdink MH, Klitsie JW. The acceptance of a 7-week cycle with a modern low-dose oral contraceptive (Minulet). *Contraception* 1993 **45**: 119–127.
27 de Voogd WS. Postponement of withdrawal bleeding with a monphasic oral contraceptive containing desogestrel and ethinylestradiol. *Contraception* 1991 **44**: 107–112.
28 Kovacs GT, Rusden J, Evans A. A trimonthly regimen for oral contraceptives. *Br J Fam Plan* 1994 **19**: 274–275.

29 Surrey ES, Halme J. Direct effects of medroxyprogesterone acetate, danazol, and leuprolide acetate on endometrial stromal cell proliferation in vitro. *Fertil Steril* 1992 **58**: 273–278.

30 Telimaa S, Apter D, Reinila M, Ronnberg L, Kauppila A. Placebo-controlled comparison of hormonal and biochemical effects of danazol and high-dose medroxyprogesterone acetate. *Eur J Obstet Gynecol Reprod Biol* 1990 **36**: 97–105.

31 Moghissi KS, Boyce CR. Management of endometriosis with oral medroxyprogesterone acetate. *Obstet Gynecol* 1976 **47**: 265–267.

32 Cornillie FJ, Puttemans P, Brosens IA. Histology and ultrastructure of human endometriotic tissues treated with dydrosgesterone (Duphaston). *Eur J Obstet Gynecol Reprod Biol* 1987 **26**: 39–55.

33 Johnston WIH. Dydrogesterone and endometriosis. *Br J Obstet Gynaecol* 1976 **83**: 77–80.

34 Roland M, Leisten D, Kane R. Endometriosis therapy with medroxyprogesterone acetate. *J Reprod Med* 1976 **17**: 249–252.

35 Luciano AA, Turksoy RN, Carleo J. Evaluation of oral medroxyprogesterone acetate in the treatment of endometriosis. *Obstet Gynecol* 1988 **72**: 323–327.

36 Kohler G, Goretzlehner G, Brachmann K. Lipid metabolism during treatment of endometriosis with the progestin dienogest. *Acta Obstet Gynecol Scand* 1989 **68**: 633–635.

37 Schlaff WD, Dugoff L, Damewood MD, Rock JA. Megestrol acetate for treatment of endometriosis. *Obstet Gynecol* 1990 **75**: 646–648.

38 Hull ME, Moghissi KS, Maygar DF, Hayes MF. Comparison of different treatment modalities of endometriosis in infertile women. *Fertil Steril* 1987 **47**: 40–44.

39 Telimaa S. Danazol and medroxyprogesterone acetate inefficacious in the treatment of infertility in endometriosis. *Fertil Steril* 1988 **50**: 872–875.

40 Telimaa S, Penttila I, Puolakka J, Ronnberg L, Kauppila A. Circulating lipid and lipoprotein concentration during danazol and high-dose medroxyprogesterone acetate therapy of endometriosis. *Fertil Steril* 1989 **52**: 31–35.

41 Nikschick S, Kohler G, Mannchen E. Carbohydrate metabolism during treatment of endometriosis with the progestin dienogest. *Exp Clin Endocrinol* 1989 **94**: 211–214.

42 Greenblatt RB, Dmowski WP, Mahesh VB, Scholer HFL. Clinical studies with an antigonadotropin, danazol. *Fertil Steril* 1971 **22**: 102–112.

43 Davison C, Banks W, Fritz A. The absorption, distribution, and metabolic rate of danazol in rats, monkeys, and human volunteers. *Arch Int Pharmacodyn Ther* 1976 **221**: 294–298.

44 Barbieri RL, Lee H, Ryan KJ. Danazol binding to rat androgen, glucocorticoid, progesterone and estrogen receptors: correlation with biological activity. *Fertil Steril* 1979 **31**: 182–186.

45 Steingold KA, Lu JKH, Judd HL, Meldrum DR. Danazol inhibits steroidogenesis by the human ovary *in vivo*. *Fertil Steril* 1986 **45**: 649–654.

46 Nilsson B, Sodergard R, Damber MG, Damber JE, Von Schouler B. Free testosterone levels during danazol therapy. *Fertil Steril* 1983 **39**: 505–509.

47 Wood GP, Wu CH, Flickinger GL, Mikhail G. Hormonal changes associated with danazol therapy. *Obstet Gynecol* 1975 **45**: 302.

48 Ahn YS, Harrington WJ, Simon SR *et al.* Danazol for the treatment of idiopathic thrombocytopenic purpura. *N Engl J Med* 1983 **308**: 1396–1399.

49 Agnello V, Pariser K, Gell J, Gelfand J, Turksoy RN. Preliminary observations on danazol therapy of systemic lupus erythematosus: effects on antibodies, thrombocytopenia and complement. *J Rheumatol* 1983 **10**: 682–687.

50 El-Roeiy A, Dmowski WP, Gleicher N *et al.* Danazol but not gonadotropin-releasing hormone agonists suppresses autoantibodies in endometriosis. *Fertil Steril* 1988 **50**: 864–868.

51 Shaw RW. An open randomised comparative study of the effect of goserelin depot and danazol in the treatment of endometriosis. *Fertil Steril* 1992 **58**: 265–272.

52 Boothroyd CV, Lepre F. Permanent voice change resulting from danazol therapy. *Aust NZ J Obstet Gynaecol* 1990 **30**: 275–276.

53 Valimaki M, Nilsson CG, Roine R, Ylikorkala O. Comparison between the effects of nafarelin and danazol on serum lipids and lipoproteins in patients with endometriosis. *J Clin Endocrin Metab* 1989 **69**: 1097–1103.

54 Bruce R, Godsland I, Stevenson J *et al.* Danazol induces resistance to both insulin and glucagon in young women. *Clin Sci* 1992 **82**: 211–217.

55 Bruce R, Lees B, Whitcroft SI. Changes in body composition with danazol therapy. *Fertil Steril* 1991 **56**: 574–576.

56 Dmowksi WP, Kaperawakis E, Scommegna A. Variable effects of danazol on endometriosis at 4 low dose levels. *Obstet Gynecol* 1982 **59**: 408–415.

57 Moore EE, Harger JH, Rock JA, Archer DF. Management of pelvic endometriosis with low dose danazol. *Fertil Steril* 1981 **36**: 15–20.

58 Dmowski WP, Cohen MR. Treatment of endometriosis with an antigonadotropin, danazol: a laparoscopic and histologic evaluation. *Obstet Gynecol* 1975 **46**: 147–154.

59 Siebel MM, Berger MJ, Weinstein FG, Taymor ML. The effectiveness of danazol on subsequent fertility in minimal endometriosis. *Fertil Steril* 1982 **38**: 534–537.

60 Venturini PL, Bertolini S, Brunengi MCM. Endocrine metabolic and clinical effects of gestrinone in women with endometriosis. *Fertil Steril* 1989 **52**: 589–599.

61 Marchini M, Fedele L, Bianchi S *et al.* Endometrial patterns during therapy with danazol or gestrinone for endometriosis: structural and ultrastructural study. *Hum Pathol* 1992 **23**: 51–56.

62 Cornillie FJ, Brosens IA, Vasquez G, Riphagen I. Histologic and ultrastructural changes in human endometriotic implants treated with the antiprogesterone steroid ethylnorgestrienone (gestrinone) during 2 months. *Int J Gynaecol Pathol* 1986 **5**: 95–109.

63 Coutinho EM, Azadian-Boulanger G. Treatment of endometriosis by vaginal administration of gestrinone. *Fertil Steril* 1988 **49**: 418–422.

64 Hornstein MD, Gleason RE, Barbieri RL. A randomized double-blind prospective trial of two doses of gestrinone in the treatment of endometriosis. *Fertil Steril* 1990 **53**: 237–241.

65 Worthington M, Irvine LM, Crook D *et al.* A randomized comparative study of the metabolic effects of two regimens of gestrinone in the treatment of endometriosis. *Fertil Steril* 1993 **59**: 522–526.

66 Fedele L, Bianchi S, Viezzoli T, Arcaini L, Candiani GB. Gestrinone versus danazol in the treatment of endometriosis. *Fertil Steril* 1989 **51**: 781–785.

67 Thomas EJ, Cooke ID. Successful treatment of asymptomatic endometriosis: does it benefit infertile women? *Br Med J* 1987 **294**: 1117–1119.

68 Fukuda Y, Tamura S, Hatanaka S. Effects of gestrinone on serum lipid and lipoprotein levels in women with endometriosis [in Japanese]. *Nippon Sanka Fujinka Gakkai Zasshi – Acta Obstet Gynaecol Japonica* 1989 **41**: 577–584.

69 Kettel LM, Murphy AA, Mortola JF *et al.* Endocrine responses to long-term administration of the antiprogesterone RU486 in patients with pelvic endometriosis. *Fertil Steril* 1991 **56**: 402–407.

70 Tjaden B, Galetto D, Woodruff JD, Rock JA. Time-related effects of RU486 treatment in experimentally induced endometriosis in the rat. *Fertil Steril* 1993 **59**: 437–440.

71 Kokko E, Janne O, Kauppila A, Vihko R. Effects of tamoxifen, medroxyprogesterone acetate, and their combination on human endometrial estrogen and progestin receptor concentrations, 17-hydroxysteroid dehydrogenase activity and serum hormone concentrations. *Am J Obstet Gynecol* 1982 **143**: 382–388.

72 Jordan VC, Fritz NF, Langan Fahey S, Thompson M, Tormey DC. Alteration of endocrine parameters in premenopausal women with breast cancer during longterm adjuvant therapy with tamoxifen as the single agent. *J Nat Cancer Inst* 1991 **83**: 1488–1491.
73 Haber GM, Behelak YF. Preliminary report on the use of tamoxifen in the treatment of endometriosis. *Am J Obstet Gynecol* 1987 **156**: 582–586.
74 Taguchi O, Nishizuka Y. Reproductive tract abnormalities in female mice treated neonatally with tamoxifen. *Am J Obstet Gynecol* 1985 **151**: 675–678.

Chapter 11
Evaluation of Treatment with Gonadotrophin-releasing Hormone Analogues

R.W. SHAW

Introduction

Endometriosis has its peak incidence between 30 and 45 years of age and is dependent for its continued growth and development upon normal ovarian function and oestrogen synthesis. The treatment of endometriosis very much depends upon the extent and site of the disease process, the current severity and range of symptoms, the patient's future childbearing expectations, her age and whether this was an initial or recurrent diagnosis. Thus treatment needs to be tailored to each individual's needs.

Medical treatments have an advantage over a primarily surgical approach in that they can be administered on a number of occasions and do not require the patient to be put at risk by the surgical intervention. There are a number of endocrine and pharmacological approaches currently utilized, which include continuous combined oral contraceptive preparations; progestogens; danazol; gestrinone and non-steroidal anti-inflammatory agents. Although these different drugs have been proved to be efficacious to varying degrees, they are associated with side-effects of variable degrees of severity. In some individuals, the severity of side-effects proves intolerable, such that the patients fail to complete the prescribed course of therapy. For these reasons, new, and hopefully more effective, treatment approaches are continually being sought. One of the most recent approaches has been the introduction of the gonadotrophin-releasing hormone analogues (GnRH-A).

For many years surgical oophorectomy has been thought to be the most effective overall treatment for endometriosis. This treatment, however, is usually reserved as the final resort in patients who no longer contemplate further pregnancies. A reversible means of achieving a 'pharmacological medical oophorectomy' would perhaps offer many advantages in younger women with significant symptoms from their endometriosis. Such an approach has been made possible by the repetitive administration of GnRH-A. Their continued administration results in desensitization or down-regulation of the pituitary GnRH receptor, with a resultant reduction in circulating serum gonadotrophin concentrations and a secondary inhibition of ovarian steroidogenesis. This potential for reversibly inducing a state of hypogonadotrophic hypogonadism has made these drugs ideal candidates in the treatment of a number of gynaecological disorders, including endometriosis, and the results of clinical trials utilizing these agents in this disorder will now be reviewed.

Structure and mode of action of GnRH analogues

Mode of action of GnRH

The structure of the hypothalamic releasing hormone (GnRH), a decapeptide which controls luteinizing hormone (LH) and follicle-stimulating hormone (FSH) synthesis and release from the pituitary, was identified in 1971 [1]. Shortly afterwards, a synthetic GnRH became available for use in physiological and clinical investigations. As a result of these studies, the mechanisms by which GnRH stimulates the release of LH and FSH from the pituitary gonadotrophes became elucidated. These data indicated that the intracellular pathways through which the GnRH stimulates biosynthesis and secretion of LH and FSH is receptor-mediated and calcium-dependent. A variety of pathways of intracellular signalling have been implicated and the ovarian steroids oestrogen and progesterone further modulate gonadotrophe sensitivity to GnRH throughout the menstrual cycle, whilst GnRH can itself have a 'self-augmenting' effect. Our current understanding of the mechanism of action of GnRH is shown in Fig. 11.1 [2] and has been reviewed recently in detail by Clayton [3] and Kiesel and Runnebaum [4].

Structure of the GnRH analogues

The native hypothalamic GnRH has a relatively short half-life when administered intravenously or subcutaneously. The half-life ($t_{1/2}$) of GnRH is 3.5 min. To try and utilize GnRH in a number of clinical situations, it became necessary to develop analogues of GnRH which had more prolonged half-lifes. Many hundreds of GnRH-A have been synthesized and these can be considered to fall into two main groups: those which are basically agonistic (stimulatory) analogues when initially given, and those that are antagonists with immediate block of receptor function. The agonistic analogues have progressed more rapidly towards introduction into clinical practice because the antagonists have induced local side-effects at the site of injection. The experimental data on agonistic analogues demonstrated that replacement of amino acids, particularly in position 6 and 10 of the native GnRH decapeptide molecule, resulted in a series of superactive agonistic analogues with a reduced susceptibility to degradation by pituitary enzymes and hence a prolonged therapeutic half-life and duration of action – half-lives of 2–5 hours. In addition, the analogues demonstrated high binding affinity for the GnRH receptor (Table 11.1).

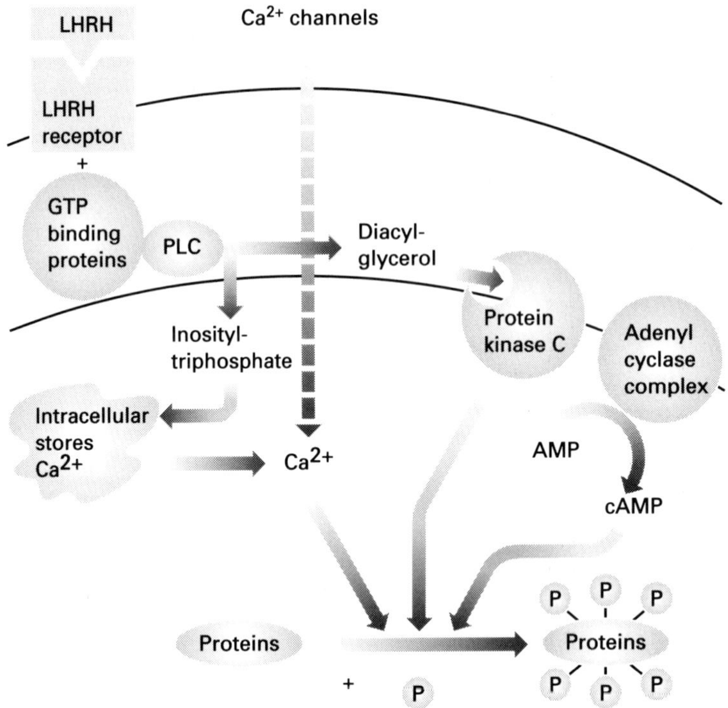

Fig. 11.1 Schematic representation of GnRH (LHRH) mechanism of action at pituitary gonadotrophe. GTP, guanosine triphosphate; PLC, phospholipase C; AMP, adenosine monophosphate; P, phosphate group; cAMP, cyclic AMP; Ca^{++}, calcium ion. Redrawn from [2] with permission.

Gonadotrophin changes following administration of GnRH-A

The physiological function of the pituitary gonadotrophe is normally dependent on pulsatile stimulation by hypothalamic GnRH at roughly 90-min intervals. Excess GnRH receptors are present on the pituitary cell surface which retain the cell's potential to respond to the next GnRH pulse whilst new receptors are being processed. The above process allows an orderly and systematic secretion of gonadotrophins in response to each GnRH pulse. However, administration of GnRH in a continuous fashion results in a very marked reduction in gonadotroph responsiveness, subsequent reduction in LH and FSH synthesis and release and a resultant suppression of gonadal function [5].

When agonistic GnRH-A are administered in the pharmacological doses used clinically, the majority of the GnRH receptors become rapidly occupied and subsequently internalized. This initially results in a supraphysiological release of LH and FSH with an associated response from the gonadotrophin

Table 11.1 Amino acid sequence of native GnRH and the major agonistic analogues used in the treatment of endometriosis

	1	2	3	4	5	6	7	8	9	10
Native GnRH	pGlu	His	Trp	Ser	Tyr	Gly	Leu	Arg	Pro	Gly-NH_2
Nonapeptide analogues										
Histrelin						D-His(Imbzl)			Pro-NEt	
Leuprolerin						D-Leu			Pro-NEt	
Buserelin						D-Ser(Bu^t)			Pro-NEt	
Decapeptide analogues										
Tryptorelin						D-Trp				
Nafarelin						$(D\text{-}Nal)_2$				
Goserelin						D-Ser(Bu^t)				Aza-Gly-NH_2

target cells and increased steroid production. A single administration of a GnRH-A therefore results in increased levels of FSH and LH above baseline for 24 hours.

Continued exposure of the gonadotrophe to the analogue results in an inability to replenish the GnRH receptors, with a gradual loss of available receptors on the surface. The pituitary cells thus have few receptors available to respond either to endogenous GnRH or to GnRH agonist. This results in a gradual reduction of LH and FSH secretion and synthesis (and a secondary suppression of ovarian gonadal steroid hormone production), with levels falling below baseline by 7–10 days.

The immediate endocrine changes seen at commencement of a GnRH-A, either in the mid-luteal phase, day 22 of the cycle, during administration of buserelin (intranasally) or on day 1 of the menstrual cycle following administration of a depot preparation of goserelin (3.6 mg), are shown in Figs 11.2 and 11.3 [6]. In both instances, an initial agonist-induced release of LH and FSH is apparent but this is rapidly followed by a subsequent reduction in gonadotrophin and steroid levels from 2–3 days after commencement of GnRH-A, down to low levels of LH and FSH. Oestradiol falls to within the menopausal range and progesterone is maintained at low levels throughout the continued administration of the drugs. These suppressed levels of gonad-

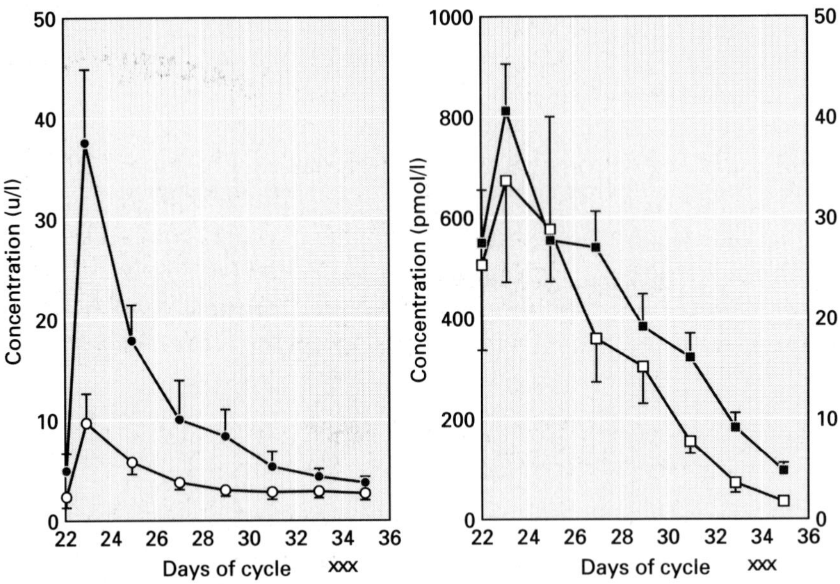

Fig. 11.2 Initial 'agonist' effect followed by 'down-regulation' following intranasal buserelin 100 μg five times daily in 16 normal women commencing therapy in the mid-luteal phase of the cycle. Menstruation was delayed by between 5 and 8 days. Black circles, luteinizing hormone; open circles, follicular stimulating hormone; black squares, oestradiol-17β (pmol/l); open squares, progesterone (nmol/l). Redrawn from [6] with permission.

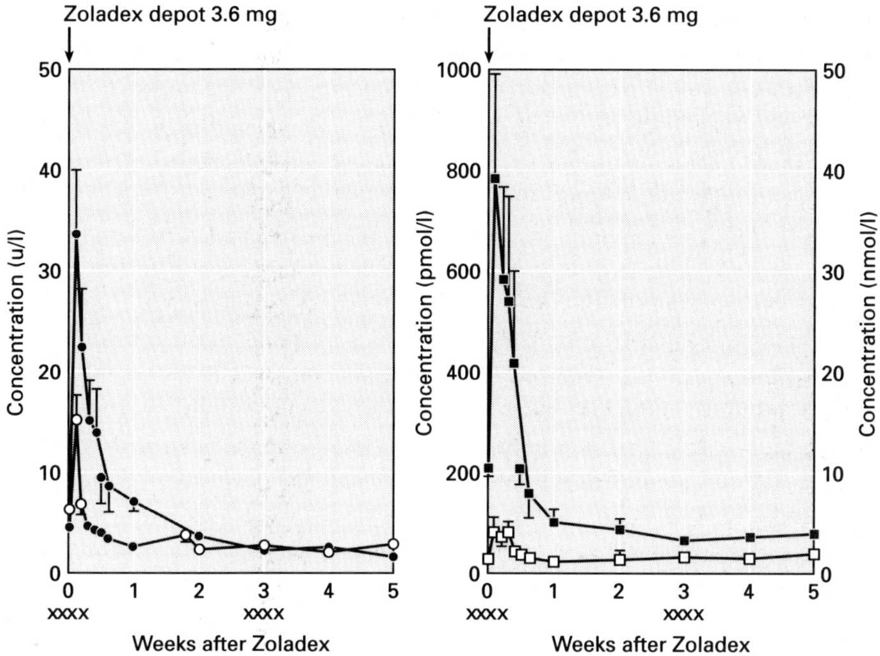

Fig. 11.3 'Agonist' initial increase in LH and FSH followed by reduced circulating levels when 'desensitization' of pituitary had occurred following administration of a goserelin (Zoladex) 3.6 mg depot on day 1 of the menstrual cycle in eight women. A menstrual bleed commonly occurs between 15 and 22 days after first depot injection only. Black circles, luteinizing hormone; open circles, follicular stimulating hormone; black squares, oestradiol-17β (pmol/l); open squares, progesterone (nmol/l). Redrawn from [6] with permission.

otrophins and ovarian steroids can be maintained for prolonged periods of time. The changes are readily reversible following removal of the GnRH-A from the circulation. Continued administration of GnRH-A thus achieves a reversible and marked suppression of the pituitary–ovarian axis with resultant hypogonadotrophic hypogonadism, which can be used endocrinologically in the treatment of a number of benign gynaecological conditions.

Other endocrine changes associated with GnRH-A administration

The suppression of ovarian function during GnRH-A administration results in levels of oestradiol within the postmenopausal range and levels of progesterone that are anovulatory, but also reduced levels of circulating testosterone arising from ovarian origin – adrenal secretion of androgens is unaffected. There is no change in sex-hormone-binding globulin (SHBG); thus free testosterone (free androgen index) will also be reduced during GnRH-A administration. This is in contrast to the alterations observed with other endocrine therapies, particularly danazol and gestrinone, where serum total testosterone is not reduced but SHBG is markedly reduced, resulting in a rise in free testosterone. There are no other endocrine-induced changes following GnRH-A administration – e.g. thyroid function, adrenal function, insulin, etc.

GnRH-A formulations

Pharmacology of GnRH-A

The biological efficiency of the GnRH-A is related to their absorption, metabolic clearance, bioavailability and affinity for the GnRH receptor. All GnRH agonistic analogues have a prolonged half-life, varying between 1.3 and 5 hours. Being small polypeptide molecules, they have to be administered parenterally since they would otherwise be readily destroyed by digestive enzymes in the stomach. The pharmacokinetics of the GnRH-A depends on the formulation and the route of administration.

Aqueous solutions

Aqueous solutions are ideal for acute administration as an assessment of pituitary function. Following subcutaneous injection the analogue is rapidly absorbed and blood concentrations are elevated for several hours. For treatment the GnRH-A are effective when given as single daily subcutaneous injections. Recommended doses vary between 100 and 500 μg daily. Other modes of administration may be preferable for long-term treatment regimes.

Intranasal

Novel formulations for intranasal delivery have been developed. The agonists are absorbed from the mucosa, with some variation between individuals, and related to the molecular size and hydrophilic/lipophilic characteristics of the individual analogue. Absorption is limited to 2–5% of the metered dose. Thus dosages of 200–400 μg need to be administered two or three times daily to maintain an effective drug serum concentration [7,8]. Such routes of administration are popular with patients because of their ease of use, but have the disadvantage of multiple daily applications.

Depots

Sustained-release formulations have been developed which allow continuous low-dose release of the agonist and hence maintain continued occupation of the GnRH receptors. A number of hydrophobic polymers and hydrogels are available as carrier vehicles for the GnRH-A. The development of biodegradable polymers of DL-L-lactide–glycolactide have been most commonly used. The depots are either microparticulate suspensions (triptorelin, leuprolerin) 3.75 mg monthly for intramuscular injection or a cylindrical rod (goserelin) 3.6 mg monthly. The current depot preparations have life expectancies of 4 weeks but longer-duration depots (6–12 weeks) are under development. Most release between 120 and 160 μg of GnRH-A per day.

The pharmacokinetics of the two sustained-release systems are different, with the microcapsule formulation inducing an initial fast release of the agonist which slowly decreases thereafter during the following weeks, compared with the goserelin implant where serum levels progressively increase during the first 2 weeks before decreasing in a mirror-like fashion for the following 2 weeks [9, 10].

Differences between formulations

Comparison of the circulating levels of oestradiol in cohorts of patients receiving danazol 600 mg daily, intranasal buserelin 1200 μg daily, intranasal nafarelin 400 μg daily or goserelin a 3.6 mg implant administered monthly show differences in the degree of suppression of serum oestradiol between these drugs. The goserelin implant and other depot preparations produce a more rapid, complete and constant suppression of oestradiol [11]. The levels of oestradiol suppression achieved by danazol 600 mg/day are to within the early follicular range (180–200 pmol/l), whilst all the GnRH agonists maintain a greater degree of oestradiol suppression, near to or within the postmenopausal range (less than 100 pmol/l).

Initial studies utilizing GnRH-A in the treatment of endometriosis

It was the initial study of Meldrum *et al.* [12] which suggested that a long course of treatment with GnRH-A may have beneficial effects on patients with endometriosis. This followed primarily an assessment of endocrine responses in a group of five women treated with D-Tryp^{6}Pro^{9}NEt-luteinizing-hormone-releasing hormone (LHRH) administered subcutaneously from day 2 of the cycle and compared with the endocrine response in a group of 12 women who had undergone surgical oophorectomy. At the end of 1 month's treatment with the GnRH-A, the serum levels of FSH had decreased below basal levels and in four of the five women serum levels of oestradiol were within the castrate range, these being maintained during the period of study. Although the treatment period was short, four patients reported an improvement or disappearance of their symptoms related to endometriosis.

Since this initial report, many non-comparative studies have been published investigating these aspects. One of the first definitive reports of an attempt to treat patients with endometriosis using a GnRH-A came from our own group in 1983 [13]. We treated six patients over a 6-month period with intranasal buserelin 200 μg three times a day (total 600 μg daily) or in one subject a single daily dose of 400 μg. The single dose of 400 μg proved to be inadequate and the patient withdrew. The remaining five patients completed 6 months of therapy and at second-look laparoscopy the endometriotic deposits had either been completely eliminated or markedly resolved in all cases, with an associated improvement in symptoms. Although the patients experienced hot flushes on therapy, there were no other reported significant side-effects from this study and histological examination of the endometrium at the end of 6 months showed poorly developed proliferative or atrophic endometrium. This paper [13] confirmed the value of the use of GnRH-A in subjects with endometriosis and pointed the way to further definitive studies. We also emphasized the caution that would be needed in the presence of ovarian endometrioma.

A number of other reports soon appeared confirming significant reductions in symptoms following either intranasal or daily subcutaneous injections, using a variety of analogues [14–17]. All of these studies confirmed the ability of analogues to suppress serum oestradiol after the first month of treatment, usually to induce amenorrhoea, to bring about marked symptomatic relief and, where second-look laparoscopies were performed, to reduce or remove completely the visible peritoneal endometriotic deposits. Hypo-oestrogenic side-effects, particularly hot flushes and sweats, were reported by the majority of patients following 6–8 weeks' administration of analogues. Other hypo-oestrogenic side-effects were less common and usually developed only after more than 3 or 4 months' treatment (e.g. atrophic vaginitis).

Comparison of dosage regimens

The 1980s saw a rapid acceptance of GnRH agonists as treatment for endometriosis, using a variety of formulations and doses. Current recommended dose regimes are aimed at establishing consistent down-regulation in the majority of patients. The endocrine effect of administration is really an 'all-or-nothing' impact on the pituitary, allowing little facility to specifically modulate the degree of pituitary desensitization achieved.

One study compared 600 and 900 μg daily of intranasal buserelin. A significantly greater degree of suppression of serum oestradiol was achieved with the 900 μg dose, with a resultant increased incidence of oestrogen deficiency side-effects as compared with 600 μg. Whilst a larger dose seemed necessary for suppression of ovarian function, there was no difference between the two doses in the degree of resolution of endometriotic deposits or suppression of symptomatology. Thus complete suppression may not be necessary for achievement of clinical response in endometriosis [15]. A similar conclusion was reached by a Japanese group [18], who evaluated 300, 600 and 900 μg of buserelin intranasally. They concluded that the 900 μg dose was necessary for consistent clinical effectiveness and suppression of ovarian function.

Comparisons of intranasal and daily subcutaneous injections of buserelin have shown no difference in efficacy or side-effects [19, 20] or between subcutaneous and intranasal nafarelin [21]. However, in a study of 100 women randomized to intranasal buserelin or a buserelin implant, it was reported that more significant suppression of the pituitary ovarian axis was achieved with the 6-weekly implant. In addition, there were greater improvements in laparoscopic scores and histological regression of endometriotic implants with the depot than with the intranasal buserelin [22].

The depot preparations have consistently been shown to achieve lower levels of circulating oestradiol than intranasal preparations [11] and this perhaps results from the greater daily dose of analogue released into the circulation from a depot (120–160 μg/day) compared with the 3–5% absorbed from intranasal doses, equivalent to 20–60 μg/day, depending on preparation and dosage of intranasal regimes. As will be seen later, however, all regimes using currently recommended doses appear to achieve equivalent efficacy of symptom relief and impact on the endometriotic deposits. It may, then, be the convenience factor of a monthly depot preparation that is more relevant than perhaps the actual analogue or its precise method or mode of administration in determining patient/physician choice.

Results of comparative clinical trials

Whilst the numerous reported open, non-randomized reports confirmed the drugs' efficacy, comparative trials were necessary to compare GnRH-A with other medical treatments. To date, these have been comparisons with danazol, which is a widely used and effective form of medical treatment for endometriosis.

Several randomized comparative or double-blind placebo-controlled studies have compared the efficacy of various GnRH agonists as against danazol [21–30]. In these studies, the efficacy of drug therapy has been evaluated by comparing the impact on the endometriotic disease by changes in the revised American Fertility Society (RAFS) scores [31] or additive diameter of implants [32]. In addition, alterations in the subjective symptom scores and evaluation of tolerability and adverse events during drug treatments have been carefully made and reported in several studies, which will now be summarized.

Symptomatic relief

Some of the commonest symptoms found in patients with endometriosis are dysmenorrhoea, pelvic pain and dyspareunia and common clinical findings would be pelvic tenderness and induration. These have been prospectively assessed in a number of comparative trials [21, 28–30]. In these trials, both GnRH agonists and danazol had significant effects in reducing the total mean symptom scores within 2 months of commencing either medication. Further improvement was observed in the majority of patients until the fourth or fifth month of treatment, at which time maximum overall response had usually been achieved.

Dysmenorrhoea is one of the first symptoms to be alleviated and usually completely. This is not surprising since the majority of the patients are rapidly rendered amenorrhoeic.

Pelvic pain is usually also effectively inhibited, as menstruation ceases. However, it may take between 3 and 4 months before a significant impact on dyspareunia is appreciated by the patient. This may reflect this symptom's association with deep-seated involvement of endometriosis in the uterosacral ligaments or fixity of the ovaries. If due to the latter, the symptom may not be relieved at all during medical therapy.

Changes in total symptom scores from one study comparing subcutaneous depot goserelin 3.6 mg monthly versus danazol 600 mg daily [29] are shown in Fig. 11.4 and the data are comparable for the other published trials [21, 28, 30].

All the above studies have followed patients up for at least 6 months post-cessation of GnRH agonists or danazol. In the follow-up period, it has been demonstrated that there has been a continued reduction in the mean subjective symptom scores compared with pretreatment values. Any increase in scores observed was usually associated with the return of dysmenorrhoea to some extent as menstruation resumed, although in most instances to a less severe degree than pretreatment.

Some studies have followed patients up for at least 12 months post-treatment [21, 27, 28, 30]. The longer-term follow-up for 12 months has shown continued benefit in terms of reduced mean symptom scores, particularly for one of the main symptoms, dysmenorrhoea. The majority of patients had no or only mild dysmenorrhoea for up to 12 months after cessation of treatment [27]. Prolonged relief of other symptoms such as dyspareunia and pelvic pain were also observed in this study [27] (Table 11.2).

To date, none of these comparative trials have shown any significant differences between the symptomatic effects of the GnRH agonists when compared with danazol at doses of 600 or 800 mg daily and both have been shown to have prolonged beneficial effects on the symptoms of endome-

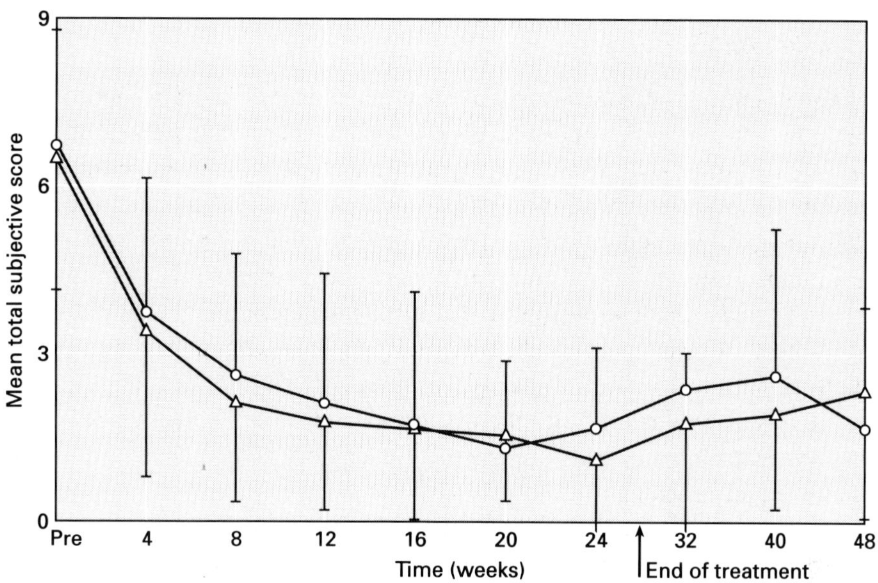

Fig. 11.4 Changes in the mean (± SD) of the total subjective symptom scores during treatment with goserelin (triangles, $n = 158$) or danazol (circles, $n = 65$) in a comparative randomized trial of goserelin 3.6 mg depot every 4 weeks versus danazol 600 mg (oral) daily for 24 weeks with 24 weeks post-treatment follow-up [29]. Shaw RW, Zoladex Endometriosis Study Team. An open randomized comparative study of the effect of goserelin depot and danazol in the treatment of endometriosis. *Fertil Steril* 1992; **58**: 265–72. Reproduced with permission of the publisher, The American Fertility Society.

triosis. Further studies are required, with larger cohorts of patients, to analyse more fully the efficacy of GnRH-A in terms of patients categorized in relationship to both initial severity of symptoms and initial diagnostic staging of the disease. Only then may the benefits of one treatment approach over another become apparent.

Impact on endometriotic implants

All the published comparative trials used patients with pelvic endometriosis proved by an initial laparoscopy before treatment was commenced and reassessed the disease at second-look laparoscopy at the end of 6 months' treatment. This was usually before the recommencement of menstruation and ovulatory function, which may overemphasize the impact on the disease. The changes in RAFS scores from three such comparative trials, utilizing buserelin, goserelin and nafarelin versus danazol are summarized in Table 11.3.

The results are in overall agreement. There are highly significant reductions in both total RAFS scores and scores resultant from the implant

Table 11.2 Symptom category at end of treatment and 12 months' follow-up

	Nafarelin 400 mg daily intranasally (% patients with symptom category)				Danazol 600 mg daily orally (% patients with symptom category)			
	Absent	Mild	Moderate	Severe	Absent	Mild	Moderate	Severe
Dysmenorrhoea	($n = 71$)				($n = 32$)			
Baseline	6	61	27	7	13	44	31	13
End treatment	7*	3*	0*	0*	0†	0†	0†	0†
12 months post-treatment	41	51	6	3	41	38	16	6
Pelvic pain	($n = 71$)				($n = 32$)			
Baseline	37	42	21	0	31	56	9	3
End treatment	77	21	1	0	75	19	6	0
12 months post-treatment	65	35	0	0	66	31	3	0
Dyspareunia	($n = 66$)				($n = 31$)			
Baseline	51	31	10	7	41	38	13	9
End treatment	87	12	2	0	93	7	0	0
12 months post-treatment	87	12	1	0	84	13	3	0

* 90% of patients and † 100% of patients amenorrhoeic and therefore excluded.
Modified from [27].

Table 11.3 Changes in RAFS scores following treatments with various GnRH analogues or danazol in comparative trials

	Henzl *et al.* [21]		Protocol 310 Study Group [28]		Shaw [29]	
	Nafarelin 400 µg intranasally	Danazol 800 mg/day	Buserelin 200 µg s.c./day 1200 µg/day intranasally	Danazol 400–800 mg orally	Goserelin 3.6 mg depot (monthly)	Danzol 600 mg/day orally
Number of patients	73	70	134	50	175	74
Total RAFS score						
Baseline	20.4	18.4	16.4	14.2	16.4	14.5
End of treatment	11.7	10.5	8.0	9.4	6.7	7.0
Difference	–43%	–43%	–51%	–34%	–59%	–52%
Score for implants alone						
Baseline	9.0	9.3	11.7	10.9	9.0	10.4
End of treatment	4.0	3.0	4.4	5.7	2.5	3.4
Difference	–56%	–68%	–62%	–38%	–73%	–67%
Score for adhesions						
Baseline	11.4	9.1	4.7	3.3	7.0	4.0
End of treatment	7.7	7.5	3.6	3.6	4.2	3.6
Difference	–32%	–18%	–23%	+9%	–40%	–15%

s.c. = Subcutaneously.

component alone ($P<0.001$). However, no trials have shown significant differences between the effect of GnRH agonists and danazol in this respect. In some studies [21, 28, 29], there have been small but apparently significant reductions in RAFS adhesion scores in patients treated with GnRH agonists. By comparison there have been smaller decreases [21, 29] or even an increase [28] in adhesion scores in patients receiving danazol in these trials. Such changes in adhesion scores have been difficult to explain since with none of the studies was laparoscopic intervention allowed at the first laparoscopy. One explanation has been that significant changes in vascularity occur during GnRH agonist administration and this may lead to an apparent visual change in adhesions, resulting in a lower score being allocated at the second-look laparoscopy when using the RAFS scoring system.

Differential responses to GnRH-A

When the RAFS scores are analysed according to the stage of classification at initial diagnosis, comparable effects are observed in each of the four stages of the RAFS system. This breakdown is available from data in two of these studies [28, 29] and is summarized in Table 11.4.

Thus it is apparent that hormonal therapy has an impact, with resolution of implants whatever the stage or severity of the disease. This is perhaps more clearly demonstrated when the additive diameter of implant (ADI) scoring system [32] is utilized. The results of one study using goserelin depot versus danazol 600 mg daily are shown in Fig. 11.5. Overall there was a highly significant reduction in total ADI score, as well as comparable reductions in ADI scores in all stages of endometriosis. The differences were significant within each group ($P<0.001$) but there was no difference between goserelin and danazol. There was a mean reduction of –81.4% in patients treated with goserelin and –73.5% in those treated with danazol. In addition, 46.3% of those receiving goserelin compared with 33.8% of those treated with danazol showed an apparent clinical 'cure' with a total ADI score of 0 at the post-treatment laparoscopy [29].

Endometriomas

Whilst there may be overall changes at all stages of disease, there appear to be differences in the type of endometriosis that responds to GnRH-A therapy, particularly in the long term. Peritoneal and superficial ovarian lesions respond extremely well. However, deep-seated disease involving the bladder or rectum, whilst achieving a significant suppression of symptoms and cessation of cyclical bleeding during therapy, tend to recur very rapidly after drug therapy. In addition, endometriomas larger than 3 cm reduce marginally in

Table 11.4 Changes in endometriotic implants as assessed by RAFS [31] scoring or additive diameter of implants [32] following GnRH analogues or danazol in comparative randomized trials (mean score for group)

	RAFS implant alone score [28]		Additive diameter of implant [29]	
Score	Buserelin 200 μg s.c./ day or 1200 μg/day	Danazol 400–800 mg/ day orally	Goserelin 3.6 mg depot monthly	Danazol 600 mg/day orally
Number of patients having both assessments	134	50	175	75
Stage 1 AFS				
Baseline	3.1	2.5	25.7	19.6
End of treatment	0.9	1.1	2.9	5.3
Difference	–71%	–56%	–89%	–73%
Stage II AFS				
Baseline	6.1	6.1	30.8	34.1
End of treatment	1.4	1.6	5.1	7.6
Difference	–77%	–74%	–84%	–78%
Stage III AFS				
Baseline	15.4	15.0	49.2	54.7
End of treatment	4.7	5.3	12.8	13.5
Difference	–69%	–65%	–74%	–75%
Stage IV AFS				
Baseline	28.1	24.6	65.9	88.8
End of treatment	10.7	13.3	13.0	34.0
Difference	–62%	–46%	–80%	–63%

s.c. = Subcutaneously.

diameter but recur rapidly and need surgical treatment subsequent to cessation or soon after the end of therapy.

The usefulness of GnRH agonist therapy for 3 months of presurgical treatment in patients with endometriosis has been suggested following publication of a recent prospective but non-randomized study from Donnez *et al.* [33]. In this study, regression of greater than 25% reduction in diameter was obtained in only 30% of the danazol-treated patients compared with 82% of patients receiving a buserelin subcutaneous implant. These data would suggest that GnRH agonist would be advantageous prior to surgery in this specific subgroup of patients.

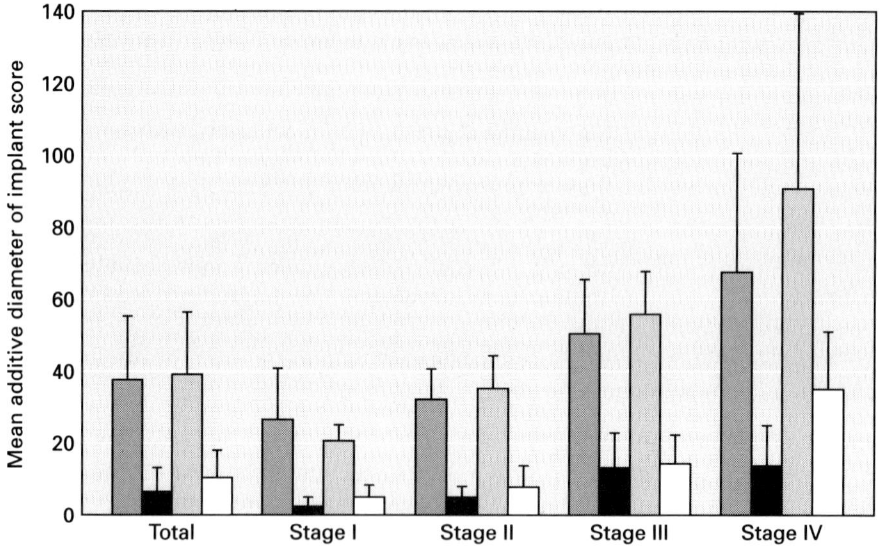

Fig. 11.5 Changes in additive diameter of implant (ADI) scores, total and ADI scores in revised AFS stages I–IV (mean ± SD) before and after treatment in patients randomized to goserelin 3.6 mg depot monthly × 6 ($n = 175$) or danazol 600 mg daily × 24 weeks ($n = 74$). Dark grey, goserelin pretreatment; black, danazol pretreatment; light grey, goserelin post-treatment; white, danazol post-treatment [29]. Shaw RW, Zoladex Endometriosis Study Team. An open randomized comparative study of the effect of goserelin depot and danazol in the treatment of endometriosis. *Fertil Steril* 1992; **58**: 265–72. Reproduced with permission of the publisher, The American Fertility Society.

Recurrence rates following GnRH agonist therapy

There have been few long-term follow-up studies published as yet studying patients who have received GnRH agonist therapy. One such study has been published by ourselves [34] and reported 130 patients who had been treated with GnRH agonists, either buserelin, nafarelin or goserelin, between 1985 and 1987 and who had been followed up for a minimum of 5 years. Patients reported were symptomatic and recurrence was confirmed either at subsequent laparoscopy or laparotomy or, in a proportion of cases, by return of severe specific symptoms of their endometriosis. The cumulative recurrence rate by the fifth year after treatment ended was 53.4%. However, the rate varied according to the initial stage at first diagnosis: 5-year recurrence rates were 36.9% for minimal disease (stages I and II) and 74.4% for severe disease (stages III and IV). The change in endometriosis stage of classification scores at second-look laparoscopy for those patients whose disease recurred after treatment was not significantly different from those whose disease did not recur during the study period. Hence patients with endometriosis who have been treated with a GnRH agonist, as with any other medical or surgical treatment for endometriosis, are highly likely to suffer recurrence of their disease, particularly if their disease is of greater severity at the outset.

Adverse effects experienced during GnRH-A therapy

In many patients receiving medical therapy for the treatment of their endometriosis, the adverse effects of the drug therapy may be as severe as, or in some instances, less desirable or tolerable than their disease symptoms. Adverse effects such as these may well lead to patients ceasing therapy before completing a desired course.

The adverse effects reported during GnRH agonist usage result from the hypo-oestrogenaemia induced. The adverse effects which may be predicted are 'menopausal-like' symptoms, particularly hot flushes, vaginal dryness, loss of libido, fatigue and headache. Depending on the relative degree of oestrogen suppression, but more probably on the population studied and specific questions asked, the incidence of the two main adverse effects of hot flushes and vaginal dryness can vary between 70 and 95% (hot flushes) and 18 and 71% (vaginal dryness). In comparative trials, it is clear that danazol causes significantly less frequent and less severe menopausal-like symptoms. However, danazol induces androgenic and anabolic changes, such as weight gain, muscle cramps, oily skin, acne and, very occasionally, hirsutism or voice changes. The relative incidence of the major side-effects from several of the comparative trials have been summarized in Table 11.5.

There are significant differences between danazol and GnRH-A but perhaps the relative severity of the adverse symptoms is best judged by the proportion of patients who discontinue therapy because of them. In most trials discontinuation before completion of treatment has been relatively low, particularly in those patients receiving GnRH agonists. In one study, the European Goserelin Trial [29], a significant difference between the number of drop-outs in patients receiving goserelin 3.6 mg depot every 28 days (2/204, 1%) compared with those randomized to danazol 600 mg daily (10/103, 9.5%) was observed ($P < 0.05$). Other studies also reported a significantly greater proportion of the patients discontinuing danazol therapy. This indicates that the hypo-oestrogenic adverse effects induced by GnRH agonists are perhaps better tolerated than the androgenic/anabolic effects induced by danazol. This may be an important factor in determining the choice of medical therapy, particularly in patients with recurrent disease who may have been intolerant to previous drug therapies.

Safety issues

The ability of GnRH agonist to induce a state of hypo- or normogonado-

Table 11.5 Commonest adverse side-effects recorded in comparative trials of GnRH analogues vs. danazol

	[27]		[28]		[29]	
	Naferelin 400 μg/day intranasally	Danazol 600 mg/day orally	Buserelin 200 μg s.c./day 1200 μg/day i.n.	Danazol 400–800 mg/day orally	Goserelin 3.6 mg depot (monthly)	Danazol 600 mg/day orally
Number	171	92	116	51	204	103
Percentage of patients with:						
Hot flushes	98	59	71	35	98	58
Vaginal dryness	18	6	29	8	71	29
Decreased libido	17	9	9	10	66	52
Headaches	9	9	23	16	5	3
Weight gain	1	38	1	43	1	27
Breast pain	11	6	n/a	n/a	5	1
Nausea	2	8	2	23	5	12
Muscle cramps	2	8	2	23	1	12
Acne	16	21	6	31	37	54
Oily skin	n/a	n/a	n/a	n/a	25	48
Mood changes (depression/emotional lability)	7	5	10	26	50	44

s.c. = Subcutaneously; n/a = not asked; i.n. = intranasally.

trophic hypogonadism and significant hypo-oestrogenaemia has implications for a number of metabolic processes. The overall ovarian steroid environment induced is comparable to that seen in postmenopausal women. One might therefore expect to see comparable symptoms and changes. Several studies have looked for any changes in electrolytes, liver enzymes and haematological/clotting systems [1, 23, 24, 28] and the results are well summarized in table form in a paper published by Kiesel and coworkers [24]. These show that there are no demonstrable changes in haemoglobin, haematocrit, erythrocytes, thrombocytes, leucocytes or prothrombin time in patients receiving GnRH-A in large multicentre studies, and likewise no changes in creatinine, proteins, albumin or liver enzymes.

Lipoprotein changes have been assessed in a number of studies but very often for only limited subfractions. However, where subfractions were analysed in depth and reported, there was no change in total cholesterol during 6 months' therapy, a slight but insignificant increase in low-density lipoprotein (LDL) cholesterol and a non-significant reduction in high-density lipoprotein (HDL). Apolipoprotein β showed an insignificant rise. These lipoprotein changes do not appear to be marked and are not deemed to be atherogenic [35, 36].

Changes in bone mineral density during GnRH-A therapy

The effective suppression of ovarian function is the key to the success of GnRH-A use in the treatment of endometriosis. However, prolonged sustained oestrogen deprivation in premenopausal women has a significant impact in accelerating the loss of trabecular bone. This side-effect is the key issue causing many drug regulatory authorities to limit the duration of GnRH-A therapy in patients with endometriosis to a period of 6 months. It is also pertinent in relationship to the time interval to re-treatment. This has stimulated the search for combination or 'add-back' regimes to counteract this predictable effect of hypo-oestrogenaemia. It is known that endometriotic patients predominantly have a recurrent disorder which may entail several courses of medical suppressive therapy during their reproductive life. Thus safety issues are paramount and appropriate add-back regimes are necessary to extend the utility of GnRH agonists for the long-term treatment of endometriosis.

Mechanisms of changes in bone mass

Bone loss induced by GnRH agonist therapy occurs through several mechanisms, but can be viewed as similar to that observed in the post-menopausal woman, who likewise has a hypo-oestrogenic state. The hypo-oestrogenaemia induced by GnRH agonists exerts its effect on the bone through three target tissue sites to bring about loss of bone mass.

The parathyroid

This stimulates calcitonin secretion and antagonizes the peripheral action of parathyroid hormones. A decrease in oestrogen levels leads to a reduction in parathyroid secretion of calcitonin, with a resultant decrease in total body calcium. This allows 'unrestrained' parathyroid hormone activity and an increase in bone resorption.

Action within bone

Oestrogen receptors are present in osteoblasts or osteoblast-like cells [37]. When oestrogen levels are reduced, there is a reduction in oestrogen-stimulated osteoblast activity. This results in decreased mineral deposition and reduced bone formation. Oestrogens are thought to stimulate transforming growth factor beta and insulin-like growth factor 1, both of which stimulate bone formation *in vitro* [38], and to inhibit prostaglandin E_2 and interleukin 1, which stimulate bone resorption. Thus with hypo-oestrogenaemia both decreased bone formation and increased bone resorption occur simultaneously.

Gut and calcium absorption

Decreased oestrogen levels lead to a decreased conversion of vitamin D to 1,25-dehydroxy vitamin D, which is an oestrogen-dependent process. This results in a reduced gut absorption of calcium. Reduced levels of 1,25-dehydroxy vitamin D have been reported during GnRH agonist therapy [39].

Changes in bone biochemistry

Amongst the earliest demonstrable changes to be found when continuing treatment with GnRH-A are rises in both urinary calcium–creatinine and hydroxyproline–creatinine ratios [40, 41]. These reflect an increase in bone resorption after withdrawal of the protective effect of oestrogen on the skeleton. In the normal bone remodelling cycle, there is a coupling between bone resorption and bone formation. Relatively soon after an increase in the bone resorption process, there is an increase in the parameters reflecting bone formation. Serum alkaline phosphatase and osteocalcin are markers of bone formation and these likewise rise during GnRH-A therapy [39, 42].

Changes in measurable bone mineral density

As long ago as 1987, Matta *et al.* [43] reported reduction in bone mineral density (BMD) as assessed utilizing computerized quantitative tomography of the predominantly trabecular bone in the lumbar spine. These data demonstrated a significant mean loss of BMD of –5.6% in the lumbar vertebrae L2–4 and a reduced loss of a mean of –0.9% in the more predominantly cortical bone of the shaft of the femur, as evaluated by dual-photon absorptiometry (DPA) following 6 months' treatment with the GnRH agonist buserelin [43]. With further follow-up of these patients some 6 months after ceasing therapy, when there had been return of ovarian function, the group subsequently reported that the loss in BMD in the majority of patients was reversible [44]. However, it may take many months for the process of bone remodelling to return to balance, and baseline BMD may never be re-established in all individuals and may be age-determined (Fig. 11.6).

The method of BMD measurement and the specific bone studied (due to the variation in the component of trabecular or cortical bone within it) give some variability of results in these studies. However, there are now abundant data from both double-blind and open comparative studies to indicate that a

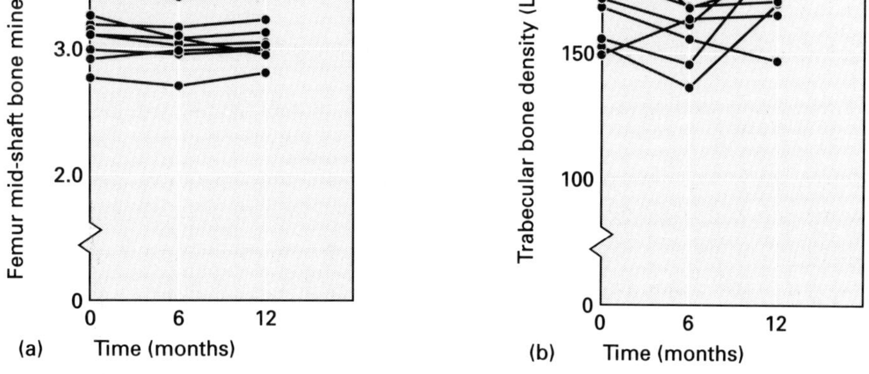

Fig. 11.6 Individual values for (a) femur cortical bone content (dual photon absorptiometry; DPA), $n = 12$, and (b) lumbar vertebral trabecular bone content L2–4 (computerized axial tomography; CAT scan), $n = 11$, in patient before, following 6 months' therapy with buserelin 400 μg t.d.s. intranasally and 6 months post-therapy. Redrawn from [44] with permission.

significant loss in trabecular bone as early as 3 months after beginning GnRH agonist therapy occurs in patients being treated for endometriosis (for review see [45, 46]). The majority of studies, using DPA or dual-energy X-ray absorptiometry (DEXA) measurement techniques, indicate a mean reduction of –5–6% BMD within the lumbar spine and –3–4% loss in Ward's triangle of the femoral neck. Follow-up studies show a return towards baseline BMD in the majority of individuals with increasing time following cessation of the GnRH agonist therapy. However, in some individuals, even 12 months off therapy, there has not been a return to baseline BMD.

This loss in BMD is greater in percentage terms than that observed during the first year in older women at the menopause, but is comparable to that observed in similar-aged women to endometriosis patients who wholly breast-feed for 6 months [47].

It should be emphasized that the bone loss from GnRH agonist treatment of endometriosis has not produced any immediate clinical dramatic effect and the patients remain asymptomatic. However, such a loss among women who, for the most part with endometriosis, have a recurrent disease and may require medical interventive treatment could induce repetitive reductions in BMD without complete replacement. It would thus have a cumulative effect with a postulated negative impact on peak bone mass when entering the menopause. For this reason, strategies to avoid or prevent such bone loss are being developed. These include selection of patients with low risk factors for osteoporosis. Women at increased risk are those with a family history, Caucasian or oriental, reduced body mass index, smokers, high alcohol intake and low dietary calcium intake (less than 800 mg/day). In addition, multi-agent 'add-back therapy' to counteract the bone depletion effects of GnRH agonists is being developed.

Development of add-back regimes in endometriosis

Whilst oestrogen replacement is known to be highly effective at preventing further reduction in BMD in postmenopausal women, the oestrogen dependence of endometriosis has resulted in reluctance to administer oestrogen add-back therapy at doses likely to be effective at preventing BMD changes.

Whilst there are limited data available to date, a number of add-back regimes have been investigated.

Sodium etidronate/calcium carbonate

Etidronate and fluoride increase bone formation and improve the radiological density of bones. One study [48] administered sodium etidronate 400 mg/

day for 14 days and calcium carbonate 500 mg/day for the next 42 days in three successive cycles, together with norethisterone 10 mg or 2.5 mg daily. This combination failed to completely reduce the bone loss induced during GnRH agonist therapy and had no impact on the other symptomatic hypo-oestrogenic symptoms (hot flushes, sweats, etc.) [48].

Norethisterone

Norethisterone at a dose of 5 mg twice a day has been shown to prevent bone loss in postmenopausal women [49]. However, in a randomized double-blind placebo-controlled study, norethisterone, in doses of 0.7–2.45 mg daily for 6 months in conjunction with the GnRH agonist nafarelin, failed to reduce the bone loss observed in the nafarelin and placebo arm of the study [50]. Norethisterone, at a higher dose of 5 mg/day for 4 weeks and then increased to 10 mg/day for a further 20 weeks in conjunction with the GnRH agonist leuprolerin in a randomized controlled study, demonstrated equivalent efficacy in reduction of RAFS scores but did not completely inhibit the bone loss in the add-back group when treated over 6 months [51]. The BMD loss was significantly less than baseline ($P < 0.05$), albeit less than the loss seen in the analogue placebo-treated group ($P < 0.001$). A further study of large doses of progesterones alone may be necessary, although, even at the doses in the above study [51], norethisterone reduced the HDL cholesterol and increased the LDL/HDL ratio.

Medroxyprogesterone acetate

Medroxyprogesterone acetate (MPA), in doses of 20–30 mg daily in an uncontrolled study in patients receiving the GnRH agonist histrelin for 6 months, was shown to prevent the bone loss observed in a group of historic controls receiving histrelin alone. This add-back regime also reduced the incidence of oestrogenic vasomotor symptoms but had an adverse impact on the endometriotic process with no change in RAFS scores post-treatment [52].

Hormone replacement therapy (HRT) regimes

Concerns over the use of combined oestrogen/progesterone HRT add-back have been expressed in that the oestrogen may well negate the impact of GnRH agonists on the endometriotic process, which is essentially oestrogen-dependent. However, in one recent study [53], with the GnRH agonist goserelin, administered in conjunction with oestradiol patches 25 μg twice weekly and MPA 5 mg daily, this concern appeared to be unfounded. This study demonstrated that the add-back HRT treatment did not negate the impact of GnRH agonist on the endometriosis process, with comparable reduction in RAFS scores to the analogue-alone-treated group. The add-back therapy did not, however, abolish hot flushes completely and was only able to reduce the bone loss to a mean of –2.5% compared with the expected –5% in the analogue-alone-treated group. It remains to be evaluated whether higher doses of HRT oestrogen replacement can be utilized to completely prevent the bone loss and yet not impair the impact of the disease process.

Tibolone

Tibolone is a synthetic steroid. The structure relates to the progestogens norethynodrel and norethisterone. It shows weak progestogenic, oestrogenic and androgenic actions. We investigated this agent in a combination add-back therapy with the GnRH agonist Decapeptyl 3.75 mg monthly in a placebo-controlled study administering tibolone in a dose of 2.5 mg daily [54]. The tibolone-treated group had significantly reduced hypo-oestrogenic side-effects with the mean of hot flushes reduced from six per day in the placebo-treated group to one per day in the tibolone group (and in 50% of patients no hot flushes at all). The combination therapy did not impair the GnRH-agonist-induced action on the endometriotic deposits and did successfully achieve a prevention in BMD reduction during the 6 months' treatment. In the tibolone-treated group, a non-significant loss of –1.1% in lumbar vertebral BMD was demonstrated compared with –5.1% in the analogue alone ($P < 0.001$) [54].

This combination, then, has for the first time achieved all the aims in the add-back regimes and warrants further investigation. As with any synthetic progestogen, a small increase in LDL cholesterol was observed, but the values were still well within the normal ranges for women of this age-group.

Conclusion

Data published to date indicate that medical treatment utilizing GnRH agonists can be highly effective in relieving the symptomatology of endometriosis, both during therapy and during 12 months of follow-up if given for 6 months. The studies have indicated a significant impact on reduction in the amount of endometriotic lesions, although this is far greater in those involving the peritoneum and the effect is less marked or negligible in deep-seated disease or with endometriotic cysts, where early recurrence following cessation of therapy can be expected.

Although hypo-oestrogenic side-effects like those seen at menopause are common whilst receiving GnRH agonists, these symptoms are in general well tolerated by patients, with few drop-outs being reported from the trials undertaken. There appear to be no significant changes in serum lipoproteins or other biochemical or haematological parameters during treatment, and the only adverse events relate to the hypo-oestrogenaemic-induced reduction in BMD. This reduction in BMD, whilst statistically significant, is not clinically significant following 6 months' therapy. In the majority of individuals, BMD returns to baseline levels within 6–12 months of ceasing a course of therapy. Currently, various add-back regimes are being investigated to determine the most appropriate combination to give with GnRH agonists to counteract this bone loss and enable these highly effective drugs to be used in long-term therapy and for repeat courses in recurrent endometriosis.

References

1 Schally AV, Arimura A, Baba Y *et al.* Isolation and properties of the FSH and LH-releasing hormone. *Biochem Biophys Res Commun* 1971 **43**: 393–399.

2 Shaw RW, Soulter WP, Stanton SL (eds). *Gynaecology*, 1992, p. 127. Edinburgh, Churchill Livingstone.

3 Clayton RN. Cellular actions of gonadotrophin-releasing hormone: the receptor and beyond. In: Shaw RW, Marshall JC (eds). *LHRH and its Analogues – Their Use in Gynaecological Practice*, 1989, pp. 19–34. London, Wright.

4 Kiesel L, Runnebaum B. Mechanisms involved in the hormonal treatment of endometriosis. In: Chandha DR, Buttram VC (eds). *Current Concepts in Endometriosis*, 1990, pp. 179–196. New York, Alan R Liss.

5 Knobil E, Plant TM, Wild L, Belchetz PE, Marshall G. Control of the rhesus monkey menstrual cycle: permissive role of hypothalamic gonadropin-releasing hormone. *Science* 1980 **207**: 1371–1374.

6 Shaw RW. LHRH analogues in the treatment of endometriosis – comparative results with other treatments. *Clin Obstet Gynaecol* 1988 **2**: 659–675.

7 Holland FJ, Fishman L, Costigan DC. Pharmacological characteristics of the gonadotrophin-releasing hormone analog D-Ser (TBU)-EA-luteinising hormone-releasing hormone (buserelin) after subcutaneous and intranasal administration in children with central precocious puberty. *J Clin Endocrinol Metab* 1986 **63**: 1065–1070.

8 Chan RL, Henzl MR, LePage ME. Absorption and metabolism of nafarelin, a potent agonist of gonadotrophin-releasing hormone. *Clin Pharmacol Ther* 1988 **44**: 275–282.

9 Happ J, Scholteib H, Jacobi GH. Pharmacodynamics, pharmacokinetics and bioavailability of the prolonged LH-RH agonist decapeptyl-SR. In: Klijn JMG *et al.* (eds). *Hormonal Manipulation of Cancer, Peptides, Growth Factors and New (Anti) Steroidal Agents*, 1987, pp. 249–253. New York, Raven Press.

10 Clayton RN, Bailey LC, Cottam J. A radioimmunoassay for GnRH agonists analogue in serum patients with prostate cancer treated with D-Ser (TBu) AZA Gly GnRH. *Clin Endocrinol* 1985 **22**: 453–462.

11 Shaw RW. GnRH analogs in the treatment of endometriosis – rationale and efficacy. In: Thomas E, Rock J (eds). *Modern Approaches to Endometriosis*, 1991 pp. 257–274. London, Kluwer Academic Publishers.

12 Meldrum DR, Chang RJ, Lu J *et al.* Medical oophorectomy using a long-acting GnRH agonist: a possible new approach to the treatment of endometriosis. *J Clin Endocrinol Metab* 1982 **54**: 1081–1083.

13 Shaw RW, Fraser HM, Boyle H. Intranasal treatment with luteinizing hormone-releasing hormone agonist in women with endometriosis. *Br Med J* 1983 **287**: 1167–1169.

14 Lemay A, Maheux R, Faure N, Jean C, Fazekas A. Reversible hypogonadism induced by a luteinizing hormone-releasing hormone (LHRH) agonist (buserelin) as a new therapeutic approach for endometriosis. *Fertil Steril* 1984 **41**: 863–871.

15 Shaw RW, Matta W. Reversible pituitary ovarian suppression induced by an LHRH agonist in the treatment of endometriosis: comparison of two dose regimens. *Clin Reprod Fertil* 1986 **4**: 329–336.

16 Schriock E, Monroe SE, Henzl M, Jaffe RB. Treatment of endometriosis with a potent agonist of gonadotrophin releasing hormone (Nafarelin). *Fertil Steril* 1985 **44**: 585–586.

17 Steingold KA, Cedars M, Lu JKH *et al.* Treatment of endometriosis with a long-acting gonadotrophin-releasing hormone agonist. *Obstet Gynecol* 1987 **69**: 403–411.

18 Minaguchi H, Vermura TL, Shitzsu K. Clinical study on finding the optimal dose of a potent LHRH agonist (Buserelin) for the treatment of endometriosis – multicentre trial in Japan. In: Rolland R, Chandha DR, Willesmen WNP (eds). *Gonadotrophin Down Regulation in Gynaecological Practice*, 1986, pp. 211–225. New York, Alan R Liss.

19 Lemay A, Maheux R, Huot C, Blanchet J, Faure N. Efficacy of intranasal or subcutaneous luteinizing hormone-releasing hormone agonist inhibition of ovarian function in the treatment of endometriosis. *Am J Obstet Gynecol* 1988 **158**: 233–236.

20 Dmowski WP, Radwanska E, Binor Z, Tummon I, Pepping P. Ovarian suppression induced with buserelin or danazol in the management of endometriosis: a randomized, comparative study. *Fertil Steril* 1989 **51**: 395–400.

21 Henzl MR, Corson SL, Moghissi K *et al.* Administration of nasal nafarelin as compared with oral danazol for endometriosis. *N Engl J Med* 1988 **318**: 455–489.

22 Donnez J, Nisolle-Pochet M, Clerckx-Braun F, Sandow J, Casanas-Roux F. Administration of nasal buserelin as compared with subcutaneous buserelin implant for endometriosis. *Fertil Steril* 1989 **52**: 27–30.

23 Matta WH, Shaw RW. A comparative study between buserelin and danazol in the treatment of endometriosis. *Br J Clin Pract* 1986 **41** (Suppl. 48): 69–73.

24 Kiesel L, Thomas K, Tempore A *et al.* Efficacy and safety of buserelin treatment in women with endometriosis – a multicentre open-label study. *Gynaecol Endocrinol* 1989 **3** (Suppl. 2): 5–19.

25 Sondheimer SJ, Klioze SS, Schreider J, Setescak L, Spiro T. A comparison of the efficacy and safety of Buserelin vs Danazol in the treatment of endometriosis. In: Chandha DR, Buttram VC Jr (eds). *Current Concepts in Endometriosis*, 1990, pp. 253–267. New York, Alan R Liss.

26 Lemay A. Comparison of GnRH analogues to conventional therapy in endometriosis. In: *International Symposium on GnRH Analogues*, Geneva, 1988. Abstract 020.

27 The Nafarelin European Endometriosis Group. A large scale danazol controlled trial of efficacy and safety with one year follow-up. *Fertil Steril* 1992 **57**: 514–522.

28 Protocol 310 Study Group. A comparison of the efficacy and safety of buserelin vs. danazol in the treatment of endometriosis. In: Chandha DR, Buttram VC Jr (eds). *Current Concepts in Endometriosis.* 1990, pp. 253–267. New York, Alan R Liss.

29 Shaw RW. An open randomised comparative study of the effect of goserelin and danazol in the treatment of endometriosis. *Fertil Steril* 1992 **58**: 265–272.

30 Rock JA, Truglia JA, Caplan RJ, the Zoladex Endometriosis Study Group. Zoladex (goserelin acetate implant) in the treatment of endometriosis: a randomised comparison with danazol. *Obstet Gynecol* 1993 **82**: 198–205.

31 American Fertility Society. Revised American Fertility Society classification of endometriosis. *Fertil Steril* 1985 **43**: 351–352.

32 Doberl A, Berqvist A, Jeppson S *et al.* Regression of endometriosis following shorter

treatment with, or lower dose of danazol. *Acta Obstet Gynaecol Scand* 1984 **123** (Suppl.): 51–58.

33 Donnez J, Nisolle M, Clerckx F. Evaluation of preoperative use of danazol, gestrinone, lynestrenol, buserelin spray and buserelin implant in the treatment of endometriosis associated infertility. In: Chandha DR, Buttram VC Jr (eds). *Current Concepts in Endometriosis*, 1990, pp. 357–382. New York, Alan R Liss.

34 Waller KG, Shaw RW. Gonadotropin-releasing hormone analogue for the treatment of endometriosis: long-term follow up. *Fertil Steril* 1993 **59**: 511–515.

35 Shaw RW. Goserelin-depot preparation of LHRH analogue used in the treatment of endometriosis. In: Chandha DR, Buttram VC Jr (eds). *Current Concepts in Endometriosis*, 1990, pp. 383–392. New York, Alan R Liss.

36 Crook D, Gardner R, Worthington M. Zoladex (ICI 118630) versus Danazol in the treatment of pelvic endometriosis: effects on plasma lipid risk factors. In: Stoll BA (ed.). *Proceedings of the International Symposium on Endocrine Therapy. Hormone Res* 1989 **32** (Suppl. 1): 157–160.

37 Eriksen EF, Colvard DS, Berg NJ *et al.* Evidence of oestrogen receptors in normal human osteoblast-like cells. *Science* 1988 **241**: 81–84.

38 Ernst M, Schmid C, Frankenfoldt C, Froesch ER. Estradiol stimulation of osteoblastic proliferation *in vitro*: mediator roles for TGF beta, PGF2 IGF1 (Abstract). *Calcif Tiss Res* 1988 **42** (Suppl.): 117.

39 Scharla HS, Minne HW, Waibel-Treber S *et al.* Bone mass reduction after oestrogen deprivation by long acting gonadotropin-releasing hormone agonists and its relation to pretreatment concentrations of 1,25-dihydroxyvitamin D3. *J Clin Endocrinol Metab* 1990 **70**: 1055–1061.

40 Bergquist C. Effects of nafarelin versus danazol on lipids and calcium metabolism. *Am J Obstet Gynecol* 1990 **162**: 589–591.

41 Gudmundsson JA, Lyunghall S, Bergquist C *et al.* Increased bone turnover during gonadotropin-releasing hormone superagonist-induced ovulation inhibition. *J Clin Endocrinol Metab* 1987 **65**: 159–163.

42 Ylikorkala O, Nilsson CG, Horvonen E *et al.* Evidence of similar increases in bone turnover during nafarelin and danazol use in women with endometriosis. *Gynecol Endocrinol* 1990 **4**: 251–260.

43 Matta WH, Shaw RW, Hesp R, Katz D. Hypogonadism induced by luteinizing hormone-releasing hormone agonist analogues: effects on bone density in premenopausal women. *Br Med J* 1987 **294**: 1523–1524.

44 Matta WH, Shaw RW, Hesp R, Evans R. Reversible trabecular bone density loss following induced hypo-oestrogenism with the GnRH analogue Buserelin in premenopausal women. *Clin Endocrinol* 1988 **29**: 45–51.

45 Fogelman I, Fentiman I, Hamed H, Studd JWW, Leather AT. Goserelin (Zoladex) and the skeleton. *Br J Obstet Gynecol* 1994 **101** (Suppl. 10): 19–23.

46 Dawood MY. Hormonal therapies for endometriosis: implications for bone metabolism. *Acta Obstet Gynecol Scand* 1994 **73** (Suppl. 159): 22–34.

47 Hayslip CC, Lein TA, Wray HL *et al.* The effect of lactation on bone mineral content in healthy postpartum women. *Obstet Gynecol* 1989 **73**: 588–592.

48 Surrey ES, Fournet N, Voigt B *et al.* Effects of sodium etidronate in combination with low-dose norethisterone in patients administered a long-acting GnRH agonist: a preliminary report. *J Endocrinol Metab* 1993 **81**: 581–586.

49 Abdalla HI, Hart DM, Lindsay R, Leggate I, Hooke A. Prevention of bone mineral loss in postmenopausal women by norethisterone. *Obstet Gynecol* 1985 **66**: 789–792.

50 Eldred JM, Haynes P, Thomas EJ. A randomised double blind placebo controlled trial of the effects on bone metabolism of the combination of nafarelin acetate and norethisterone.

Clin Endocrinol 1992 **37**: 354–359.
51 Surrey ES, Tud HL. Reduction of vasomotor symptoms and bone mineral density loss with combined norethisterone and long-acting gonadotrophin-releasing hormone agonist therapy of symptomatic endometriosis: a prospective randomised trial. *J Clin Endocrinol* 1992 **75**: 558–563.
52 Cedars MI, Lu JKH, Meldrum DR, Judd HL. Treatment of endometriosis with a long-acting gonadotropin-releasing agonist plus medroxyprogesterone acetate. *Obstet Gynecol* 1990 **75**: 641–645.
53 Edmonds DK, Howell R. Can hormone replacement therapy be used during medical therapy of endometriosis? *Br J Obstet Gynaecol* 1994 **101** (Suppl. 10): 24–26.
54 Lindsay P, Shaw RW. The effect of livial on GnRH agonist induced bone loss (Abstract). 7th International Congress on the Menopause, Stockholm, 20–24 June 1993.

Part 4
Surgical Treatments

Chapter 12
Conservative Laparoscopic Treatment of Ovarian Endometriosis

M. NISOLLE AND J. DONNEZ

Introduction

It has been proved that ovarian endometriomas respond less well to medical therapy than does peritoneal endometriosis [1–3]. Therefore, surgical therapy is required. Conservative microsurgery has nowadays been replaced by endoscopic procedures [4–7]: vaporization of the cyst wall, fulguration and/or ovarian stripping. Drainage alone is still suggested by some authors [8], but we have recently proved that this procedure is completely ineffective [9].

In our department, advanced operative laparoscopy techniques for laser adhesiolysis and vaporization of endometriotic implants have been developed. There are at least three advantages of laser laparoscopy over conventional operative laparoscopy: precise destruction of diseased tissue, minimal bleeding and minimal damage to the adjacent normal tissue. Tissue reaction and postoperative adhesion formation have been shown to be minimal.

Although laparoscopic treatment of benign ovarian cysts is an effective technique involving little risk of complications [10, 11], several criteria must be taken into account before performing this procedure.

Classification of ovarian endometriosis

Three different types of ovarian endometriosis [11, 12] can be classified, as follows:

1 Superficial haemorrhagic lesions.
2 Haemorrhagic cysts (endometriomas).
3 Deep-infiltrating ovarian endometriosis (infrequent).

Superficial lesions

Superficial ovarian lesions are small, vesicular lesions covering the ovarian cortex, or small implants, usually found on the lateral surface of the ovary. Adhesions between the ovary and the broad ligament are often observed. From a histopathological point of view, the endometrial cyst may be lined by free endometrial tissue, similar histologically and functionally to eutopic endometrium. Active ectopic endometrial tissue can cover the inner surface of a small cavity in the ovary. In some instances, atypical epithelium and ciliated cells are found [2, 13].

Endometriomas

The term 'chocolate cyst' was applied by Sampson [14] to describe the endometrial cysts of the ovary. In large endometriomas, the cyst is often lined by a flattened endometrial epithelium. The cyclical changes of these enclosed lesions are less significant than those in free-growing lesions, and late secretory changes and menstrual bleeding are absent. The mobilization of the cysts from their fixed position provokes the rupture and subsequent spillage of contents.

As pointed out by Hughesdon [15], the internal surface of a chocolate cyst is really the external surface of the ovary; the ovarian cortex is identifiable by the presence of primordial follicles.

The appearance on ovarioscopy [16] is as dark, fibrotic areas with haemosiderin pigmentation which alternate with highly vascularized areas with focal bleeding. The vessels in these areas are often congested, and tend to be larger at the hilus of the ovary.

Three months after drainage of the endometrioma and gonadotrophin-releasing hormone agonist (GnRH-a) therapy (which provokes amenorrhoea), chocolate-coloured fluid is still present [9]. This fact proves that endometrial shedding is not responsible for chocolate-coloured fluid formation. In the authors' opinion, the origin of this fluid could be from cyst wall exudation, congested cyst wall blood-vessels or inflammation around persistent intracystic endometrial foci which are resistant to medical therapy.

Preoperative evaluation

In all cases, a preoperative evaluation of the cyst has to be made. This includes transvaginal sonography, which determines the size of the endometrioma (Plate 12.1, facing p. 242), and, in some cases, the presence of multiple small endometriomas. The transvaginal Doppler ultrasound with colour flow imaging permits the evaluation of pulsatility and/or the resistance index. This must certainly be performed in women >40 years who are suffering from infertility and endometriomas to exclude ovarian carcinomas.

A preoperative evaluation of serum CA-125 levels must be made before endoscopic surgery, especially in cases of large or multilocular endometriomas.

Computerized tomography (CT) provides high-quality images of the ovaries but does not give any more information than the ultrasound except in cases of large or multilocular endometriomas (Fig. 12.1).

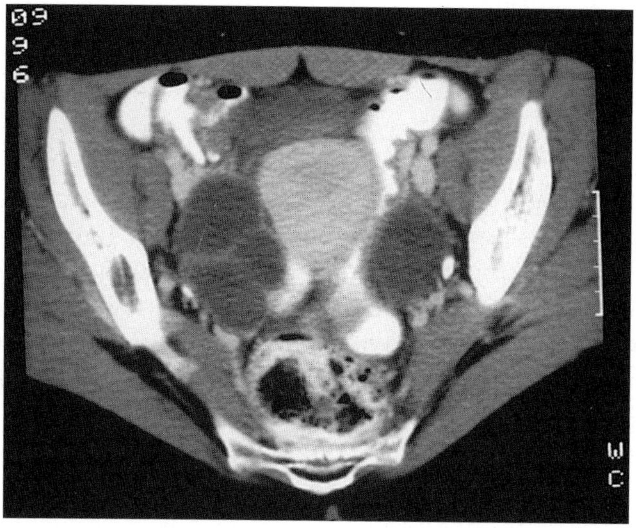

Fig. 12.1 Computerized tomography: multilocular endometriomas.

The accuracy, convenience, relatively low cost and availability of high-resolution ultrasound equipment have resulted in it remaining the principal and usually only imaging modality in assessing pelvic masses.

Endoscopic techniques

Laser surgery

The endoscopic use of the laser is not new in medicine, and several types of operative procedures have been carried out with the CO_2 laser laparoscope for the treatment of reproductive pathology. The most frequent indication is endometriosis, which can be vaporized by CO_2 laser laparoscopy with highly satisfactory postoperative pregnancy rates [4–7, 10, 11]. Laser surgeons have removed endometriosis from the reproductive structure with great precision, but vaporization of peritoneal endometriotic lesions or the endometriotic cyst wall provokes residual carbon charring. Expensive high-power operating lasers are thus required for the vaporization of tissue without residual carbon charring.

Instruments

The Swiftlase [17] allows char-free ablation, even when using a 30 W operating laser. The Swiftlase (Sharplan Model 757) is a miniature optomechanical scanner compatible with any CO_2 laser (Plate 12.2, facing p. 242). It consists of two almost, but not exactly, parallel folding mirrors. Optical reflections of the CO_2 laser optical beam from the mirrors cause the beam to deviate from its original direction by an angle θ (Fig. 12.2). The mirrors constantly rotate at slightly different angular velocities, thereby rapidly varying with time between zero and a maximum value, θ_{max}. By attaching the laparoscope focusing coupler of focal length F to the Swiftlase, the CO_2 laser generates a focal spot which rapidly and homogeneously scans and covers a round area of diameter $2F \tan \theta_{max}$ at the distal end of the laparoscope. For a single-puncture laparoscope $F = 300$ mm, θ_{max} is selected to provide a round treatment area of 2.5 mm diameter. The rapid movement of the beam over the tissue ensures a short duration of exposure on individual sites within the area and a very shallow ablation.

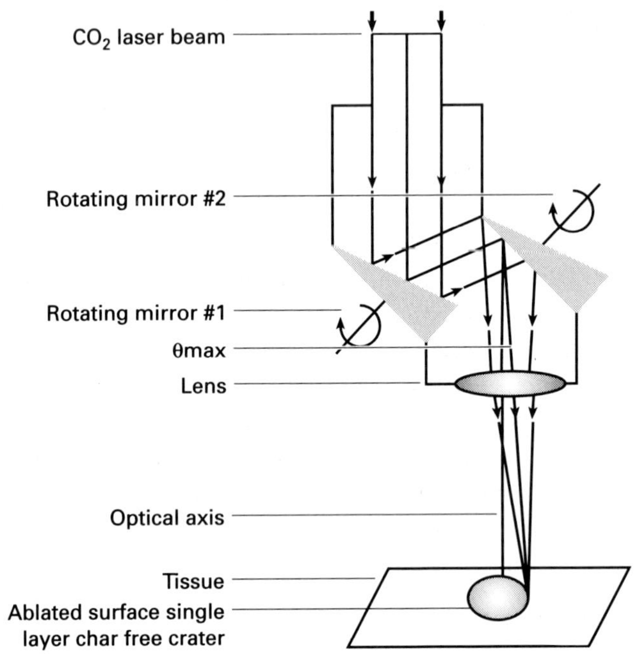

Fig. 12.2 Swiftlase consists of two almost, but not exactly, parallel folding mirrors. The mirrors constantly rotate at slightly different angular velocities. The rapid movement of the beam provides a char-free ablation.

Since therapeutic CO_2 medical lasers typically generate a focused beam of less than 0.9 mm diameter at the laparoscope working distance, using the Swiftlase with a laser power level of 30 W will generate an optical power density of more than 50 W/mm^2 on tissue. This is considerably higher than the threshold for vaporization of tissue without residual carbon charring. The time required for the Swiftlase to homogeneously cover a 2.5 mm round area is about 100 ms. During this time, the 30 W operating laser will deliver

3000 mJ to the tissue. Since the typical energy required to completely ablate tissue is about 3000 mJ/mm^3, keeping the laparoscope precisely on a single site for 0.1 s will generate a clean char-free crater of 0.2 mm depth.

However, the laparoscope can also be smoothly and evenly moved across an extended lesion intended for treatment, consequently ablating a tissue layer as thin as 0.05–0.1 mm.

Laser techniques

The procedure is performed under general anaesthesia. After induction of a pneumoperitoneum, a 12 mm trocar is inserted subumbically. The laparoscope is connected to a video camera. Three 5 mm trocars are systematically inserted suprapubically: one in the mid-line, approximately 3 cm above the symphysis pubis, and the two others a few centimetres on either side, taking care to avoid the epigastric vessels.

The initial phase of the laparoscopy is purely an evaluation of the severity of the endometriotic lesions according to the American Fertility Society (AFS) classification. For this purpose, all peritoneal lesions are noted and the ovarian endometriomas, which are often adherent to the ovarian fossa, are mobilized. The endometrioma is grasped with an atraumatic forceps, and the cyst is incised in order to aspirate the chocolate-coloured material, to wash out the cyst with irrigation fluid and, finally, to carefully examine the interior wall of the cyst. The ovarian cystoscopy permits the exclusion of papillary vegetation or other evidence suggesting malignancy. Thereafter, treatment of the endometrioma according to its size is carried out using the CO_2 laser equipped with the Swiftlase. From 1982 to 1993, 6250 laser laparoscopies were carried out in our department. In this series, 2912 patients underwent laparoscopy for endometriosis.

Ovarian endometriomas < 3 cm

Ovarian endometriomas are treated during first-look laparoscopy if a penetration of no more than 3 cm into the ovary is observed and if the cyst diameter is no greater than 3 cm.

Small (< 1 cm in diameter) endometriotic implants of the ovary were vaporized, using the CO_2 laser equipped with the Swiftlase, until follicles containing fluid were encountered or no further pigmented tissue was seen. Larger (< 3 cm in diameter) endometriomas were destroyed as follows: the cyst wall was incised, the chocolate-coloured material was aspirated and the cyst was washed out with irrigation fluid. After washing, the interior wall of the cyst was carefully examined to confirm the absence of any suspected intracystic lesions (ovarian cystoscopy) and a biopsy was taken for histologic evaluation. With a power setting of 40 W and continuous-mode application, the interior wall of the cyst was then vaporized using the CO_2 laser equipped with the Swiftlase (Plate 12.3, facing p. 242). The vaporization continued until no further pigmentation could be seen. After copious irrigation, the ovaries were left open.

Ovarian endometriomas > 3 cm

In our series of patients with endometriosis, ovarian endometriomas larger than 3 cm in diameter were found in 481 patients. A three-step therapy was proposed because of the size of the endometriomas: drainage of the cyst, interval therapy with GnRH analogues for 3 months, followed by laparoscopic surgery and CO_2 laser vaporization of the cyst lining with closure of the ovary.

During diagnostic laparoscopy, the endometrial cyst was washed out with irrigation fluid (saline solution) (Plate 12.4a facing p. 242) and a biopsy was taken. In cases of multilocular endometrial cysts, all the endometriomas must be opened and rinsed carefully. Then, GnRH-a (goserelin, Zoladex) therapy was given for 12 weeks to reduce the cyst size. A decrease of 50% in cyst diameter was observed after drainage when followed by 12 weeks' GnRH-a therapy (Fig. 12.3). Drainage alone (if not associated with GnRH-a) was found to be ineffective [9]. Indeed, 12 weeks after drainage, the ovarian cyst diameter was unchanged, when compared with the diameter observed before drainage.

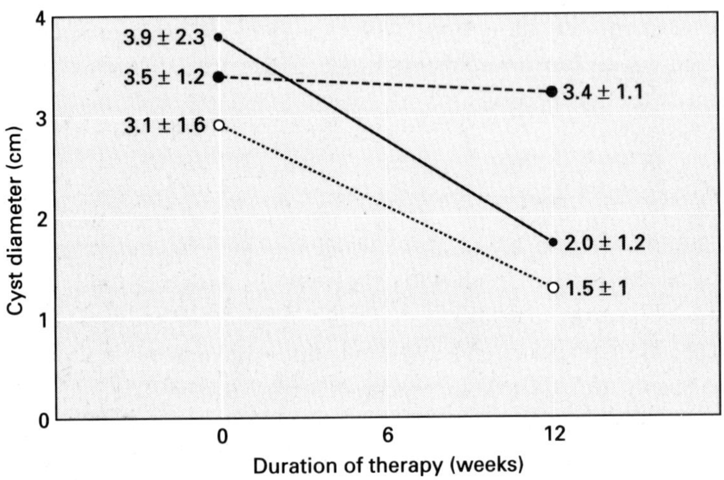

Fig. 12.3 A decrease of 50% in cyst diameter was observed after drainage followed by a 12-week GnRH-a therapy. Drainage alone is ineffective: the ovarian cyst diameter is unchanged. Dashed line, no therapy ($n = 36$, 2% reduction); dotted line, GnRH-a ($n = 67$, 49.8% reduction); solid line, GnRH-a/MPA ($n = 18$, 41.7% reduction). MPA = medroxyprogesterone acetate.

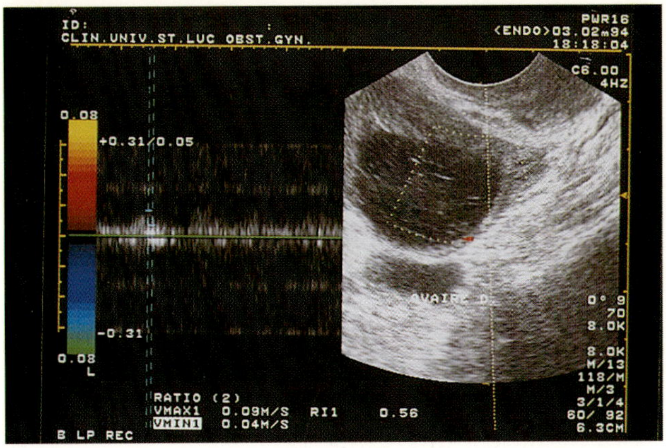

Plate 12.1 Transvaginal Doppler ultrasound with colour flow imaging: typical endometriotic cyst (proved later by laparoscopy).

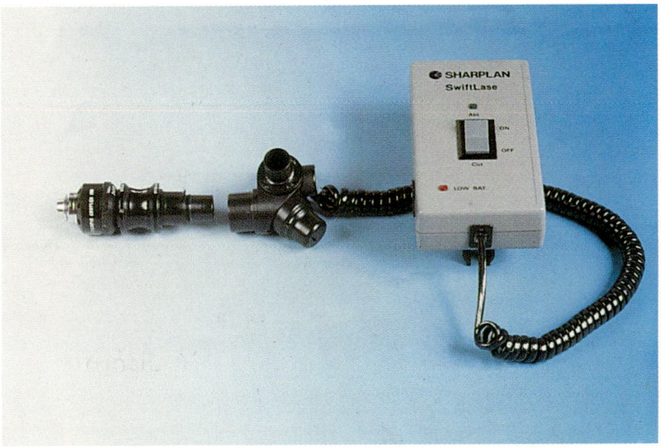

Plate 12.2 Swiftlase: miniature optomechanical scanner compatible with any CO_2 laser.

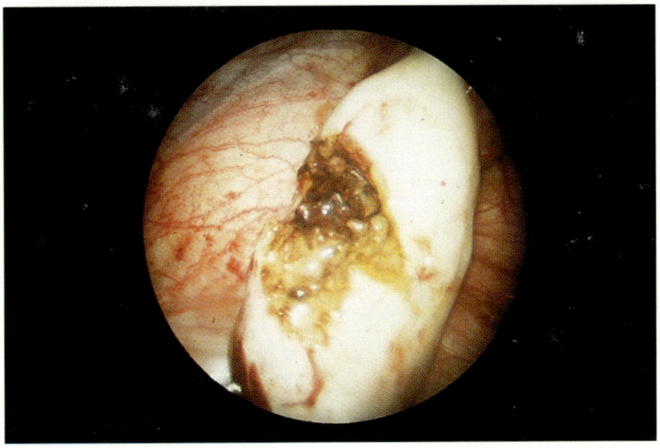

Plate 12.3 Endometrioma less than 3 cm in size: the interior wall of the cyst is vaporized using the CO_2 laser.

[*facing page 242*]

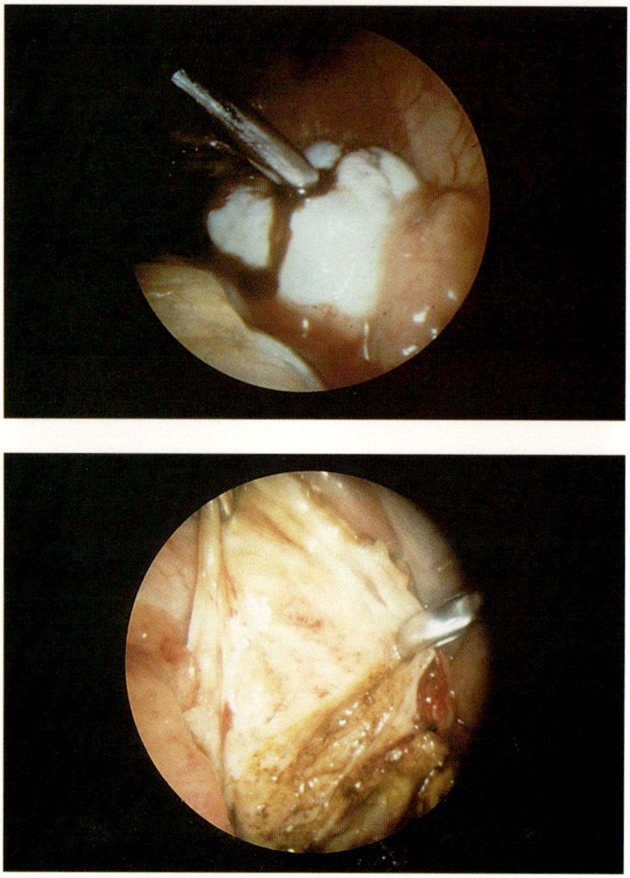

(a)

(b)

Plate 12.4 Endometrioma > 3 cm. (a) First step: drainage and washing out with saline solution. (b) Second step: after 12-weeks GnRH agonist, the atrophic interior cyst wall is easily vaporized with the Swiftlase.

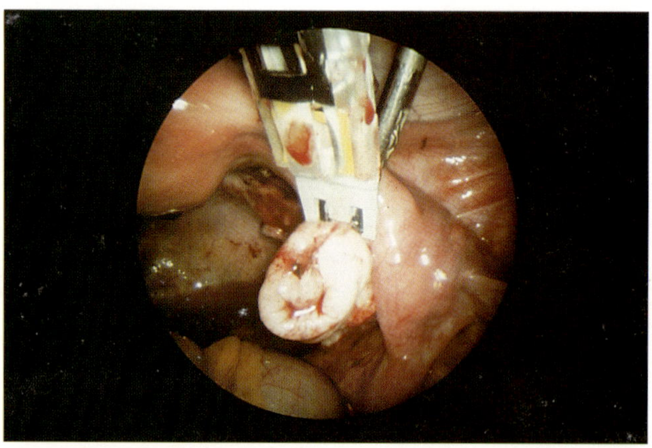

Plate 12.5 Ovarian closure with an 'Endohernia' titanium clip.

In this series, the ovarian cysts ranged from 3 to 8 cm in size. A partial cystectomy of the protruded portion of the ovarian cyst was then carried out with the CO_2 laser. Ovarian cystoscopy was performed for an evaluation of the interior cyst wall and a biopsy was taken. The residual endometrial cyst wall was then vaporized with the CO_2 laser, equipped with the Swiftlase (Plate 12.4b, facing p. 242).

In cases of multilocular endometrial cysts, all the residual endometriomas must be vaporized.

Ovarian closure

In cases of large cysts treated by laser surgery, closure must be suggested in order to decrease the risk of postoperative adhesions between the vaporized area and other pelvic structures [18].

Suturing [19]. The ability to suture during laparoscopy was initially developed by Semm and Mettler [19]. Loop ligation using the Endoloop or Roeder loop is mostly used as an adjuvant to haemostasis, and as a classic ligature in the case of salpingo-oophorectomy or oophorectomy.

With the advent of endoligature and the intra- and extracorporeal operative knotting techniques, classic methods used at laparotomy were introduced into endoscopic surgery and have become a mainstay. The intracorporeal knotting technique has been recommended by Semm and Mettler [19] for fine ovarian sutures. Two lower abdominal puncture sites are necessary and, through these, laparoscopic needle-holders are introduced to manipulate suture, needle and involved tissue. The suture material used is 4/0 or 6/0 polydioxanone (PDS).

Fibrin sealant [7, 18]. Fibrin sealant is useful in controlling microvascular or capillary bleeding from ruptured or surgically dissected tissues. It is particularly beneficial for patients with increased bleeding tendencies while undergoing surgery. It might also be used to seal tissue with different kinds of biomaterials. Thus, fibrin sealant has a place in all surgical disciplines for the purposes of tissue sealing, haemostasis and support of wound healing. There seem to be a few drawbacks, such as the risk of viral transmittance; however, the benefits of combining fibrin sealing with modern-day surgery far outweigh any known risks. In our series, Tissucol (fibrin sealant) (Immuno AG, Vienna, Austria) was injected transabdominally into the intraovarian vaporized area, and the edges of the ovarian cyst were approximated with atraumatic forceps for 2–3 min. After clotting occurs, further mechanical stress should be avoided for 3–5 min. At the end of the procedure, copious irrigation of the pelvic cavity was carried out to prevent deposits of carbon and glue. Thereafter, 100–200 ml of 32% Dextran 70 was instilled into the peritoneal cavity in all patients.

Clips. Clips can also be used for closing the ovarian cortex after cystectomy. The clip is of medium to large size and made of titanium, an inert, non-reactive metal (Autosuture (Endohernia^{R}); Ethicon). Three to four clips were applied using the 10 mm clip applicator; this was usually sufficient to achieve the ovarian closure (Plate 12.5, facing p. 242). For ovarian surgery, a titanium clip was preferred to one made of PDS material.

Ovarian cystectomy

Ovarian cystectomy, a frequently performed procedure for benign ovarian cysts, will be described in Chapter 13. The procedure begins with adhesiolysis between the posterior wall of the endometrioma and the broad ligament. Once the cyst is mobilized, the cortex is grasped with a forceps introduced through a second trocar. The cortex is incised using laser or scissors. The cyst wall is then exposed.

The incision is enlarged with scissors and, by traction and countertraction, the dissection is carried out. The surgeon must constantly observe tissue tension, and the grasping forceps must often be moved in order to apply the traction in just the right place to avoid tearing the ovary. At the ovarian hilus, the dissection is often more difficult, but nevertheless the dissection should continue until the cyst is completely removed from the ovary. Aquadissection can be used to facilitate the dissection. Injection of dilute vasopressin between the capsule and the ovarian cortex can also be used to create a tissue plane dissection and to reduce oozing in the ovarian bed. If the cyst is opened and spillage occurs, peritoneal irrigation must be performed in order to remove the chocolate-coloured fluid. Ovarioscopy and careful evaluation of the internal cyst wall allow the surgeon to exclude the presence of malignant lesions. Thereafter, the interior ovarian surface is examined and rinsed.

Haemostasis is usually achieved spontaneously but, if necessary, bipolar coagulation can be used. But aggressive electrocoagulation can be the cause of ovarian destruction and premature ovarian failure.

Because normal ovarian tissue was often removed together with the cyst wall, the technique of ovarian cystectomy was abandoned in our department for the treatment of endometriomas associated with infertility.

Results

The operating time varied from 45 to 80 min. Vaporization of the mucosal lining was facilitated by the preoperative therapy (GnRH-a administered subcutaneously) [9, 20]. Indeed, the interior wall of the endometrial cyst seen during ovarian cystoscopy was found to be less haemorrhagic and more atrophic than before therapy. These data were confirmed by ovarian biopsy. An endometriotic lesion was considered 'active' when typical glandular epithelium appeared either proliferative or completely unresponsive to hormonal therapy with typical stroma. Such a lesion was found significantly more often (84% of cases) ($P < 0.001$) before GnRH-a therapy than after GnRH-a therapy (44% of cases) [2, 5, 7, 9, 20].

Pregnancy rates

The cumulative pregnancy rates were analysed in a consecutive series of 407 patients with ovarian endometriosis (AFS moderate $n = 305$; AFS severe $n = 102$). A pregnancy rate of more than 55% was achieved in moderate endometriosis and 44% in severe endometriosis (Fig. 12.4). The majority of pregnancies occurred during the first 10 months following surgery.

Recurrence rate

Laparoscopic stripping of ovarian endometriomas may be difficult in cases of very large cysts and/or friable cyst walls. Fayez and Vogel [8] reported a 22% incidence of deep ovarian endometriosis at second-look laparoscopy after this procedure. Using the same laparoscopic procedure, Canis *et al.* [21] reported a 7% incidence of deep ovarian endometriosis at second-look laparoscopy in

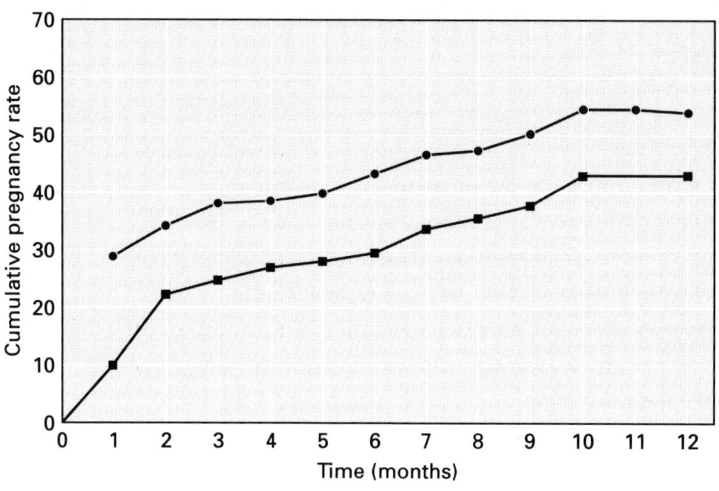

Fig. 12.4 Cumulative pregnancy rate after combined (medical and surgical) therapy in moderate and severe endometriosis. Circles, moderate, first study GnRH ($n = 305$); squares, severe, first study GnRH ($n = 102$).

cases of endometriomas of > 3 cm. They suggest an additional vaporization or fulguration when the ovarian stripping is not satisfactory. In our series of 814 patients with ovarian endometriomas treated with the combined (GnRH-a and laser surgery) therapy, 560 patients were followed up for 2–10 years. A recurrence of ovarian endometriomas was observed in 41 cases (7%).

Conclusion

The CO_2 laser laparoscopy offers several advantages over cautery. With the CO_2 laser, the laparoscopist is able to control the process of vaporization by visualizing the three-dimensional boundaries of the lesion.

In a previous study [6], significantly different pregnancy rates according to the stage of endometriosis were found. Severe endometriosis had the poorest prognosis in terms of pregnancy rates. For this reason, a preoperative hormonal (GnRH-a) therapy was given to patients with very large ovarian endometriomas (> 3 cm). The release of a GnRH-a by a biodegradable implant is effective in reducing endometriotic size to a greater extent than other drugs and permits a decrease in pelvic inflammation. Treatment by sustained release is an effective alternative to using steroid hormones before laser laparoscopy. A subcutaneous GnRH-a implant permits a substantial reduction in large ovarian cyst diameter and a decrease in pelvic inflammation, so that a second-look laser laparoscopy could be carried out for laser vaporization of residual endometriomas. During ovarian cystoscopy, the interior ovarian wall was found to be atrophic. The cyst vascularity was decreased, and the vaporization was thus facilitated.

References

1 Donnez J, Lemaire M, Karaman Y, Nisolle M, Casanas-Roux F. Combined (hormonal and microsurgical) therapy in infertile women with endometriosis. *Fertil Steril* 1987 **48**: 239.

2 Nisolle M, Casanas-Roux F, Donnez J. Histologic study of ovarian endometriosis after hormonal therapy. *Fertil Steril* 1988 **49**: 423–426.

3 Donnez J, Nisolle M, Casanas-Roux F. Endometriosis-associated infertility: evaluation of preoperative use of danazol, gestrinone and buserelin. *Int J Fertil* 1990 **42**: 128.

4 Nezhat C, Crowgey SR, Garrison CP. Surgical treatment of endometriosis via laser laparoscopy. *Fertil Steril* 1986 **45**: 778–783.

5 Donnez J. CO_2 laser laparoscopy in infertile women with adhesions or endometriosis. *Fertil Steril* 1987 **48**: 390–394.

6 Donnez J, Nisolle M, Casanas-Roux F. CO_2 laser laparoscopy in infertile women with adnexal adhesions and women with tubal occlusion. *J Gynecol Surg* 1989 **5**: 47–53.

7 Donnez J, Nisolle M. Laparoscopic management of large ovarian endometrial cysts: use of fibrin sealant. *J Gynecol Surg* 1991 **7**: 163–167.

8 Fayez JA, Vogel MF. Comparison of different treatment methods of endometriomas by laparoscopy. *Obstet Gynecol* 1991 **78**; 660–665.

9 Donnez J, Nisolle M, Gillerot S *et al.* Ovarian endometrial cysts: the role of gonadotropin-releasing-hormone agonist and/or drainage. *Fertil Steril* 1994 **62**: 63–66.

10 Nezhat C, Nezhat F, Silfen SL. Video laseroscopy: the CO_2 laser for advanced operative laparoscopy. *Obstet Gynecol Clin North Am* 1991 **18**: 585–604.

11 Donnez J, Nisolle M, Casanas-Roux F. Endoscopic surgery. *Ballière's Clin Obstet Gynaecol* 1993 7: 839–848.

12 Donnez J, Nisolle M, Casanas-Roux F, Clerckx F. Endometriosis: rationale for surgery. In: Brosens I, Donnez J. (eds). *The Current Status of Endometriosis: Research and Management*, 1993, pp. 385–395. Carnforth, Parthenon Publishing.

13 Nisolle M, Paindaveine B, Bourdon A *et al.* Histologic study of peritoneal endometriosis in infertile women. *Fertil Steril* 1990 **53**: 984–988.

14 Sampson JA. Peritoneal endometriosis due to dissemination of endometrial tissue into the peritoneal cavity. *Am J Obstet Gynecol* 1927 **14**: 422–469.

15 Hughesdon PE. The structure of endometrial cysts of the ovary. *J Obstet Gynaecol Br Empire* 1957 **64**: 481–487.

16 Brosens IA, Puttemans PJ. Double-optic laparoscopy: salpingoscopy, ovarian cystoscopy and endo-ovarian surgery with the argon laser. *Baillière's Clin Obstet Gynaecol* 1989 **3**: 595–608.

17 Donnez J, Zair E, Nisolle M, Slatkine M. Swiftlase: a new technology for endoscopic peritoneal endometriosis and endometriotic cyst management. *J Gynecol Surg* 1994 (submitted for publication).

18 Donnez J, Nisolle M, Karaman Y *et al.* CO_2 laser laparoscopy in peritoneal endometriosis and in ovarian cyst. *J Gynecol Surgery* 1990 **5**: 391.

19 Semm K, Mettler L. Technical progress in pelvic surgery via operative laparoscopy. *Am J Obstet Gynecol* 1980 **138**: 121–127.

20 Donnez J, Nisolle M, Clerckx F, Sandow J, Casanas-Roux F. Administration of nasal buserelin as compared with subcutaneous buserelin implant for endometriosis. *Fertil Steril* 1989 **52**: 27–30.

21 Canis M, Mage G, Wattiez A *et al.* Second-look laparoscopy after laparoscopic cystectomy of large endometriomas. *Fertil Steril* 1992 **58**: 617–619.

Chapter 13
Techniques for Ablation and Excision of Endometriosis

M.J. CANIS, S. BOUGHIZANE, F.H. LOH, J.L. POULY, A. WATTIEZ, H. MANHES, G. MAGE AND M.-A. BRUHAT

Introduction

The goals in the surgical treatment of endometriosis are complete ablation and/or excision of the active endometriotic tissue and correction of anatomical distortion induced by the adhesions and the cystic lesions [1]. This treatment should be achieved with minimal tissue damage. Over the last few years, laparoscopic surgery has been accepted as a valuable alternative to the conventional and the microsurgical approaches by laparotomy. The advantages of laparoscopy are so obvious that one may consider any laparoscopic procedure as valuable. Discussion and debates comparing the most effective laparoscopic technique (excision, coagulation, vaporization) and instruments (CO_2 laser, electrocautery or scissors) are not crucial to the outcomes. One should be able to identify the disease and to use the most effective surgical modality for each location and each patient, in order to obtain the desired postoperative result, which may be pain relief, intrauterine pregnancy or both. Surgical and medical treatments have their own indications, taking into account the limits of each approach. For instance, medical treatments have no effect on dense pelvic adhesions, whereas microscopic peritoneal disease cannot be treated surgically.

Despite the development of laparoscopic surgery, which is becoming the gold standard for treatment of endometriosis, many questions, such as the activity of the implants, postoperative adhesion re-formation and recurrence of endometriosis, have still to be answered. Endometriosis remains enigmatic and poorly understood.

Patient preparation

As for any surgical procedure, perfect exposure is the key to satisfactory treatment, and adequate laparoscopic 'retractors' are the key to exposure. We think that the first 'retractor' is the bowel preparation, which is given to each patient on the day before surgery. The patient lies in a modified dorsal lithotomy position, with legs slightly flexed (15–20°) and abducted to form a 45° angle. This position allows easy manipulation of the uterus, intraoperative examinations, easy access to the vagina and to the rectum and proper insertion of second-puncture trocars. A shoulder brace is placed on the left side. The left arm (on the operator's side) is fixed alongside the patient's body.

The pneumoperitoneum is the second laparoscopic 'retractor'; it should be maintained using an automatic insufflator capable of delivering up to 9 l/min [2, 3]. Uterine canulation is the third 'retractor'. We use a long curette taped to a tenaculum or the Valtchev apparatus. This device, which also allows uterine anteflexion, may be very helpful to treat posterior cul-de-sac endometriosis. The Trendelenburg position is the fourth 'retractor'. The correct angle, about 10°, is required to push all the bowel loops over the superior pelvic brim. Prophylactic antibiotics are routinely administered in patients with ovarian endometriomas or deep infiltrating peritoneal implants, or with a previous history of pelvic inflammatory disease.

Laparoscopic diagnosis of endometriosis: a 'staging' procedure

Laparoscopic diagnosis is a staging procedure. Our technique is described in Chapter 9. It should be achieved by accounting for atypical, typical and deeply invasive peritoneal implants [4–6]. Routine puncture of enlarged ovaries has recently been advocated again by Candiani *et al.* [7]. The vagina and the posterior cul-de-sac are assessed using vaginal examination and/or vaginal and rectal probes [8]. If an ovarian endometrioma is found, a biopsy is required to rule out malignancy and to differentiate endometriomas from functional cysts [9].

The treatment

General principles

Basically endometriotic implants can be treated using excision or *in situ* destruction achieved by coagulation or vaporization. Although excision seems more dangerous, injuries to the ureters and the rectum might occur during vaporization as well as during excision. As endometriosis is an invasive disease, when all the endometriotic tissue is treated, ablation is as dangerous and as difficult as excision. A complete treatment is a retroperitoneal procedure, often dissecting close to the ureter, the uterine vessels or the rectum.

Endometriosis is surrounded by fibrotic tissue. Active glands and stroma will often be identified during pathologic examination of tissues which appeared 'fibrotic' at laparoscopy; therefore complete treatment of fibrotic tissue is required whenever possible. Most authors agree that excisional techniques improve tissue recognition when compared with vaporization and/or coagulation. As it may be difficult to distinguish normal coagulated tissue from abnormal tissue, a cutting effect should be used when outlining the limits of lesions to be excised. When using a CO_2 laser, a very high-power density is required to avoid carbonization.

Irrespective of the procedure, prior identification of the tissue is the key to safe surgery. Cutting or vaporizing without prior identification is a blind procedure. Identification is achieved by inspection in simple cases or by dissection with hydrodissection and/or scissors. This old surgical rule is still essential at laparoscopy. Careful haemostasis and frequent peritoneal lavages are required. To allow better visualization, one should proceed from the lower to the upper part and from the posterior to the anterior part of the pelvis so that bleeding induced by the first steps do not obscure the operative field.

Laparoscopic surgery should follow the principles of microsurgery: magnification obtained when the endoscope is close to the tissue, constant irrigation of the operative field, minimal and gentle tissue handling, avoiding grasping, precise tissue dissection and careful and meticulous haemostasis, using bipolar coagulation and avoiding thermal damage to adjacent healthy tissue. Trauma to the visceral peritoneum, deperitonealized areas, sutures and postoperative drainage should be avoided.

Adhesiolysis

Adhesiolysis is the most difficult step and the main limit of laparoscopic treatment of endometriosis. The adhesions should be sectioned only when put under tension. One should proceed from the simple adhesions to the more complex dissections. As uterine cannulation is an essential means of laparoscopic retraction, the posterior cul-de-sac should be freed as early as possible. Laparoscopic adhesiolysis may be performed using hydrodissection, scissors, atraumatic forceps or CO_2 laser. It is mandatory to first dissociate the tissues and then cut identified structures. If the dissection is difficult, curved scissors are the best instruments. Mechanical section is as effective as electrical or laser section, but does not induce any thermal effects so identification of the tissue is easier. Hydrodissection is useful when beginning the cleavage of surgical planes; it can generate high enough pressure to dissociate normal tissues but not fibrotic tissue and vessels. Our own practice is not to use any medical pretreatment or intraperitoneal adjuvant aimed at preventing postoperative adhesion formation.

Treatment of superficial peritoneal implants

Excision

The lesion margins are identified and outlined with a cutting instrument, with or without previous coagulation of the adjacent normal peritoneum. The implant is lifted up with atraumatic forceps, and separated from the normal underlying tissue using dissection and traction. Excision may be easy or extremely difficult depending on the location, thickness and size of the implant.

Vaporization

Vaporization is achieved using a high-power density delivered over a short time. The rapid expansion of water to vapour results in transformation of thermal energy to mechanical energy, thus causing tissue separation and significant smoke production. Vaporization is precise when performed without carbonization. Since the power density decreases in a Gaussian distribution from the middle of the beam to the periphery, a very high-power density is required to avoid carbonization in the periphery of the shot. Most CO_2 lasers are actually used in the superpulse or even ultrapulse mode, allowing a high-power density with minimal thermal damage. The CO_2 laser is obviously the best instrument to vaporize peritoneal implants. The extinction length of this laser is very short so that 'what you see is what you get'.

Coagulation

Coagulation occurs with lower energies and results in lower temperature at the tissue level. Between 60 and 80°C, blanching is obtained, with the loss of intracellular water and coagulation of proteins. Using coagulation it is almost impossible to control the depth of the tissue effect. Although the blanching effect may appear limited, thermal damage to adjacent structures may occur when using large instruments and long duration of contact. The blanching of the surface of black lesions does not ensure complete destruction of the lesion, and, when opening the cyst, chocolate fluid will be found, demonstrating that coagulation of the deeper part of the cyst is necessary.

On the other hand, to treat superficial peritoneal lesions, blanching is effectively achieved using coagulation with a defocused CO_2 laser beam or a bipolar forceps. These instruments should be moved fast enough to avoid unnecessary thermal damage.

Treatment of deep infiltrating peritoneal implants

To treat deep infiltrating endometriotic implants, most experts would agree that complete excision of endometriotic and fibrotic tissue is required. Therefore laparoscopic excision resembles an 'oncologic procedure'. Although complete excision might require rectal resection and/or total abdominal hysterectomy, these invading lesions should be managed performing a radical but still realistic procedure. Hysterectomy is not acceptable in a young patient!

An assistant trained in operative laparoscopy and in the clinical diagnosis of deep endometriosis should stand between the legs. He/she will expose the operative field by performing rectovaginal examination and moving rectal and vaginal probes. It is wise to begin the dissection in an uninvolved area to allow easier identification of adjacent structures. Adhesiolysis may be necessary to identify the organs involved by the implant, but it is time-consuming since excision of both points of attachment of the adhesion is required. Therefore, whenever possible, it is faster to first dissect the implants from adjacent organs such as the rectum. In this way, adhesiolysis and identification are performed in the same step so that excision may begin at once. Once the rectum has been fully dissected, the pelvis is filled with warm Ringer lactate solution and the rectum with air or methylene blue, looking for incidental rectal lacerations. In the same way, ureters should be routinely visualized and fully dissected up to the uterus whenever the uterosacral ligaments are involved. The excision of deep implants should be performed towards the uterus, allowing an easier identification of the ureters. The nodule is then outlined anteriorly and the excision is completed. A vaginal incision is often but not routinely required [10]. When the vagina is opened, the procedure may be completed vaginally or laparoscopically.

Extensive peritoneal lavage is used to minimize the consequences of vaginal contamination. Haemostasis is also checked when the uterus is back in its normal situation, allowing identification of bleeders masked by the tension on the vessels when the uterus is held in anteversion. These procedures will result in very large deperitonealized areas which cannot be sutured. Although we have performed very few routine second-look laparoscopies in such patients, we are convinced that adhesion re-formation in the posterior cul-de-sac is decreased by uneventful complete excision of abnormal tissue. Treatment of complete cul-de-sac obliteration is impossible without perfect co-operation between the surgeon and the assistant.

To excise uterosacral nodules, the peritoneum is incised lateral to the uterosacral ligament. The ureter is first identified, dissected and protected. Thereafter the uterosacral ligament is resected, beginning posteriorly and working towards the uterus. When the nodule has been freed from the underlying tissue, the anterior part of the ligament is cut. Most deep uterosacral implants can be treated without vaginal incision.

In patients with pelvic pain, a postoperative medical treatment is given for 3–6 months to attempt to reduce the recurrence rate. Deep infiltrating bowel, rectal or ureteral endometriosis should be excised. Most of these cases are still treated by laparotomy.

Treatment of ovarian endometriomas

When treating ovarian endometriomas we should have four goals:

1 To rule out malignancy, using our previously reported protocol, as when dealing with any ovarian cystic masses [11].

2 To remove all the ovarian ectopic endometrium; in older patients complete excision is required as malignant transformation may occur in ovarian endometriomas [12].

3 To minimize the ovarian trauma in order to preserve ovarian follicules.

4 To minimize postoperative adhesion formation or re-formation, since postoperative adhesions are common after ovarian surgery [13].

In 1957 Hughesdon showed that in more than 90% of ovarian endometriomas the cyst wall represents an inverted anterior ovarian cortex with adhesions and implants on its surface [14]. This hypothesis may explain why most endometriomas are located on the anterior ovarian surface and are often fixed to the broad ligament. The ovary should be freed from all adhesions to allow complete dissection of the cyst. Frequently, during ovariolysis, the endometrioma will be opened spontaneously, since the cyst is usually fixed to the broad ligament. Consequently, we think that the cyst cannot be removed entirely without complete ovariolysis and without an anterior ovarian incision. A posterior incision does not allow complete treatment and may induce adhesions in an area not commonly involved by adhesions.

Ovarian cystectomy [15, 16] or stripping of the lining, laser vaporization [17] or excision [18] have been described for treatment of ovarian endometriomas.

At laparoscopy, CO_2 laser vaporization is time-consuming and requires a preoperative medical treatment. Consequently we treat most ovarian endometriomas by intraperitoneal cystectomy. This ovarian incision is essential to obtain a good approximation of the ovary after the dissection. When the cyst has not ruptured during the adhesiolysis, the ovary is incised on the ovarian antemesenteric border [15]. When the cyst is opened accidentally when freeing the ovary, an anterior vertical incision is performed, starting from the location of the rupture. This incision is only grossly approximated at the end of the procedure. The adhesions potentially induced with this incision will be located on a site where adhesion re-formation is quite common. The incision should be large enough to avoid a difficult dissection. On the most dependent part, the ovarian cortex may be so thin that the cleavage plane cannot be identified; in such cases a partial resection of the ovarian cortex or an enlarged incision is necessary to identify the cleavage. The cyst wall and the ovarian cortex are grasped with atraumatic grasping forceps and the plane is developed by pulling these forceps slowly in opposite directions. The forceps are frequently repositioned near the cleavage plane so as to allow permanent visual control of the dissection and prevent tearing of tissue and associated bleeding.

In difficult cases, three suprapubic instruments are necessary. Two grasping forceps are used to expose the plane developed with scissors, hydrodissection or bipolar coagulation. Difficulties are encountered with small and large endometriomas, in patients who received a preoperative medical treatment as well as in those who did not. During the dissection, these difficulties should be recognized early enough to avoid unnecessary ovarian damage and the diffuse oozing which would prevent an effective CO_2 laser ablation. Once the dissection is completed, additional haemostasis is achieved using bipolar coagulation. When the spontaneous ovarian shape is unsatisfactory, it is approximated with 4/0 intraovarian sutures [19].

As one of our patients had an abdominal wall endometrioma located at a previous suprapubic trocar site, we think that abdominal wall contamination should be avoided using a laparoscopic bag or a 10 mm trocar when extracting the cyst wall. When using a 10 mm trocar, one should use a 5 mm external reducer, so that the cyst can be grasped with a 5 mm forceps and easily brought inside the trocar. The 5 mm external reducer is essential; indeed, if a 10 mm forceps is inserted in a 10 mm trocar, it is impossible to bring the cyst inside the trocar.

Laparoscopic laser vaporization is used to treat endometriomas less than 3 cm in diameter or the remaining part of larger cysts when a complete dissection is not possible. Laser treatment of endometriomas is easier and faster when performed after a 3-month course of medical treatment [20]. The CO_2 laser is the best instrument for treatment of superficial ovarian endometriotic lesions.

Reviewing our data, we found that adhesions are the main limiting factors of complete treatment (Table 13.1). Complete treatment was achieved in 89%

Table 13.1 Laparoscopic treatment of ovarian endometriomas, according to the size of the cyst and the overall adhesion score

		Partial treatment		Complete treatment	
	N	*n*	%	*n*	%
Cyst < 3 cm	54	12*	22.2	42	77.8
Cyst ⩾ 3 cm	118	13*	11.0	105	89.0
Adhesion score ⩽ 50	127	13†	10.2	114	89.8
Adhesion score > 50	45	12†	26.7	33	73.3

* NS

† $P < 0.01$.

of the cysts of more than 3 cm, but in only 73.3% of the cysts diagnosed in patients with an overall adhesion score of more than 50 (including all the adnexal adhesions and the posterior cul-de-sac obliteration). The efficacy of laparoscopic treatment of ovarian endometriomas, including large ones, has been confirmed from data obtained at second-look laparoscopy (SLL) before 1991 (Table 13.2).

Table 13.2 Results of second-look laparoscopy (lap.) after complete treatment of an ovarian endometrioma. The ovarian score is the American Fertility Society (AFS) ovarian score

Group	No. of cases	First lap.	Second lap.	*P**
Cyst < 3 cm	13	16	2.3 ± 5.4	< 0.002
Cyst ⩾ 3 cm	61	20	1.7 ± 2.4	< 0.001
Total	74	19.3 ± 1.5	2.1 ± 5.0	< 0.001
Severe endometriosis	55	19.2 ± 1.5	2.3 ± 5.1	< 0.001
Moderate endometriosis	19	19.6 ± 1.3	1.8 ± 4.8	< 0.001
Ovarian adhesion < 16	58	19.2 ± 1.6	2.0 ± 4.7	< 0.001
Ovarian adhesion = 16	16	19.8 ± 1.0	2.75 ± 6.1	< 0.001

* Statistical comparison used the Wilcoxon signed rank test.

In a previous report [16], we found that adhesion formation occurred in 21% of the adnexa treated by intraperitoneal cystectomy; furthermore, complete or partial recurrence of adhesions treated at laparoscopy occurred in 82.3% of the cases. To study contralateral adhesions, contralateral adnexa without deep ovarian endometriosis were selected, including adnexa with an initial adnexal adhesion score ⩽ 4. In both groups, the mean adnexal adhesion was different at SLL (Table 13.3). Three adnexa with an initial adnexal adhesion score ⩽ 4 had an adnexal adhesion score of 8 at SLL. One of these failures was explained by a postoperative haematoma. As expected, postoperative adhesions can be induced by poor laparoscopic procedures. Strict guidelines should be followed to minimize postoperative adhesions [2,21,22].

Recurrence rates were studied retrospectively, including 163 patients followed for more than 1 year. The incidence of pathologically confirmed recurrences was 15.9% (25 cases). Most recurrences occurred within the first postoperative year or after the end of the second postoperative year. Early recurrences were attributed to incomplete treatment whereas late recurrences might result from the natural history of the disease.

We confirmed that ovarian function was not impaired by laparoscopic dissection of ovarian endometriomas. We found no difference when comparing patients who had had prior treatment of ovarian endometriomas with patients with tubal infertility or those treated for endometriosis but without

Table 13.3 Results of second-look laparoscopy (lap.): comparison of adnexal adhesion scores after complete treatment of an ovarian endometrioma of more than 3 cm. The adhesion scores were obtained by adding the American Fertility Society (AFS) scores attributed to ovarian and tubal adhesions

Group	No. of cases	First lap.	Second lap.	P*
Cyst > 3 cm	72	12.5 ± 10.6	11.2 ± 11.2	> 0.3
Severe endometriosis	51	15.9 ± 10.4	13.8 ± 12.0	> 0.3
Moderate endometriosis	21	4.4 ± 5.1	4.5 ± 4.9	> 0.9
Ovarian adhesion = 16	17	26.3 ± 6.6	16.0 ± 12.3	< 0.02
Ovarian adhesion $\leqslant 4$	24	3.0 ± 3.9	4.9 ± 6.6	> 0.2
Ovarian adhesion > 4 and < 16	30	12.8 ± 6.7	13.5 ± 11.8	> 0.7
Contralateral adnexa				
All cases	32	5.6 ± 9.9	3.9 ± 6.9	> 0.4
Adnexal adhesion score $\leqslant 4$	23	0.6 ± 1.4	1.7 ± 2.9	> 0.1

* Statistical comparison used the Wilcoxon signed rank test.

Table 13.4 Mean number of oocytes obtained during IVF pick-up according to the indication and to previous surgical procedures

Indication	No. of cases	No. of oocytes
Tubal infertility	253	8.43
Endometriosis		
Without endometrioma	83	8.22
With an endometrioma	67	8.49
Endometrioma treated by ovarian cystectomy	34	7.96

ovarian endometriomas (Table 13.4). However, significant ovarian damage can be induced by poor procedures since endometriomas are often close to the ovarian vessels.

Associated and radical procedures

Section of the uterosacral ligaments, presacral neurectomy and uterine suspension can be performed laparoscopically [2, 23, 24]. These procedures, proposed to relieve chronic pelvic pain, are probably more valuable in the treatment of dysmenorrhoea and central pelvic pain than in the treatment of lateral pain [25]. However, the efficacy of these techniques in patients treated for endometriosis has never been evaluated prospectively. Moreover, damage to the ureter has been reported during laser uterosacral nerve ablation [26], and presacral neurectomy is a potentially dangerous procedure since it requires dissection of common iliac veins [27]. Consequently, further prospective randomized trials are required to study these procedures. Uterosacral ligament should be excised when infiltrated by deep implants. Presacral neurectomy should be performed only in patients with central pelvic pain, particularly central dysmenorrhoea.

Appendectomy is not routinely indicated during laparoscopic treatment of endometriosis; however, macroscopic appendicular endometriotic implants should be removed.

Finally, radical procedures such as oophorectomy, adnexectomy or hysterectomy can be achieved laparoscopically [2, 28]. These radical procedures might be indicated in pain patients over 40 years old who have undergone several operations before. Endometriosis is likely to be one of the major indications for laparoscopic hysterectomy or laparoscopically assisted vaginal hysterectomy, since the vaginal approach is difficult in these patients.

Results and complications

The results obtained in infertile patients [29] are presented in Table 13.5. Over the last 4 years, our management of infertile patients has been changed following the good results obtained in our *in vitro* fertilization–embryo transfer (IVF-ET) programme. In this way, most patients with endometriosis and male infertility are treated with IVF immediately or less than 9 months after the laparoscopic diagnosis of endometriosis. It can be seen from Table 13.6 that the treatment of infertility is quite effective in patients with endometriosis. Using laparoscopic treatment and IVF, the pregnancy rates are similar, whatever the extent of the disease and in patients with and without male infertility. Our management is summarized in Fig. 13.1. Preoperative medical treatment after ultrasonographic-guided puncture of large ovarian endometriomas appears to be an attractive approach, which needs to be carefully evaluated. In patients without pain, we have to treat infertility, not endometriosis, and our objective should be a term pregnancy with minimal cost and as soon as possible. As endometriosis often recurs after surgical treatment, the surgical treatment does not have, as in patients with tubal disease, the advantage of allowing a second pregnancy without additional treatment.

Complications of laparoscopic treatment are uncommon in our experience. Three patients underwent reoperation because of postoperative bleeding. One was reoperated on postoperative day 2, one on postoperative day 10 and one 3 weeks later. All three patients had large cysts. In two cases, the procedure was described as difficult, as several endometriomas were removed from one ovary. In our opinion the cause of this complication was the conservative management rather than the laparoscopic approach. The third postoperative haemorrhage was attributed to a coagulation disorder, induced by non-steroidal anti-inflammatory drugs and low-molecular-weight heparin.

Table 13.5 Fertility after treatment of endometriosis

	N	IUP	%
After laparoscopic treatment all cases			
All patients	255	94	36.8
Stage I	78	31	39.7
Stage II	43	15	34.8
Stage III	71	23	32.4
Stage IV	63	25	46.4
Stage IV RAFS score $\leqslant$ 70	33	19	57.6
Stage IV RAFS score > 70	30	6	20.0
Excluding immediate IVF and lost to follow-up			
All patients	198	94	47.5
Stage I	62	31	50.0
Stage II	36	15	41.7
Stage III	57	23	40.3
Stage IV	43	25	58.1
Stage IV and AFS score $\leqslant$ 70	28	19	67.8
Stage IV and AFS score > 70	15	6	40.0
After laparoscopic treatment and/or IVF lost to follow-up excluded			
All patients	227	143	63.0
Stage I	67	42	62.7
Stage II	39	26	66.6
Stage III	65	35	53.8
Stage IV	56	40	71.4
Stage IV $\leqslant$ 70	32	24	75.0
Stage IV > 70	24	16	66.7

RAFS = revised American Fertility Society; IUP = intrauterine pregnancy.

Two patients who sustained a rectal laceration during the excision of a rectovaginal nodule were managed by immediate laparotomy. One patient had a vaginal haemorrhage 10 days after the excision of a rectovaginal nodule; the haemostasis was achieved vaginally.

Discussion

Endoscopic surgery has several advantages over laparotomy. By reducing physical stress and avoiding abdominal incision, the duration of the hospital stay and postoperative recovery and the associated costs are dramatically reduced. More importantly, laparoscopy avoids peritoneal drying, thus reducing peritoneal trauma and the potential for adhesion formation. This is essential in patients with an inflammatory disease such as endometriosis.

Table 13.6 Endometriosis and infertility: male infertility

	Male infertility			
	Yes		No	
	n	IUP (%)	*n*	IUP (%)
After laparoscopic treatment (immediate and lost to follow-up and IVF excluded)				
All cases	46	15 (32.6)*	152	79 (52.0)*
Stage I	18	6 (33.3)	44	25 (56.8)
Stage II	9	3 (33.3)	27	12 (44.4)
Stage III	11	2 (18.2)	46	21 (45.7)
Stage IV	8	4 (50.0)	35	21 (60.0)
After laparoscopic treatment and/or IVF, including lost to follow-up				
All cases	57	30 (52.6)†	170	114 (67.1)†
Stage I	20	9 (45.0)	47	33 (70.1)
Stage II	10	7 (70.0)	29	21 (72.4)
Stage III	16	6 (37.5)	49	29 (59.8)
Stage IV	11	8 (72.7)	45	32 (71.0)

* $\chi^2 = 4.4$, $P < 0.02$.
† $\chi^2 = 3.24$, $P > 0.07$.
IUP = intrauterine pregnancy.

However, a laparoscopic microsurgical technique is required to ensure complete treatment and optimal results.

Provided that complete treatment is achieved, there are no scientific data to demonstrate that any laparoscopic technique or instrument is better than the others. Fortunately (or unfortunately!), the surgeon's experience and expertise are much more important. One should be able to use all the instruments and techniques as appropriate, according to the size, location and thickness of the implant and the desired postoperative effect. Undertaking large studies to compare instruments and techniques appears useless, as it seems almost impossible to demonstrate that one instrument is better than another. We have indications for excision and indications for vaporization, which are summarized in Table 13.7.

As regards ovarian endometriomas, we would stress that, in experienced hands, the laparoscopic management of large endometriomas is a valuable alternative to the conventional approach by laparotomy, but that operative difficulties will often be encountered [30], since persistent endometriomas and postoperative *de novo* adhesion formation have been found at SLL. The three-step medical and surgical treatment, initially proposed by Mettler and Semm [31] and re-evaluated by Donnez *et al.* [20], may need to be recon-

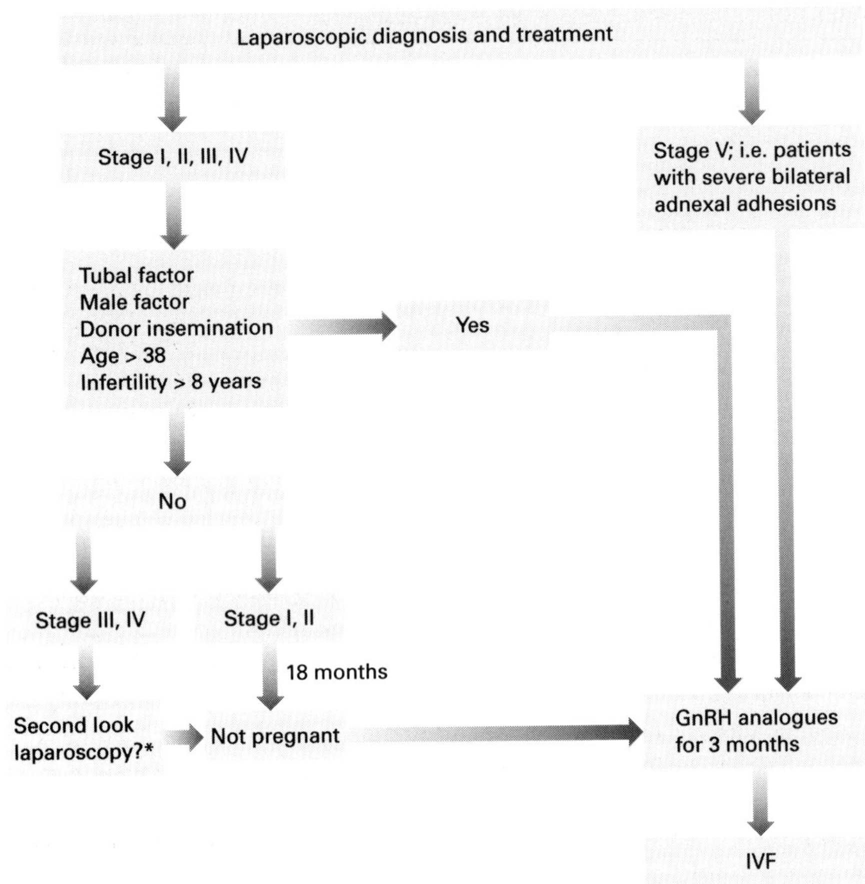

Fig. 13.1 Management of infertility associated with endometriosis.

sidered in young or infertile patients with endometriomas of more than 8 cm and/or with very active and inflammatory disease. Prospective randomized studies are required to compare all the plans of management, including IVF, which can be proposed for patients with severe endometriosis so that the surgeons of the year 2000 will be able to manage their patients according to scientific data rather than empirical feelings and clinical impressions. In patients with large endometriomas, careful preoperative and laparoscopic examinations are required to rule out malignancy, and consent for a possible laparotomy should be obtained.

Adhesiolysis remains the main limit of the surgical treatment of endometriosis. This limit will obviously differ according to the laparoscopic surgeon's experience and operating-room environment. Preoperative and intraoperative patient selection should be managed according to the

Table 13.7 Indications for excision and vaporization

Coagulation
Superficial peritoneal implant
Vaporization
1–3 mm deep peritoneal implants in safe areas
Superficial ovarian implants
Deep ovarian endometriomas < 3 cm
Large endometrioma after preoperative medical treatment
Excision
> 3 mm deep peritoneal implants
Any endometrioma in patients > 40 years old
1–3 mm deep peritoneal implants close to the ureter
Bowel, bladder, abdominal wall and vaginal disease

surgeon's experience and the patient's age, complaints and physical signs. By way of example, the management of a very severe unilateral adnexal involvement may differ according to clinical data. Once the diagnosis of a benign endometrioma has been confirmed, the adequate management may be: (i) a unilateral adnexectomy using a retroperitoneal approach and a routine dissection of the ureter in a patient over 40; (ii) a complete adhesiolysis with excision of all active disease in a young patient who complains of severe chronic pelvic pain; or (iii) biopsy and laser vaporization of the endometrioma without complete adhesiolysis in an infertile patient who has normal contralateral adnexa. Other plans of management might also be valuable in differing circumstances. Hence the same surgeon may be able to treat adequately the infertile but not the pain or the older patients. Under no circumstances, however, should the surgeon's inexperience or the technical limits of laparoscopic surgery be proposed as a valid indication for approximate, incomplete or unnecessarily radical procedures.

Postoperative adhesion re-formation appears to be one of the main limiting factors to good outcomes after laparoscopic surgery. Postoperative adhesions are related to the surgical procedure and to the natural history of the disease. As we recently found a 92.5% intrauterine pregnancy rate in patients who had been treated laparoscopically for a non-endometriotic ovarian cyst, we are convinced that adhesion formation is more common following laparoscopic treatment of endometriomas [15]. Laparoscopic surgery does not seem to improve the treatment of dense adhesions. Since IVF pregnancy rates obtained in patients with severe endometriosis and adhesions have been improved by transvaginal ultrasound-guided oocyte retrieval, such infertile patients should be treated by IVF.

To treat deep peritoneal implants, appropriate instruments, trained nurses and anaesthetists and extensive experience and expertise in endoscopic surgery are prerequisites. Endoscopic surgery is only a new surgical approach, not a new treatment based on a better understanding of the disease, so that many clinical questions have still to be answered despite the introduction of the so-considered 'magic' laparoscopy.

References

1 Cook AS, Rock JA. The role of laparoscopy in the treatment of endometriosis. *Fertil Steril* 1991 **55**: 663–680.

2 Bruhat MA, Mage G, Pouly JL *et al. Operative Laparoscopy*, 1992. New York, McGraw Hill.

3 Canis M, Mage G, Manhes H *et al.* Laparoscopic treatment of endometriosis. *Acta Obstet Gynecol Scand* 1989 **68** (Suppl). 150: 15–20.

4 Jansen RPS, Russell P. Non pigmented endometriosis: clinical, laparoscopic and pathologic definition. *Am J Obstet Gynecol* 1986 **155**: 1154–1159.

5 Martin DC, Hubert GD, Vander Zwaag R, El-Zeky FA. Laparoscopic appearances of peritoneal endometriosis. *Fertil Steril* 1989 **51**: 63–67.

6 Konninckx PR, Meuleman C, Demeyere S, Lesaffre E, Cornillie FJ. Suggestive evidence that pelvic endometriosis is a progressive disease, whereas deeply infiltrating endometriosis is associated with pelvic pain. *Fertil Steril* 1991 **55**: 759–765.

7 Candiani GB, Vercellini P, Fedele L. Laparoscopic ovarian puncture for correct staging of endometriosis. *Fertil Steril* 1990 **53**: 994–997.

8 Reich H, McGlynn F, Salvat J. Laparoscopic treatment of cul de sac obliteration secondary to retrocervical deep fibrotic endometriosis. *J Reprod Med* 1991 **36**: 516–522.

9 Martin DC, Berry JD. Histology of chocolate cysts. *J Gynecol Surg* 1990 **6**: 43–46.

10 Martin DC. Laparoscopic and vaginal colpotomy for the excision of infiltrating cul de sac endometriosis. *J Reprod Med* 1988 **33**: 806–808.

11 Canis M, Mage G, Pouly JL *et al.* Laparoscopic diagnosis of adnexal cystic masses: a 12-year experience with long term follow up. *Obstet Gynecol* 1994 **83**: 707–712.

12 Heaps JM, Nieberg RK, Berek JS. Malignant neoplasms arising in endometriosis. *Obstet Gynecol* 1990 **75**: 1023–1028.

13 Pittaway DE, Daniell JF, Maxson WL. Ovarian surgery in an infertility patient as an indication for a short-interval second-look laparoscopy: a preliminary study. *Fertil Steril* 1985 **44**: 611–614.

14 Hughesdon PE. The structure of endometrial cysts of the ovary. *J Obstet Gynaecol Br Empire* 1957 **44**: 481–487.

15 Canis M, Bassil S, Wattiez A *et al.* Fertility following laparoscopic management of benign adnexal cysts. *Hum Reprod* 1992 7: 529–531.

16 Canis M, Mage G, Wattiez A *et al.* Second look laparoscopy after laparoscopic cystectomy of large ovarian endometriomas. *Fertil Steril* 1992 **58**: 617–619.

17 Nezhat C, Crowgey S, Nezhat F. Videolaseroscopy for the treatment of endometriosis associated with infertility. *Fertil Steril* 1989 **51**: 237–240.

18 Fayez JA, Vogel MF. Comparison of different treatment methods of endometriomas by laparoscopy. *Obstet Gynecol* 1991 78: 660–665.

19 Martin DC. Laparoscopic treatment of ovarian endometriomas. *Clin Obstet Gynecol* 1991 **34**: 452–459.

20 Donnez J, Nisolle M, Karaman Y *et al.* CO_2 laser laparoscopy in peritoneal endometriosis and in ovarian endometrial cyst. *J Gynecol Surg* 1989 **5**: 361–366.

21 Luciano AA, Maier B, Koch EI, Nulsen JC, Whitman GF. A comparative study of post-operative adhesions following laser surgery by laparoscopy versus laparotomy in the rabbit model. *Obstet Gynecol* 1990 **74**: 220–224.

22 Nezhat CR, Nezhat FR, Metzger DA, Luciano AA. Adhesion reformation after reproductive surgery by videolaseroscopy. *Fertil Steril* 1990 **53**: 1008–1011.

23 Perez JJ. Laparoscopic presacral neurectomy: results of the first 25 cases. *J Reprod Med* 1990 **35**: 625–630.

24 Lichten EM, Bombard J. Surgical treatment of primary dysmenorrhea with laparoscopic uterine nerve ablation. *J Reprod Med* 1987 **32**: 37–41.

25 Tjaden B, Schlaff WD, Kimball A, Rock JA. The efficacy of presacral neurectomy for the relief of midline dysmenorrhea. *Obstet Gynecol* 1990 **76**: 89–91.

26 Grainger DA, Soderstrom RM, Schiff SF *et al.* Ureteral injuries at laparoscopy: insights into diagnosis, management and prevention. *Obstet Gynecol* 1990 **75**: 839–843.

27 Nezhat C, Nezhat F. A simplified method of laparoscopic presacral neurectomy for the treatment of central pelvic pain due to endometriosis. *Br J Obstet Gynaecol* 1992 **99**: 659–663.

28 Canis M, Mage G, Chapron C *et al.* Laparoscopic hysterectomy: a preliminary study. *Surg Endosc* 1993 **7**: 42–45.

29 Chassagnard F. External endometriosis: results of laparoscopic treatment of endometriosis in pain and in infertile patients. Indication and results for IVF in endometriosis (Medical thesis). Clermont Ferrand, 1990.

30 Vancaillie T, Schenken RS. Laparoscopic treatment. In: Schenken RS (ed.). *Endometriosis: Contemporary Concepts in Clinical Management*, 1989, pp. 251–266. Philadelphia, JB Lippincott.

31 Mettler L, Semm K. Three step medical and surgical treatment of endometriosis. *Ir J Med Sci* 1983 **152**: 26–28.

Chaper 14
Surgical Treatment of Deeply Infiltrating Endometriosis

P.R. KONINCKX AND D. MARTIN

Introduction

Endometriosis was described early in this century as a severe pathology necessitating radical surgery [1,2]. Endometriosis was defined morphologically as endometrial glands and stroma outside the uterine cavity. Until the 1960s, only adenomyosis in the rectovaginal septum and chocolate cysts in the ovary were thus recognized as endometriosis.

As a consequence of the introduction of laparoscopy in the late 1960s, the awareness that endometriosis is a very frequent disease has progressively increased. Initially, typical lesions, such as black puckered lesions and cystic ovarian endometriosis, which in their most severe form are associated with extensive pelvic adhesions, were described. In the early 1980s, laparoscopic scrutiny led to the recognition of a whole variety of small white vesicles, red vesicles, flame-like lesions, polypoid lesions and brown lesions as subtle forms of endometriosis [3–5]. Even a normal peritoneum was sometimes found to hide microscopic endometriosis [6–8]. In the late 1980s, CO_2 laser excision techniques confirmed the observation that some lesions infiltrate deeper than expected into the subperitoneal stroma [9–13], leading to the recognition of deeply infiltrating endometriosis.

Deeply infiltrating endometriosis and cystic ovarian endometriosis are the most severe forms of endometriosis and in this chapter will be called endometriotic disease [14, 15], to contrast them with minimal endometriosis and subtle endometriosis, for which arguments will be given to consider them a common condition occurring intermittently in all women.

The final diagnosis of deep endometriosis is confirmed during surgical excision. The implications of deep endometriosis for the management of endometriosis, infertility and pelvic pain will be discussed, together with the pitfalls and complications of treatment.

Definition and types of deep endometriosis

Endometriosis infiltrating deeper than 5 mm has been defined as deep endometriosis [12, 13]; this depth of 5 mm has been chosen because of epidemiological and morphological observations. Morphologically, superficial endometriosis, such as subtle or non-pigmented lesions, is very active, whereas typical lesions, which infiltrate for a few millimetres only, are frequently inactive lesions. To our surprise, deep lesions were very active, with a transition zone around 5 mm of depth. A second argument was derived from the frequency distribution of the depth of infiltration, which showed a nadir of around 5 mm of depth. Both the morphological and the epidemiological observations are consistent with the concept that the development of endometriosis is inhibited by peritoneal fluid (Fig. 14.1). These data suggest that most endometriotic lesions only infiltrate for a few millimetres and end as inactive lesions, stopped by the defence mechanisms of the body. It is suggested that endometriosis which has infiltrated more than 5 mm has an aggressive behaviour, with progressive development into a deep endometriotic lesion.

Because of this concept, we propose to call all lesions which are situated more than 5 mm under the peritoneal surface deep endometriosis. This concept does not rule out, however, that different physiological mechanisms can lead to this condition, but it emphasizes the physiopathological differ-

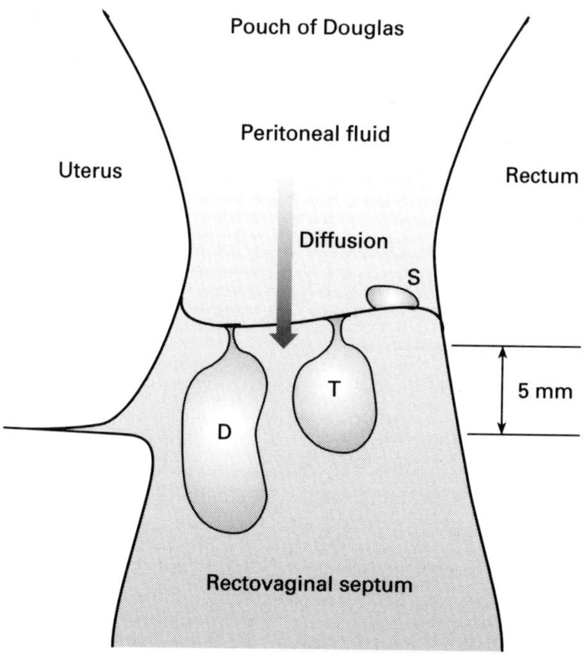

Fig. 14.1 Deeply infiltrating endometriosis is defined as endometriosis infiltrating deeper than 5 mm under the pelvic peritoneum (D). It is suggested that subtle (S) and typical (T) lesions are mainly controlled by peritoneal fluid, whereas deep lesions are influenced by plasma hormones. Medical therapy could shrink deep lesions and bring them back under peritoneal fluid control. Redrawn from [10] with permission.

ences between deep and superficial endometriosis. It has been shown that superficial pelvic endometriosis secretes CA-125 and placental protein 14 (PP-14) mainly towards the peritoneal cavity, whereas deep endometriosis secretes CA-125 and PP-14 mainly towards the bloodstream [16]. It thus seems logical to postulate that superficial pelvic endometriosis is hormonally influenced mainly by the peritoneal fluid microenvironment, whereas deep endometriosis is mainly influenced by plasma concentrations. A transition zone at a depth of some 5 mm, i.e. where diffusion from the peritoneal cavity would become less important, seems theoretically acceptable. Deep endometriosis would thus become endometriosis which has escaped from the direct influence of peritoneal fluid (Fig. 14.1).

Three types of deep endometriosis have been described [17] (Fig. 14.2).

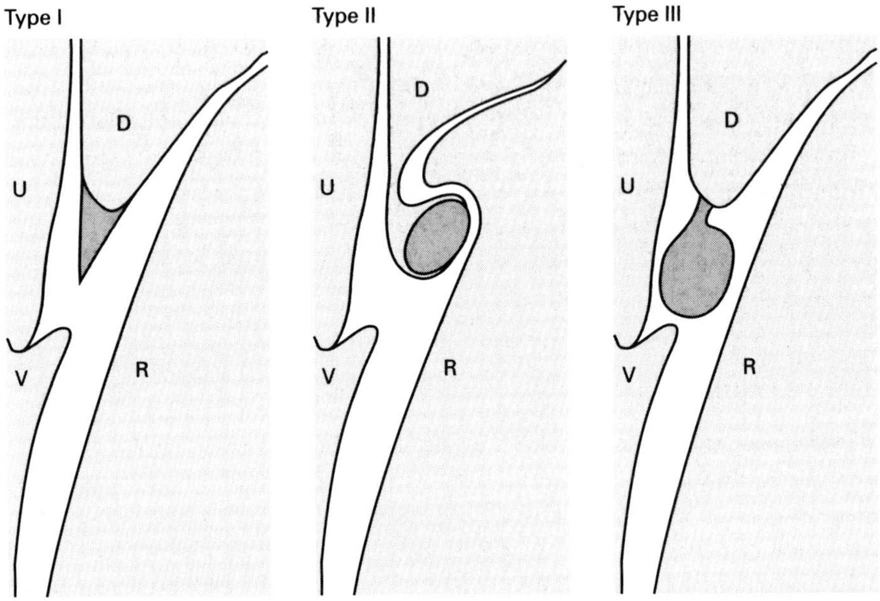

Fig. 14.2 Types of deep endometriosis: type I is suggested to be a consequence of infiltration and type II of retraction, whereas type III could be considered as adenomyosis externa. D, pouch of Douglas; R, rectum; U, uterus; V, vagina. Redrawn from [13] with permission.

Type I

Type I is characterized by a large pelvic area of typical and sometimes subtle endometriotic lesions surrounded by white sclerotic tissue. Only during excision is it seen that the endometriotic lesion infiltrates deeper than 5 mm. Typically, the endometriotic area becomes progressively smaller as it grows deeper, the lesion being cone-shaped. This lesion, therefore, was suggested to be caused by infiltration.

Type II

These lesions are mainly formed by retraction of the bowel. Clinically, they are recognized by bowel retraction around a small typical lesion. In 2–5% of women, however, no endometriosis can be seen through the laparoscope, and bowel retraction is the only clinical sign. Diagnosis is generally not too difficult, since during laparoscopy the retraction under which induration is felt is visible. During excision, the endometriotic nodule becomes rapidly apparent.

Type III

These lesions are spherical endometriotic nodules in the rectovaginal septum. In their most typical manifestation, they are felt as painful nodularities in the rectovaginal septum. At laparoscopy, they generally present as a small typical lesion, and in some women a careful vaginal examination reveals some dark blue cysts (3–4 mm) in the posterior fornix. Type III are the most severe lesions; they often spread laterally around the uterine artery and sometimes around the ureter, causing sclerosis. The spread along the uterine artery is an indirect argument for the hypothesis that deep endometriosis has escaped from the inhibitory influence of peritoneal fluid and thus is mainly under the control of factors in the peripheral circulation.

Deep endometriosis as a specific pathology

We proposed the concept that retrograde menstruation occurs in many if not all women, that implantation of these regurgitated cells occurs intermittently in almost all women, but that these implants are cleared by the immunologic defence mechanisms of the peritoneal cavity and the body [14, 15, 18]. This concept is fundamentally different from the actually prevailing concept that minimal endometriosis is not necessarily a pathology. In some women it may be equivalent to no disease. This means that future studies should consider whether women without endometriosis and women with minimal endometriosis should be treated separately, or as one group. The incidence of minimal endometriosis may reflect only the percentage of women having implants at a certain moment, or, considering that endometriosis is a dynamic disease with active remodelling, the percentage of time that each woman will have implants. It is important to realize that there is no contradiction between this concept and the fact that certain groups of women have a higher incidence of endometriosis. If those women have implants more frequently or for longer periods, it could explain why these women are more prone to develop deep endometriotic disease.

A key argument for this concept is the active remodelling of endometriosis. In young fertile baboons, spontaneous endometriosis – almost all subtle lesions – was found in 23% [19]. During subsequent laparoscopies, some of the initial lesions had disappeared, whereas new lesions had formed [20]. More important, however, was the observation that some animals with endometriosis had become normal, whereas others that had been normal at the first laparoscopy had developed endometriosis. Also, an active remodelling between typical black powderburn lesions and subtle lesions was documented. Spontaneous resolution of typical lesions, however, was not observed. Also, in women, arguments for a similar remodelling can be found [21, 22], reinforcing the concept that subtle endometriosis should not be considered as a stable but as a very dynamic situation (Fig. 14.3).

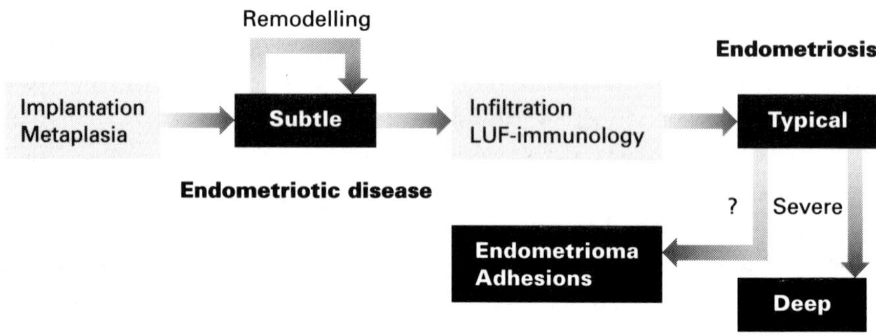

Fig. 14.3 A model for endometriosis which emphasizes intermittent subtle endometriosis in (almost) all women and active remodelling. Infiltration superficial to burnt-out typical lesions is rather frequent but in some women endometriosis develops into an endometriotic disease with severe lesions, either cystic ovarian endometriosis or deep endometriosis, or both. Redrawn from [10] with permission.

The crucial question in understanding endometriosis would thus become why endometriosis develops into a pathological condition, i.e. endometriotic disease, by forming adhesions or chocolate cysts in the ovary, or infiltrating deeply into the underlying tissues to form deep endometriosis, and why this occurs in some women only. Whereas progression of subtle lesions to typical lesions and ultimately to deep lesions or to cystic ovarian endometriosis seems logical, the evidence to support this is rather scarce. In the baboon, D'Hooghe *et al.* [20] demonstrated that 91% of baboons had additional lesions at second-look laparoscopy. In the human, Thomas and Cooke [23] found a slight increase in typical lesions over a 6-month period, and recently Hoshiai *et al.* [21] demonstrated progression of disease in four out of seven women, whereas in three the lesions remained unchanged or had decreased. The best argument in favour of progression of disease in some women can be derived from the observation that the incidence of subtle lesions decreases with age [13, 24], whereas the incidence of typical lesions, of deep lesions and of cystic ovarian endometriosis increased with age [13]. The relative incidence of lesions suggests that in many women superficial lesions start to infiltrate, but that this infiltration is generally controlled by the defence mechanisms of the body. These lesions will show as morphologically inactive, typical, black, puckered lesions surrounded by sclerosis. In a minority of women (perhaps 10–20%), deeper infiltration occurs or cystic ovarian endometriosis develops.

Whereas it has been speculated that growth factors and other macrophage secretion products in peritoneal fluid could promote the growth of endometriosis, the observation that the extent of endometriotic implants correlates inversely with markers of peritoneal inflammation [25] suggests that peritoneal fluid actually has an inhibiting effect, instead of a stimulating effect, on the development and growth of endometriosis. This has led to the hypothesis that superficial endometriotic implants are mainly under inhibitory peritoneal fluid control, whereas deeper lesions have escaped from the influence of peritoneal fluid [18]. Once free of this inhibitory effect, they become more active and grow more rapidly and deeper. This could explain the biphasic frequency distribution [13] with a transition zone around 5–6 mm, which is interpreted as where the influence shifts from the peritoneal fluid to the peripheral circulation. This hypothesis is consistent with the observation that superficial lesions secrete CA-125 and PP-14 mainly towards the peritoneal cavity, whereas deep lesions secrete mainly towards the bloodstream [16]. This concept could also explain the decreased cellular immunity [26] and natural killer (NK) cell activity in plasma of women with cystic ovarian endometriosis or with deep endometriosis [27], whereas in women with minimal endometriosis the cellular immunity is comparable to that of women without endometriosis. Finally, it is also important to realize that cystic ovarian endometriosis has escaped from peritoneal fluid control, and thus could be considered as deeply situated.

The clinical aspects of deep endometriotic disease, i.e. cystic ovarian endometriosis and deeply infiltrating endometriosis, are two clearly distinct manifestations of the same disease. They do not occur in the same women: whereas women with cystic ovarian endometriosis are scored in the revised American Fertility Society (RAFS) classes III and IV, women with deeply infiltrating endometriosis are found predominantly in classes II and I and to a lesser extent in classes III and IV [13, 18]. Deeply infiltrating endometriosis and cystic ovarian endometriosis are two independent variables, both being predictive of an increased plasma concentration of CA-125 and PP-14 [16], a decreased plasma NK cell activity [27] (DJ Oosterlynck, C Meuleman, M Waer, PR Koninckx, personal communication), pelvic pain and the subsequent infertility [28]. Cystic ovarian endometriosis is strongly associated with pelvic adhesions, whereas deeply infiltrating endometriosis is not [29]. If deeply infiltrating endometriosis and cystic ovarian endometriosis are two distinct entities, the model for the progression of endometriosis should be described as follows. Instead of progressing to 'severe disease', endometriosis progresses in some women to cystic ovarian disease and pelvic adhesions and in other women to deeply infiltrating disease and sometimes to both stages of severe disease in the same woman. It remains unknown which mechanisms control the development of endometriosis in one or both directions.

Diagnosis of deep endometriosis

Women with deep endometriosis present with severe pelvic pain, dysmenorrhoea, deep dyspareunia and chronic pelvic pain. The specific association of deep endometriosis and infertility has not yet been proved but it should be realized that the association between endometriosis and infertility is not universally accepted. Only in women with severe adhesions and gross pelvic distortions is the cause of the 'associated' infertility easily understood. In women with minor forms of endometriosis, several mechanisms, such as the luteinized unruptured follicle syndrome [30] and peritoneal macrophages [31], have been suggested. Although the diagnosis of minimal endometriosis may be associated with decreased fecundity, neither medical nor surgical therapy has been proved to reverse this decrease (Fig. 14.4).

The diagnosis of severe forms of deep endometriosis is clinically apparent by painful nodularities in the pouch of Douglas. This form of deep disease,

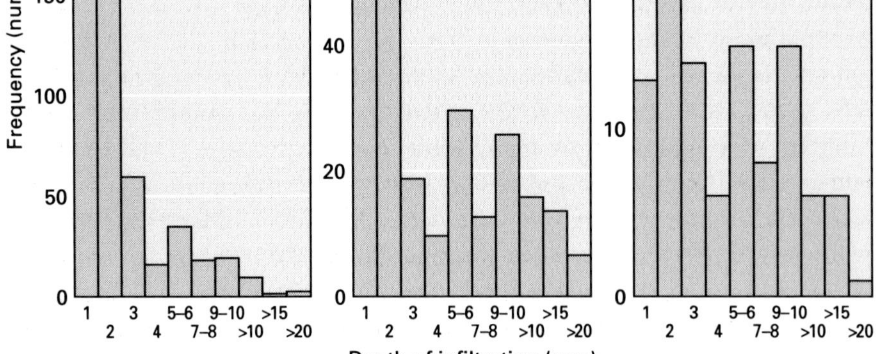

Fig. 14.4 Frequency distribution of depth of infiltration of endometriosis in women with infertility and pain and in women with pain.

generally larger type II or type III lesions, is well known to gynaecologists as 'rectovaginal endometriosis' or as endometriosis causing bowel stenosis and menstrual bleeding per anum. This disease is often considered to be an indication for hysterectomy, for anterior resection of the rectum and/or for partial resection and reanastomosis. Only recently, we realized, however, that the incidence of deep endometriosis is much more frequent than generally thought (PR Koninckx, C Meuleman, D Oosterlynck, FJ Cornillie, personal communication). Deep endometriosis is found in Leuven in over 15% of women with pelvic pain and/or infertility. Even taking into account the bias because of active referrals from all over Flanders, it remains a high number. Most of the deep lesions are, however, relatively small, and we have realized over the last years that they are easily missed, both at laparoscopy and at clinical examination.

Diagnosis of deep endometriosis is clinically important since these women will not receive specific treatment and can end up with a hysterectomy performed for chronic pain of unknown origin. Worse is that in some women the deep nodule will be left in place. These women can continue to have pain, even if the ovaries have been removed and they avoid hormone replacement therapy [32–36]. Not only is it important to recognize deep endometriosis during surgery, but it is equally important to make a tentative diagnosis before surgery in order to know in which women a bowel pretreatment should be given. The diagnostic efficacy of clinical examination, CA-125 concentrations, ultrasound, computer-aided tomography (CAT) scan and magnetic resonance imaging (MRI) can be summarized as follows.

Clinical examination

Clinical examination during the menstrual cycle is unreliable in the diagnosis of deep disease. In a retrospective study of 212 women with deep endometriosis, only 36% had been detected by clinical examination. Clinical examination during menstruation, however, is highly reliable to detect deep endometriosis, with a sensitivity and specificity of 81% and 92%, respectively (PR Koninckx, C Meuleman, D Oosterlynck, FJ Cornillie, personal communication). During menstruation, painful nodularities are not only found in women with deep disease, but also in women with cystic ovarian endometriosis and in women with severe cul-de-sac adhesions. We strongly recommend that all women scheduled for laparoscopy and complaining of pelvic pain should undergo a clinical examination during menstruation. If painful nodularities are found, it seems wise to prepare them for bowel surgery by giving a bowel pretreatment.

Measurement of CA-125

Plasma CA-125 concentrations are higher in women with endometriotic disease, both in women with cystic ovarian endometriosis and in women with deeply infiltrating endometriosis [37]. Plasma CA-125 concentrations can predict deep disease with a sensitivity of 67% and specificity of 94% [16]. CA-125 concentrations should, however, preferentially be used in combination with a clinical examination during menstruation. Both used together can diagnose reliably deep disease with a sensitivity of over 90% and a specificity of over 95% (PR Koninckx, C Meuleman, D Oosterlynck, FJ Cornillie, personal communication). CA-125 concentrations can optimally be assayed in mid-follicular samples, whereas menstrual or luteal samples, or the ratios of menstrual/follicular or menstrual/luteal samples have a lower discriminative power (PR Koninckx, C Meuleman, D Oosterlynck, FJ Cornillie, personal communication).

Radiological diagnostic techniques

Ultrasound, CAT scan or MRI is unreliable in the diagnosis of deep disease [38]. Only very large lesions can be detected, whereas these imaging techniques do not add anything to the combination of a clinical examination and a plasma CA-125 concentration. These techniques are of little value in detecting small lesions, and they cannot predict the lateral spread or extent of the disease with any reliability.

Definitive excision

The final diagnosis is made during surgical excision. Whereas larger lesions are generally visible at laparoscopy, smaller lesions can easily go unnoticed. Therefore it is important that, besides the visual inspection, the pelvis is scrutinized for induration, especially underlying even smaller endometriotic lesions. It can be very helpful for these women that a clinical examination during menstruation has been performed since otherwise in some women smaller lesions of deep endometriosis will be missed.

Surgical excision and complications

Diagnosis of deep endometriosis is confirmed during surgical excision only (PR Koninckx, B Timmermans, C Meuleman, F Penninckx, unpublished data). Although smaller lesions can be excised by electrosurgery and scissors, we prefer to use a CO_2 laser together with a high-flow insufflator [39], a three-puncture technique (one 12 mm and two 5 mm trocars) and an operative endoscope with a 7 mm operating channel (Storz, Tüttlingen, Germany). This insufflator allows the surgeon to excise endometriotic lesions with a continuous laser beam (15 W superpulse) without visible smoke. Excision is guided visually, endometriosis glowing yellowish under the laser beam, and helped by feeling for the indurations with, for instance, an irrigation cannula. Care is taken to remain at the healthy side of the border between the endometriotic nodule and normal healthy tissue. Although it can occasionally be difficult to distinguish endometriosis from normal tissue, especially when endometriosis is close to the cervix, the difference between the harder nodule and the soft tissue of the pelvis is generally apparent. Complete excision implies that endometriosis has to be resected from the rectum wall, which will occasionally be opened, that dissection of the rectovaginal septum has sometimes to be performed up to 3–4 cm below the posterior vaginal fornix, which sometimes has to be excised, and that endometriosis has, eventually, to be resected from around the ureter and the uterine artery. This can be especially difficult, since endometriosis has a tendency to infiltrate specifically along the uterine artery. Therefore, in severe cases, at the end of surgery both ureters should always be identified, and 120 ml of air should be insufflated in the rectum with 1 l of fluid in the pouch of Douglas, in order not to miss unnoticed bowel injuries.

Since the depth and the lateral spread of the endometriosis cannot be evaluated before surgery by clinical examination, laparoscopic inspection, ultrasound or MRI, a complete bowel preparation should be given in order to permit a complete excision. In women with larger lesions, a preoperative contrast enema, an intravenous pyelogram (IVP) and a sigmoidoscopy should be performed. If gross distortion of the ureter is present, ureteric stents are recommended by some or merely ureter dissection by others. When part of the rectal wall has to be removed, or when the rectum is accidentally opened, the pelvis is rinsed with a 1% hibitane or heparinized Ringer solution and the wall is sutured endoscopically with two layers of 3 × 0 Vicryl (Ethicon, USA). A defect in the posterior vaginal fornix is sutured either vaginally or endoscopically. Care is taken to suture these defects in a watertight manner. Thus surgical excision of deep endometriosis is difficult surgery since it often necessitates dissection far laterally around the ureter and uterine artery. Also the excision from the bowel wall is difficult, since in 10% of women part of the bowel wall will have to be resected. In 20% of women, especially those with rectovaginal endometriosis, i.e. type III lesions, excision has to be performed up to and including the posterior vaginal fornix [40, 41]. It is important that neither resection of part of the bowel wall nor resection of the vaginal fornix should be considered as complications of surgery but rather as a frequent necessity for appropriate surgical treatment. Our postoperative follow-up has been uneventful in a series of over 300 women.

Complications of surgery, in a series of 225 patients, have been the transection of the uterine artery in two women, necessitating clipping, a ureter injury in one woman and a late bowel perforation in six women. A ureteric lesion is a serious complication, and therefore we advocate a preoperative intravenous pyelogram, a careful dissection of the ureter from its landmarks at the pelvic brim and a liberal preventive stenting if necessary. This is judged even more important, since we realized that a ureter which is only half cut can rather easily be sutured endoscopically over a double T-tube [42]. A late bowel perforation is an even more serious complication. It occurred in six women: two women with a type II lesion and one with a type III lesion were readmitted after a week with progressively increasing symptoms of peritonitis; one woman with a type I lesion and a history of pouch anastomosis for ulcerative colitis was observed for 1 week with atypical symptoms, which later proved to be a rectal perforation; and two women with a type II lesion had acute pelvic pain 12 hours following surgery and 2 days following surgery, respectively. Although symptoms of peritonitis were minimal, an immediate laparoscopy revealed a bowel perforation in both.

It is important to realize that bowel perforations can occur during the first postoperative days, thus necessitating a low-fibre diet and eventually hospitalization. A perforation generally occurs during straining, with acute pelvic pain as the only symptom. Disturbingly, this pain disappears over the next hours and a slight peritoneal irritation can be the only symptom. A liberal use of early second-look laparoscopies is advocated in these women before symptoms of peritonitis develop. Recently we demonstrated in two women that even a bowel perforation can safely be sutured endoscopically, thus avoiding a colostomy.

In conclusion, surgical excision of deep endometriosis can be performed endoscopically with training and experience. It may require dissection of the ureter and uterine artery and bowel surgery. Occasionally, even ureter surgery might be necessary.

Medical therapy in deep endometriosis

Preoperative

Medical therapy before surgery has been discussed for many years and surgeons have claimed that deep lesions were less vascularized following medical therapy. We have demonstrated that pretreatment for 3 months with a gonadotrophin-releasing hormone (GnRH) agonist could reduce the volume of deep lesions [30]. Indeed, in our series decapeptyl (3.75 mg/month) has been given specifically to women with the most severe disease, especially deep lesions. Analysis of data showed that women pretreated with a

GnRH agonist had a much higher RAFS score at surgery than those without treatment, confirming the selection bias. Similarly, pretreated women had more and larger cystic ovarian endometriomas, also confirming a selection bias. As expected, women with pretreatment had a smaller pelvic area of endometriosis. Pretreated women had, however, a smaller volume of deep endometriosis, notwithstanding the fact that, because of the selection bias, they must have had a much higher volume before treatment. For this reason, we strongly advocate that women with severe deep endometriosis receive 3 months' pretreatment with a GnRH agonist. We have the impression that danazol might be equally effective, but our series was too small to prove this statistically. Other medical therapies have not been used frequently enough to be evaluated in this situation.

Postoperative

Medical treatment following excision of deep endometriosis has not been evaluated in any appropriately constructed trial to date. If excision has been performed completely, medical treatment is probably not necessary. Medical therapy, however, should be considered instead of repeat or more radical surgery for recurring symptoms or failures of excision.

Medical treatment instead of surgery

Medical treatment alone has not been addressed specifically in any study because of a lack of a clear-cut diagnosis of deep endometriosis without excision. Medical treatment, either by danazol, GnRH agonists or gestrinone [43, 44] does not cure endometriosis. Such treatments inactivate the endometriotic lesions, which reappear rapidly after treatment has been stopped [45]. In addition, none of these therapies have an important beneficial effect on subsequent fertility [46], but they all improve pelvic pain and the effect often persists for many months after therapy has been stopped [47, 48]. Since deep endometriosis is strongly associated with pelvic pain and since cystic ovarian endometriosis does not respond well to medical therapy, it is suggested that the observations and conclusions concerning severe pelvic pain are probably related to deep endometriosis.

Results of treatment

Pregnancy rates

Nezhat *et al.* [49] reported 25 pregnancies in 67 women following excision of deep endometriosis. We evaluated cumulative pregnancy rates in a consecutive series of 900 women with primary or secondary infertility without severe tubal damage or a severely subfertile husband [28]. Cumulative pregnancy rates were slightly lower in advanced stages of endometriosis according to the RAFS classification, being 62 and 44% in classes I and IV, respectively. When, however, the duration of infertility – which was the strongest predictor of subsequent conception – was taken into account the differences in cumulative pregnancy rates between classes I and IV disappeared. This suggests that the differences found between mild and severe endometriosis were mainly a consequence of differences in duration of infertility and possibly in the age of the women. The only group with a significantly higher cumulative pregnancy rate following surgery were women with deep endometriosis. Using a Cox multivariate stepwise regression analysis, pregnancy was predicted most strongly by a shorter duration of infertility and additionally by the surgical treatment of cystic ovarian endometriosis or of deep endometriosis, or both.

From these results it can be concluded that aggressive and complete excision of deep endometriosis can be advocated, with subsequent spontaneous pregnancy rates up to 60% within 1 year. These results can be considered excellent, taking into account the severity of disease and the large denuded area in the pelvis following excision of deep endometriosis. It remains unclear whether those women who do not conceive after 1 year should be orientated towards *in vitro* fertilization or a second-look laparoscopy. Medical treatment alone is probably not the treatment of choice for deep endometriosis and infertility. As has been pointed out, medical pretreatment seems to be useful to facilitate surgery (PR Koninckx, B Timmermans, C Meuleman, F Penninckx, unpublished data), as has been suggested for cystic ovarian endometriosis [50].

Pelvic pain

Both surgical and medical treatment are reported to be highly successful in treating pelvic pain. Candiani *et al.* [51] reported absence of dyspareunia and dysmenorrhoea in six and four women, respectively, out of 10, after 40 months. Nezhat *et al.* [49] reported moderate to complete pain relief in 162 out of 175 women, but, in some, two or more laparoscopies had been necessary. Preliminary analysis of our results in 250 women, in whom deep endometriosis was excised with a CO_2 laser, showed a cure rate of pelvic pain in 70%, with a recurrence rate of less than 5%, in a follow-up period up to 5 years (Fig. 14.5). These data should be interpreted carefully, since the completeness of excision has steadily increased. The results in the more recent years strongly suggest an almost complete cure rate without recurrences: however, this could be an over-optimistic clinical impression, which will have

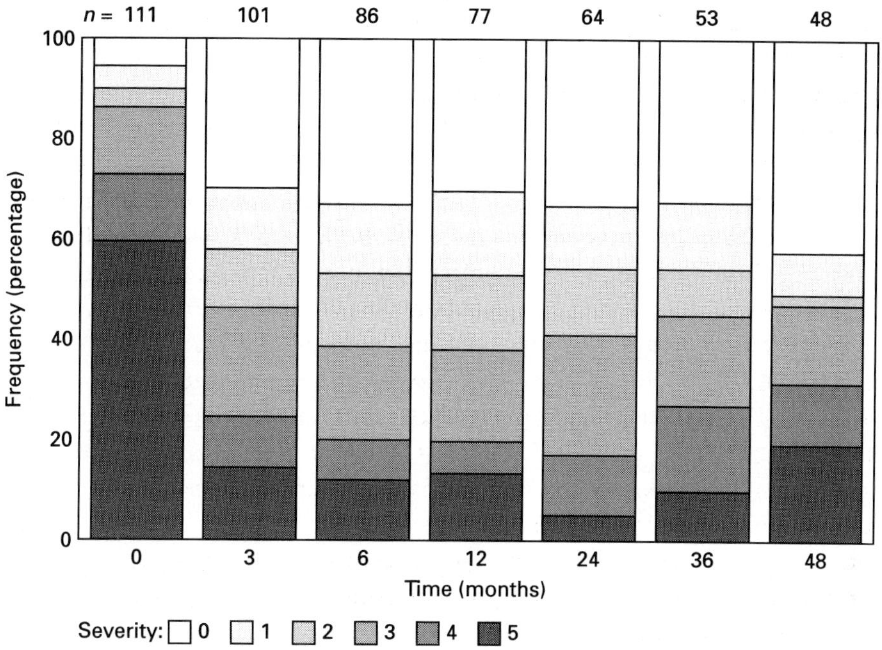

Fig. 14.5 Pain following endoscopic surgery for deeply infiltrating endometriosis.

to be proved by careful analysis of the data and long-term follow-up. Also, medical treatment of pelvic pain is highly efficient, and the effect of treatment often persists after treatment has been stopped [43, 47].

Conclusion

Deep endometriosis has been defined as endometriosis situated more than 5 mm under the peritoneal surface. This definition is important since it emphasizes the concept that deep endometriosis has escaped from the influence of peritoneal fluid. Several mechanisms may lead to this condition, such as infiltration (type I lesion), retraction of bowel (type II lesion = deeply situated) or adenomyosis externa and rectovaginal endometriosis (type III lesions).

Deep endometriosis is clinically important since it is a frequent cause of pelvic pain and probably infertility.

The diagnosis is apparent in the most severe cases, but is usually difficult, with more than 70% being missed at routine clinical examination. Therefore a clinical examination during menstruation and a plasma CA-125 concentration are recommended since they have a sensitivity of more than 90% and a specificity of more than 95% in their ability to diagnose deep endometriosis.

This will help the surgeon to identify and localize the lesion during laparoscopy.

Surgical excision is the treatment of choice, with excellent results for subsequent fertility and relief of pelvic pain. Recurrences following complete excision are rare to date in our series.

Surgical excision is difficult surgery, necessitating bowel surgery in some 10%, dissection, including excision, of the posterior vaginal fornix in over 20% and frequently dissection of the ureter. Complications of ureter lesions are avoidable and rare but late bowel perforations occur in 2–3%. This could be prevented by preventive suturing. It is most important to recognize the early symptoms of perforation since this could permit the suture of the bowel perforation by an endoscopic approach, thus avoiding a colostomy.

Acknowledgements

Past and present coworkers and coauthors are sincerely thanked for their help and discussions: Dr Sc. Freddy Cornillie (Centocor Diagnostics Europe, Heverlee), Dr Stephan Demeyere (AZ St Lucas, Brugge), Dr Karine Stukkens (H.-Hartkliniek, Asse), Dr Marc Muyldermans (AZ Virga Jesse, Hasselt), and Dr Jan Deprest (Center for Endoscopic Technologies, Leuven), Dr D. Oosterlynck (UZ Gasthuisberg, Leuven) and Dr Thomas D'Hooghe (UZ Gasthuisberg, Leuven). Prof. Dan Martin (Memphis, TN), Dr Chandrit Bambra (Institute of Primate Research, Nairobi) and Prof. Markku Seppälä, together with Dr Leena Riittinen (Helsinki University, Finland), are thanked for the opportunity of collaborative studies. The help of Dr Stefan Lempereur and Dr Stefaan Wens (Ipsen NV, Sint-Denijs-Westrem) is greatly appreciated, as well as that of Mrs Christine Dewit and Mrs Marie-Josée Vanderheyden in the laboratory and of Mrs Marleen Craessaerts as a research nurse. We also thank Mrs Diane Wolput for her secretarial efficiency.

References

1 Sampson JA. Perforating hemorrhagic (chocolate) cysts of the ovary: their importance and especially their relation to pelvic adenomas of the endometrial type ('adenomyoma' of the uterus, rectovaginal septum, sigmoid, etc.). *Arch Surg* 1921 **3**: 245–323.

2 Cullen TS. The distribution of adenomyomata containing uterine mucosa. *Am J Obstet Gynecol* 1919 **80**: 130.

3 Jansen RPS, Russell P. Nonpigmented endometriosis: clinical, laparoscopic and pathologic definition. *Am J Obstet Gynecol* 1986 **155**: 1154–1159.

4 Redwine DB. The distribution of endometriosis in the pelvis by age groups and fertility. *Fertil Steril* 1987 **47**: 173–175.

5 Martin DC, Hubert GC, Vander Zwaag R, El-Zeky FA. Laparoscopic appearances of peritoneal endometriosis. *Fertil Steril* 1989 **51**: 63–67.

6 Murphy AA, Green WR, Bobbie D, dela Cruz ZC, Rock JA. Unsuspected endometriosis documented by scanning electron microscopy in visually normal peritoneum. *Fertil Steril* 1986 **46**: 522–524.
7 Redwine DB, Yocum LB. A serial section study of visually normal pelvic peritoneum in patients with endometriosis. *Fertil Steril* 1990 **54**: 648–651.
8 Nezhat F, Allan CJ, Nezhat C, Martin DC. Nonvisualized endometriosis at laparoscopy. *Int J Fertil* 1991 **36**: 340–343.
9 Moore JG, Binstock MA, Crowdon WA. The clinical implications of retroperitoneal endometriosis. *Am J Obstet Gynecol* 1988 **158**: 1291–1298.
10 Martin DC, Vander Zwaag R. Excisional techniques for endometriosis with the CO_2 laser laparoscope. *J Reprod Med* 1987 **32**: 753–758.
11 Martin DC, Hubert GD, Levy BS. Depth of infiltration of endometriosis. *J Gynecol Surg* 1989 **5**: 55–60.
12 Cornillie FJ, Oosterlynck D, Lauweryns JM, Koninckx PR. Deeply infiltrating pelvic endometriosis: histology and clinical significance. *Fertil Steril* 1990 **53**: 978–983.
13 Koninckx PR, Meuleman C, Demeyere S, Lesaffre E, Cornillie F. Suggestive evidence that pelvic endometriosis is a progressive disease, whereas deeply infiltrating endometriosis is associated with pelvic pain. *Fertil Steril* 1991 **55**: 759–765.
14 Koninckx PR. Is mild endometriosis a natural condition instead of a disease? *Fertil Steril* 1994 (in press).
15 Koninckx PR, Oosterlynck D, D'Hooghe T, Meuleman C. Deeply infiltrating endometriosis is a disease whereas mild endometriosis could be considered a non-disease. *Ann N Y Acad Sci* 1994 (in press).
16 Koninckx PR, Riittinen L, Seppala M, Cornillie FJ. CA-125 and placental protein 14 concentrations in plasma and peritoneal fluid of women with deeply infiltrating pelvic endometriosis. *Fertil Steril* 1992 **57**: 523–530.
17 Koninckx PR, Martin DC. Deep endometriosis: a consequence of infiltration or retraction or possibly adenomyosis externa? *Fertil Steril* 1992 **58**: 924–928.
18 Koninckx PR, Martin D. Treatment of deeply infiltrating endometriosis. *Curr Opin Obstet Gynecol* 1994 **6**: 231–241.
19 D'Hooghe TM, Bambra CS, Cornillie FJ, Isahakia M, Koninckx PR. Prevalence and laparoscopic appearance of spontaneous endometriosis in the baboon (*Papio anubis, Papio cynocephalus*). *Biol Reprod* 1991 **45**: 411–416.
20 D'Hooghe TM, Bambra CS, Isahakia M, Koninckx PR. Evolution of spontaneous endometriosis in the baboon (*Papio anubis, Papio cynocephalus*) over a 12-month period. *Fertil Steril* 1992 **58**: 409–412.
21 Hoshiai H, Ishikawa M, Sawatari Y, Noda K, Fukaya T. Laparoscopic evaluation of the onset and progression of endometriosis. *Am J Obstet Gynecol* 1993 **169**: 714–719.
22 Wiegerinek MAHM, Van Dop PA, Brosens IA. The staging of peritoneal endometriosis by the type of active lesion in addition to the revised American Fertility Society classification. *Fertil Steril* 1993 **60**: 461–464.
23 Thomas EJ, Cooke ID. Successful treatment of asymptomatic endometriosis: does it benefit infertile women? *Br Med J* 1987 **294**: 1117–1119.
24 Redwine DB. Age-related evolution in color appearance of endometriosis. *Fertil Steril* 1987 **48**: 1062–1063.
25 Haney AF, Jenkins S, Weinberg JB. The stimulus responsible for the peritoneal fluid inflammation observed in infertile women with endometriosis. *Fertil Steril* 1991 **56**: 408–413.
26 Dmowski WP, Steel RW, Baker GF. Deficient cellular immunity in endometriosis. *Am J Obstet Gynecol* 1981 **141**: 377–383.
27 Oosterlynck DJ, Cornillie FJ, Waer M, Vandeputte M, Koninckx PR. Women with endo-

metriosis show a defect in natural killer activity resulting in a decreased cytotoxicity to autologous endometrium. *Fertil Steril* 1991 **56**: 45–51.

28 Koninckx PR, Deprest J, Janssens G, Oosterlynck D, Meuleman C. Cumulative pregnancy rates following CO_2 laser endoscopic excision of deeply infiltrating endometriosis (Abstract). 49th Annual Meeting American Fertility Society/39th Annual Meeting Canadian Fertility and Andrology Society, Montreal, Quebec, Canada, 9–14 October, 1993.

29 Koninckx PR, Cornillie FJ. Infiltrating endometriosis: infiltration, retraction or adenomyosis externa? In: Martin D. (ed.). *Appearances of Endometriosis*, 1992, pp. 9.1–9.8. London, Gower Medical Publications.

30 Koninckx PR, Ide P, Vandenbroucke W, Brosens IA. New aspects of the pathophysiology of endometriosis and associated infertility. *J Reprod Med* 1980 **24**: 257–260.

31 Evers JLH. The pregnancy rate of the no-treatment group in randomized clinical trials of endometriosis therapy. *Fertil Steril* 1989 **52**: 906–907.

32 Kempers RD, Dockerty MB, Hunt AB, Symmonds RE. Significant postmenopausal endometriosis. *Surg Gynecol Obstet* 1960 **111**: 348–356.

33 O'Connor DT. Pain in endometriosis. In: O'Connor DT (ed.). *Endometriosis* 1987, pp. 11–12. Melbourne, Churchill Livingstone.

34 Taylor PJ (ed.). Canadian Consensus Conference on Endometriosis. *J SOGC Suppl* 1993, April.

35 Metzger DA, Lessay BA, Soper JT, McCarty KS Jr, Haney AF. Hormone-resistant endometriosis following total abdominal hysterectomy and bilateral salpingo-oophorectomy: correlation with histology and steroid receptor content. *Obstet Gynecol* 1991 **78**: 946–950.

36 Redwine DB. Endometriosis persisting after castration: clinical characteristics and results of surgical management. *Obstet Gynecol* 1994 **83**: 405–413.

37 Koninckx PR, Muyldermans M, Meulman C, Cornillie FJ. CA 125 in the management of endometriosis. *Eur J Obstet Gynaecol Reprod Biol* 1993 **49**: 109–113.

38 Deprest J, Marchal G, Koninckx PR. MRI in the diagnosis of deeply infiltrating endometriosis (Abstract). 22nd Annual Meeting of the American Association of Gynecologic Laparoscopists (AAGL), San Francisco, Marriott, CA, 10–14 November 1993.

39 Koninckx PR, Vandermeersch E. The persufflator: an insufflation device for laparoscopy and especially for CO_2-laser-endoscopic surgery. *Hum Reprod* 1991 **6**: 1288–1290.

40 Martin DC. Laparoscopic and vaginal colpotomy for the excision of infiltrating cul-de-sac endometriosis. *J Reprod Med* 1988 **33**: 806–808.

41 Davis GD, Brooks RA. Excision of pelvic endometriosis with the carbon dioxide laser laparoscope. *Obstet Gynecol* 1988 **72**: 816–819.

42 Neven P, Vandeursen H, Baert L, Koninckx PR. Ureteric injury at laparoscopic surgery: the endoscopic management. Case review. *Gynaecol Endoscopy* 1993 **2**: 45–46.

43 Shaw RW. Endometriosis: current evaluation of management and rationale for medical therapy. In: Brosens IA, Donnez J. (eds). *The Current Status of Endometriosis*, 1993, pp. 371–383. New York, Parthenon Publishing.

44 Fedele L, Bianchi S, Bocciolone L, Dinola G, Franchi D. Buserelin acetate in the treatment of pelvic pain associated with minimal and mild endometriosis – a controlled study. *Fertil Steril* 1993 **59**: 516–521.

45 Evers JLH. The second-look laparoscopy for evaluation of the result of medical treatment of endometriosis should not be performed during ovarian suppression. *Fertil Steril* 1987 **47**: 502–504.

46 Hughes EG, Fedorkow DM, Collins JA. A quantitative overview of controlled trials in endometriosis-associated infertility. *Fertil Steril* 1993 **59**: 963–970.

47 Shaw RW. Nafarelin in the treatment of pelvic pain caused by endometriosis. *Am J Obstet Gynecol* 1990 **162**: 574–576.

48 Waller KG, Shaw RW. Gonadotrophin-releasing hormone analogues for the treatment of

endometriosis – long-term follow-up. *Fertil Steril* 1993 **59**: 511–515.
49 Nezhat C, Nezhat F, Pennington E. Laparoscopic treatment of infiltrative rectosigmoid colon and rectovaginal septum endometriosis by the technique of videolaparoscopy and the CO_2 laser. *Br Obstet Gynaecol* 1992 **99**: 664–667.
50 Donnez J, Nisolle M, Casanas-Roux F, Clerckx E. Endometriosis: rationale for surgery. In: Brosens IA, Donnez J. (eds). *The Current Status of Endometriosis*, 1993, pp. 385–395. New York, Parthenon Publishing.
51 Candiani GB, Vercellini P, Fedele L *et al.* Conservative surgical treatment of rectovaginal septum endometriosis. *J Gynecol Surg* 1992 **8**: 177–182.

Chapter 15
Role of Assisted Reproduction in Endometriosis

N.N. AMSO

Introduction

Assisted reproduction methods are here defined as involving a combination of superovulation therapy and delivery of prepared spermatozoa to the eggs. They include *in vitro* fertilization (IVF), gamete intrafallopian transfer (GIFT) and other variants such as tubal embryo transfer (TET) and direct intraperitoneal insemination (DIPI). With their advent, more patients with endometriosis failing to conceive with conventional therapy (medical and/or surgical) have been treated with one or other of these techniques. The willingness of clinicians to employ these techniques depends on the severity of endometriosis, the age of the patient and the duration of the infertility. When endometriosis or any associated scarring causes mechanical distortion of the pelvic viscera, there is little controversy regarding the optimal course of management. However, where the only finding is endometriotic implants without any distortion, the therapeutic recommendations remain controversial. Even though mild endometriosis may be associated with subfertility [1–3], it cannot be said to be a cause of infertility unless there is a mechanical disruption or impairment of embryo transport in the tube [4]. The precise relationship between endometriosis and subfertility is unclear and is discussed in Chapter 8.

In this chapter the impact of endometriosis on the reproductive outcome of infertile women and the role of different management strategies, with particular emphasis on assisted reproduction techniques, are evaluated. Whether such treatment exerts deleterious effect on the disease is also considered.

Management options

Expectant management

Endometriosis is not an absolute inhibition to conception but rather a relative reduction in fertility potential. Thus, in looking at the various therapies available, whether medical, surgical or in the form of assisted reproduction techniques, the standard against which we must measure success is the background pregnancy rate in this group of women. Such data may be estimated by evaluating studies treating such women with an approach termed 'expectant management', which is commonly employed and is surprisingly 'effective'. The most commonly used ways to evaluate and report the outcome of expectant management or the effectiveness of therapy are: (i) the crude pregnancy rate; and (ii) the life table analysis method. The crude pregnancy rate (the number of pregnancies divided by the number of patients treated) is simple to obtain but presents several major drawbacks. It does not correct for a sample bias where confounding variables may affect fertility. Secondly, it is dependent upon the length of follow-up and the pregnancy rate will invariably be increased by prolonging the follow-up period, and conversely can be artificially lowered by a brief interval of follow-up [5]. Life table analysis, on the other hand, adjusts for variability in the follow-up period and calculates the probability of pregnancy at any follow-up interval, while mathematically correcting for variable duration of follow-up.

A number of reports have examined the occurrence of pregnancies following expectant management after the diagnosis of early-stage disease at laparoscopy [6,7]. Inoue *et al.* [8] examined whether the presence and severity of endometriosis affect the reproductive outcome of infertile women and compared retrospectively the conception rates in women who had endometriosis and those who did not. The conception rates were virtually identical following expectant management or conventional therapy, regardless of the presence or absence of endometriosis. However, the conception rates declined as the stage of disease progressed, showing a statistically significant difference between stage I and stage IV disease. Similarly, they were unable to detect any influence of endometriosis in patients undergoing IVF and embryo transfer (ET). In minimal or mild endometriosis, the chance of natural conception is on average only 3% per cycle, considerably less than that of the general population [3]. However, pregnancy may still occur after a period of observation of about 2 years, with or without prior treatment, up to 50% of couples achieving a pregnancy during this period [3]. As with unexplained infertility, the chance of natural conception will be inversely related to the duration of infertility and after more than 3 years will be well below average. It is likely that the preservation of tubo-ovarian function, at least on one side, may be more important than the stage or total endometriosis score. Data on expectant management in moderate and severe endometriosis are sparse, with pregnancy rate and monthly fecundity rate lower than in women with mild endometriosis, but clearly showing a significant chance of pregnancy without treatment [2,7]. It has been estimated that approximately 10% of these couples achieve a pregnancy after 2 years of observation [3].

Medical or surgical treatments for endometriosis-related infertility have been proposed in a variety of combinations. With the addition of assisted reproduction techniques, pretreatment with either medical or surgical approaches has also been suggested. In this chapter, treatment modalities specifically intended to alleviate infertility are discussed.

Medical treatment

A number of retrospective analyses, as well as randomized controlled trials, have shown that, although medical treatment for endometriosis using a variety of drugs is effective in altering the histological manifestation, it does not increase fertility, conception rates or monthly fecundity rate. Most of these studies have assessed medical therapy in mild endometriosis and no randomized clinical trials are available which evaluate medical intervention in moderate or severe disease [9–12]. Equally, early publications, which included heterogeneous populations, suffered from inconsistent or absent staging and from incomplete reporting of data [5]. The introduction of new medications, such as dydrogesterone and gonadotrophin-releasing hormone agonists (GnRH-a), in the treatment of endometriosis-associated infertility are currently under investigation. Due to the lack of any definitive evidence, there is no rationale for the use of medical treatment for asymptomatic disease in infertile women. This is especially true as current medications are potent inhibitors of fertility and can have significant side-effects. For this reason, women with minimal/mild disease should be managed in the same way as those with unexplained infertility.

Surgical treatment

A surgical approach to enhancing fertility in women with endometriosis is probably the most commonly utilized form of therapy. In performing conservative surgery, clinicians attempt: (i) to remove active endometriotic implants using cauterization or laser vaporization; and (ii) to restore and maintain normal anatomy by division of adhesions and mobilization of tubes/ovaries, preserving or even enhancing fertility potential. In the presence of anatomic distortion secondary to adhesion formation, surgical intervention is crucial to enhance conception rates. However, the value of removal of endometriotic implants only is questionable. The use of conservative surgery specifically in mild/moderate endometriosis does not show any advantages to either medical or expectant treatment [13–15]. In severe endometriosis, conception occurs significantly more readily after surgery [16] and laser vaporization may also raise fertility [17]. Combinations of surgical and medical treatments have been reported but the data are conflicting and no benefit has been demonstrated in mild disease [14].

Assisted reproduction

Pelvic endometriosis refractory to medical or surgical therapy currently accounts for between 7 and 35% of patients undergoing IVF procedures [18, 19]. Several groups have reported varying degrees of success following IVF treatment in women with different stages of endometriosis [20–25]. Further expansion of IVF technology has resulted in the development of GIFT and TET as additional modalities in the treatment of these women. This section will review the current indications for assisted reproductive technology, the impact of severity of endometriosis on follicular response, oocyte recovery, fertilization rates, pregnancy rates, outcome of treatment and the effect of prior medical treatment or aspiration of endometriotic cysts on the overall outcome.

Indications

All stages of endometriosis have increasingly been viewed as suitable indications for assisted reproduction treatment. Its timing is dependent on the severity of disease and previous therapy, as well as other factors, such as the female age and duration of infertility. In women with severe endometriosis with mechanical blockage and where surgical therapy is inappropriate, IVF should be expedited. Such treatment is recommended 1–2 years after previous unsuccessful medical or surgical therapy, with the prognosis depending on the factors outlined above. In minimal or mild endometriosis, the balance of choice seems to be clearly in favour of IVF or GIFT treatment after more than 2 years of expectant management.

Outcome of treatment with assisted conception

Early experience of IVF treatment in women with endometriosis was very encouraging [20, 22, 26]. The pregnancy rate in women who had been pretreated with danazol was similar to that in other groups of infertile women [20]. Prospective [27] and retrospective [24, 26] studies have reported high pregnancy rates in women with minimal/mild endometriosis irrespective of prior treatment, and implantation (= 12%) as well as pregnancy rates (= 27%) per transfer compatible with tubal disease and unexplained infertility. Disappointing pregnancy rates in women with severe disease [22, 26] (< 10% per embryo transfer) were attributed to a reduction in the number of oocytes obtained at laparoscopic egg collection, resulting in fewer embryos being replaced in this group. Interestingly, the presence or degree of endometriosis did not appear to affect the fertilization or embryo cleavage rates, which were similar in all stages of endometriosis to those in women with tubal disease. It was also speculated that the reproductive performance of women with mild and moderate disease following IVF is excellent and perhaps even better than in other categories of infertility [26]. Retrospective studies [24, 25] utilizing ultrasound-guided techniques for oocyte collection have reported no significant effect of aetiology on the total number of clinical pregnancies. However, in one study [24], the clinical pregnancy rate per ET was significantly higher in patients with mild as compared with severe endometriosis (26.5% versus 13.3%, respectively). Others were unable to detect any influence of ovarian endometriosis (superficial or deep) on the oocyte recovery rate or pregnancy rate per ET [28] and concluded that the pregnancy and live birth rates were not reduced with advanced degrees of endometriosis [23, 25] but positively correlated with a shorter infertility duration [25]. In contradiction to the above studies, Simon *et al.* [29] recently reported poor IVF outcome for all stages of endometriosis in comparison with tubal infertility, manifested by significant reduction of pregnancy and implantation rates, but not fertilization rates. Further, when the results of their oocyte donation programme were classified according to the origin of the oocytes donated, patients who received embryos derived from endometriotic ovaries showed a significantly reduced implantation rate as compared with the other groups. The authors concluded that infertility in endometriosis patients may be related to alterations within the oocyte, resulting in embryos with decreased ability to implant. Large national registers [18, 30, 31] have repeatedly reported similar pregnancy rates for women with endometriosis in comparison with other categories, following IVF or GIFT treatments. These figures should be interpreted with care as these registers include women with different grades of the disease, undergoing a variety of stimulation protocols and in different centres.

The effectiveness of assisted reproduction treatment appears to be maintained in successive cycles, giving rise to favourable cumulative pregnancy and live birth rates. In a group of 168 women with endometriosis undergoing IVF treatment, the pregnancy and live birth rates per cycle were similar to those of other groups. The cumulative pregnancy and live birth rates (47% and 35%, respectively) after five treatment cycles were also comparable with those in tubal (52% and 38%) and unexplained (56% and 42%) infertility, and were significantly higher than those in male (28% and 18%) or multiple factor (38% and 30%) infertility [32]. Unfortunately, there was no attempt to subdivide the results according to the severity of the endometriosis.

Miscarriage rate

An early report [28] showed a significantly higher miscarriage rate in moderate/severe endometriosis, resulting in lower ongoing pregnancy and take-home baby rates. However, an expanded study by the same group [23] showed no difference in the ongoing pregnancy rate per cycle or ET between the different stages of endometriosis and the authors concluded that women with stage III/IV disease did not have a compromised take-home baby rate. Similarly, other investigators were unable to detect any difference in the rate of spontaneous abortion among the different stages of endometriosis following GIFT [33] or IVF [25].

The influence of endometriosis on fertilization rate

The evidence from the published literature has been conflicting. Whereas early reports [21, 34] suggested reduction in the fertilization rate in comparison with tubal damage (33% versus 68%), subsequent publications consistently showed comparable fertilization rates with other infertility categories (mild endometriosis = 71–86%; severe endometriosis = 72–88%; tubal = 69–80% and unexplained infertility = 59–67%) [20, 22–24, 27]. The discrepancy is difficult to explain but may be due to pretreatment of endometriosis with danazol [20], the type of stimulation protocol employed, the methodology of gamete handling, laboratory conditions or a combination of these. The balance of current opinion suggests that fertilization rate is not affected in early or advanced endometriosis.

GnRH-a stimulation protocols

The use of GnRH-a in combination with gonadotrophin for IVF was first reported in 1984 [35]. Indeed, in the USA 74% of all stimulation cycles utilize a combination of GnRH-a and gonadotrophin [36]. In women with endometriosis undergoing IVF treatment, a paired analysis of patients receiving identical gonadotrophin stimulation with or without GnRH-a [23] showed a higher number of preovulatory oocytes retrieved and transferred, no cancellation of treatment cycles and a higher pregnancy rate in the GnRH-a group (42% versus 17%). Analysis of the data according to the severity of endometriosis showed that significant effects were only present in advanced-stage disease (III and IV). The type of stimulation protocol in women with minimal endometriosis undergoing GIFT did not affect the pregnancy rate, but the long down-regulation protocol resulted in a slightly, though not significantly, increased pregnancy rate [37]. More appropriately designed studies are required to confirm the above results and to determine the role of GnRH-a, if any.

GIFT or IVF? Tubal or uterine embryo transfer?

While IVF is frequently recommended for all women who have not succeeded with conventional fertility treatment, GIFT is frequently advocated as the first choice for those women with endometriosis and patent Fallopian tubes. Since its introduction, GIFT has been shown to be as effective as IVF for the treatment of women with endometriosis [33, 38]. More recently, TET has also been successful in the treatment of women with minimal/mild endometriosis and has achieved similar rates to GIFT and IVF with uterine transfer [39, 40]. Many of the studies comparing uterine with tubal transfers following IVF contain small numbers of patients and do not stratify the results according to the cause of infertility [39–41]. There is no clear evidence in the literature that tubal gamete transfer or TET is superior to conventional IVF-ET in the treatment of endometriotic patients with healthy patent tubes.

Pretreatment suppression of endometriosis with danazol or GnRH-a

Several groups have reported disappointing results with IVF in women with endometriosis [21, 42] and proposed pre-IVF suppression of the disease. The severity of endometriosis in women treated for 6–9 months with danazol (400–800 mg/day) or gestrinone (2.5 mg twice weekly) was reported to be reduced in all cases at the time of laparoscopic oocyte collection [43]. Pretreatment also resulted in an improved fertilization rate, an increased proportion of women undergoing ET and higher pregnancy and implantation rates. Similarly, suppression of moderate or severe endometriosis with GnRH-a (buserelin 900 μg daily intranasally) for 6 months prior to IVF resulted in reduction in the severity of the disease, improved ovarian accessibility, a significant increase in the number of oocytes retrieved and embryos replaced, and an overall pregnancy rate per transfer of 35% in women who had failed to conceive with previous IVF treatment [44]. Other reports [25] could not demonstrate any association between prior therapy of endometriosis and improved IVF results. Instead, there was an association between a shorter duration of infertility and an improved outcome. It must be noted that none of the above studies was randomized, they included relatively small numbers of patients in the different subgroups and, in one [25] pretreatment was completed on average 24 months before IVF and was not aimed specifically at improving IVF results. All the above discrepancies highlight the need for properly designed and randomized studies to determine the impact of pre-IVF suppression of endometriosis on the overall outcome.

Pre-IVF aspiration of endometriomas

Aspiration of endometriomas prior to IVF with the aim of improving follicular response, fertilization and pregnancy rates has been reported [45]. Patients with endometriosis who had failed to conceive following previous conventional IVF treatment were included, and all other fertility factors were excluded. Aspiration was carried out under local anaesthetic with transvaginal ultrasound guidance and the patients subsequently underwent IVF. Significantly higher numbers of oocytes were obtained and more embryos were replaced, resulting in a 28% pregnancy rate per transfer. However, no difference in the fertilization or cleavage rates was noted in the treatment cycles before or after aspiration. Possible explanations are that the endometriomas may exert mechanical effects on the ovarian blood supply, resulting in poor response, or that, due to their presence, oocyte recovery becomes more difficult. Alternatively, their presence within the ovary may impair the normal intraovarian mechanisms of follicle and oocyte maturation, which may affect the quality of oocytes retrieved. This, however, does not seem to influence their fertilization and cleavage capacity but results in functionally abnormal embryos with defective implantation potential. Based on this evidence, it would appear that aspiration of endometriomas could enhance the chances of successful outcome with IVF treatment.

Does assisted reproduction treatment influence the course of endometriosis?

It is tempting to think that assisted reproduction treatment with its associated changes in the hormonal milieu may adversely affect the course and severity of endometriosis. There is evidence to suggest that endometriosis is a progressive disease and that atypical implants may evolve spontaneously into classical powderburn implants. However, the natural history is not clearly understood and the disease seems to progress in most untreated women although spontaneous regression has been described in mild cases. Similarly, evidence is accumulating to suggest: (i) that endometriosis is a systemic disease, with visible endometrial implants representing a local manifestation of this process [46]; and (ii) the presence of a link between endometriosis and alterations in both humoral and cell-mediated immunity [47]. Pregnancy is thought to induce involution of endometriotic implants. However, McArthur and Ulfelder [48] showed that the behaviour of endometriosis during the gravid state was highly variable and regression of disease seemed to be due to decreased tissue responsiveness to hormonal stimulation rather than necrosis of lesions. A non-invasive test that reliably correlates with the extent of disease would be useful in determining its progression or regression. However, no such test is available clinically at present, nor do any effective screening markers exist [4], and any assessment would require laparoscopic evaluation of the pelvis. Not surprisingly, there is scant evidence in the literature evaluating the course of the disease in women who have undergone assisted reproduction treatment. The issues that need consideration are:

1 Do endometriotic implants contain a similar amount of oestrogen receptors (ER) and progesterone receptors (PR) to the intrauterine endometrium and do they undergo cyclical changes in response to endogenous hormones?

2 What parameters should be employed to assess progression of disease: symptomatic assessment, revised American Fertility Society scoring or, more logically, the occurrence of spontaneous pregnancy following unsuccessful assisted reproduction treatment?

Several studies have examined ER and PR content in endometriotic tissue and endometrium during the menstrual cycle or following medical treatment [49–51]. Endometriotic implants contain specific ER and PR in both glandular epithelium and stroma. In contrast to the intrauterine endometrium, the intensity of immunostaining was less in the endometriotic biopsies [50] and more heterogeneous in distribution and did not undergo the predictable changes in response to endogenous hormones, with some implants containing few or no receptors at all [49]. Differences in ER and PR levels in primary and recurrent endometriosis indicate that possibly different mechanisms of hormonal regulation for the two forms of the disease exist [51]. It is possible that factors such as the site of implantation may influence the behaviour of endometriosis, as well as affecting alterations in a putative paracrine response. Poor vascularity, surrounding fibrosis or exposure to inflammatory cells may also be responsible. Implants on the ovary may be exposed to a different hormonal milieu and hence behave differently. Further, the receptor content in women who had been treated with danazol, medroxyprogesterone acetate or oral contraceptives was significantly reduced and virtually non-detectable [49]. All the above factors should be taken into consideration when deciding the effect of assisted reproduction treatment on endometriosis.

To the author's knowledge, there are no reports in the literature of long-term follow-up of endometriotic women who have undergone multiple attempts of assisted reproduction. Wardle *et al.* [43] assessed the pelvis during laparoscopic egg collection in women who were pretreated for endometriosis immediately prior to IVF and reported reduction in the severity of disease in all cases, despite the level of hormones achieved during the ovulation induction phase. In other studies [25, 32], women underwent up to five IVF attempts, but no mention was made of the effect of such treatment on the progression or severity of the disease or its symptomatology. In a prospective randomized study comparing uterine and laparoscopic tubal transfer (N.N.

Table 15.1 Clinical details of endometriosis patients, year of diagnosis and laparoscopic findings at tubal embryo transfer

Patient		History (endometriosis treatment)	Assisted reproduction treatment and laparoscopic assessment
(1)	KS	Active endometriosis; February 1987 (GnRH-a), laparoscopy January 1988, reduced severity	TET December 1989 (1st attempt), normal-looking pelvis, no endometriosis noted
(2)	AM	Minimal endometriosis; February 1988 (GnRH-a), laparoscopy October 1988, endometriosis uterovesical peritoneum and both pelvic side walls	TET January 1991 (1st attempt), old endometriosis at uterovesical peritoneum, puckering in pouch of Douglas and left tube slightly tethered to the ovary
(3)	AS	Active mild endometriosis; March 1989 (danazol)	TET February 1991, normal-looking pelvis, no endometriosis noted
(4)	MN	Active mild endometriosis; 1986 (danazol), laparoscopies 1987 and 1988, no endometriosis. GIFT March 1989	TET August 1989, normal-looking pelvis, no endometriosis noted, TET March 1991, normal-looking pelvis, no endometriosis noted
(5)	NM	Active mild endometriosis; July 1988 (gestrinone), laparoscopy 1989, no residual disease	TET September 1990, normal-looking pelvis, no endometriosis noted, TET June 1991, normal-looking pelvis, no endometriosis noted
(6)	BN	Active mild endometriosis; 1987 (GnRH-a), laparoscopy 1990, minimal endometriosis	IVF-UT September 1990 and February 1991, TET June 1991, normal-looking pelvis, no endometriosis noted
(7)	JF	Active minimal endometriosis; 1988 (treated)	TET June 1991, normal-looking pelvis, no endometriosis noted
(8)	CT	Active minimal endometriosis; December 1987 (danazol)	TET May 1990, normal-looking pelvis, no endometriosis noted
(9)	KR	Active mild endometriosis; 1985 (danazol), laparoscopy February 1988, peritoneal and ovarian endometriosis persists (GnRH-a); laparoscopy August 1988, reduced severity	TET April 1990, findings similar to August 1988 laparoscopy
(10)	AM	Minimal endometriosis; July 1988 (no treatment), laparoscopy May 1989, minimal, old and inactive endometriosis	TET October 1990, normal-looking pelvis, no endometriosis noted
(11)	PW	Minimal endometriosis; 1989 (no treatment)	TET July 1990, normal-looking pelvis, no endometriosis noted
(12)	CH	Mild endometriosis; 1986, ovaries adherent to pelvic side wall, pouch of Douglas endometriosis (progestagen), no check laparoscopy	TET July 1990, ovaries remain adherent to pelvic side walls and pouch of Douglas endometriosis, normal Fallopian tubes
(13)	MH	Minimal endometriosis; 1987 (danazol)	TET September 1990, normal-looking pelvis, no endometriosis noted

IVF-UT = *in vitro* fertilization with intrauterine transfer.

Amso and R.W. Shaw, unpublished observations), the pelvis was assessed thoroughly during TET. In 13 patients with well-documented endometriosis undergoing 15 TETs, pelvic appearance was compared to the original or most recent laparoscopic findings. The pelvis appeared normal with no evidence of endometriosis during 12 procedures and in two patients the pathological findings were similar to the most recent laparoscopic assessment. In one patient, there was a new finding in that the left Fallopian tube was slightly tethered to the corresponding ovary, but other features were unchanged. The severity of the disease, year of diagnosis, treatment received and second laparoscopy findings, whenever available, are depicted in Table 15.1. Although the number of patients is small, these observations suggest that one or repeated superovulations for assisted reproduction treatment had minimal deleterious effect in this group of patients. Furthermore, during this study, two patients with endometriosis conceived spontaneously within 6 months of an unsuccessful IVF attempt. It should be recognized, however, that the stimulation protocol in all patients utilized GnRH-a (long regimen) before addition of gonadotrophin, and this may have contributed to the continued suppression of the endometriotic lesions.

Conclusion

In summary, assisted reproduction treatment is an effective modality for infertility associated with both early and advanced endometriosis. Its role is more clearly defined than either medical or surgical treatments, especially in early disease. Combination therapy, medical or surgical, in conjunction with assisted reproduction, needs appropriate evaluation with well-designed studies, using cumulative pregnancy or live birth rates and not histological or laparoscopic findings as end-points. Further, the long-term effects of assisted reproduction treatment on endometriosis need evaluation.

References

1 Badawy SZA, Elbakry MM, Samuel F, Dizer M. Cumulative pregnancy rates in infertile women with endometriosis. *J Reprod Med* 1988 **33:** 757–760.

2 Olive DL, Stohs GF, Metzger DA, Franklin RR. Expectant management and hydrotubations in the treatment of endometriosis-associated infertility. *Fertil Steril* 1985 **44:** 35–41.

3 Hull MGR. Infertility treatment: relative effectiveness of conventional and assisted conception methods. *Hum Reprod* 1992 **7:** 785–796.

4 Audebert A, Backstrom T, Barlow DH *et al.* Endometriosis 1991: a discussion document. *Hum Reprod* 1992 **7:** 432–435.

5 Olive DL, Haney AF. Endometriosis-associated infertility: a critical review of therapeutic approaches. *Obstet Gynecol Surv* 1986 **41:** 538–555.

6 Portuondo JA, Echanjauregui AD, Herran C, Alijarte I. Early conception in patients with untreated mild endometriosis. *Fertil Steril* 1983 **39:** 22–24.

7 Hull MGR. Indications for assisted conception. *Br Med Bull* 1990 **46:** 580–595.

8 Inoue M, Kobayashi Y, Honda I, Awaji H, Fujii A. The impact of endometriosis on the reproductive outcome of infertile patients. *Am J Obstet Gynecol* 1992 **167:** 278–282.

9 Bayer SR, Seibel MM, Saffan DS, Berger MJ, Taymor ML. Efficacy of danazol treatment for minimal endometriosis in infertile women. *J Reprod Med* 1988 **33:** 179–182.

10 Telimaa S. Danazol and medroxyprogesterone acetate inefficacious in the treatment of infertility in endometriosis. *Fertil Steril* 1988 **50:** 872–875.

11 Fedele L, Bianchi S, Arcaini L, Vercellini P, Candiani G. Buserelin versus danazol in the treatment of endometriosis-associated infertility. *Am J Obstet Gynecol* 1989 **161:** 871–876.

12 Thomas EJ, Cook ID. Successful treatment of asymptomatic endometriosis: does it benefit infertile women? *Br Med J* **294:** 1117–1119.

13 Schenken RS, Malinak LR. Conservative surgery versus expectant management for the infertile patient with mild endometriosis. *Fertil Steril* 1982 **37:** 183–186.

14 Chong AP, Keene ME, Thornton NL. Comparison of three modes of treatment for infertility patients with minimal pelvic endometriosis. *Fertil Steril* 1990 **53:** 407–410.

15 Guzick DS, Rock JA. A comparison of danazol and conservative surgery for the treatment of infertility due to mild or moderate endometriosis. *Fertil Steril* 1983 **5:** 580–583.

16 Olive DL, Lee KL. Analysis of sequential treatment protocols for endometriosis associated infertility. *Am J Obstet Gynecol* 1986 **154:** 613.

17 Olive DL, Martin DC. Treatment of endometriosis-associated infertility with CO_2 laser laparoscopy: the use of one and two parameter exponential models. *Fertil Steril* 1987 **48:** 18–23.

18 HFEA. *Human Fertilization and Embryology Authority Annual Report*, 1993, pp. 17–24. London, HFEA.

19 Damewood MD. The role of the new reproductive technologies including IVF and GIFT in endometriosis. *Obstet Gynecol Clin North Am* 1989 **16:** 179–191.

20 Mahadevan MM, Trounson, AD, Leeton JF. The relationship of tubal blockage, infertility of unknown cause, suspected male infertility, and endometriosis to success of *in vitro* fertilization and embryo transfer. *Fertil Steril* 1983 **40:** 755–762.

21 Wardle PG, Mitchell JD, McLaughlin EA *et al.* Endometriosis and ovulatory disorder: reduced fertilisation *in vitro* compared with tubal and unexplained infertility. *Lancet* 1985 **ii:** 236–239.

22 Matson PL, Yovich JL. The treatment of infertility associated with endometriosis by *in vitro* fertilization. *Fertil Steril* 1986 **46:** 432–434.

23 Oehninger S, Rosenwaks Z. *In vitro* fertilization and embryo transfer: an established and successful therapy for endometriosis. *Prog Clin Biol Res* 1990 **323:** 319–335.

24 Sharma V, Riddle A, Mason BA, Pampiglioni J, Campbell S. An analysis of factors influencing the establishment of a clinical pregnancy in an ultrasound-based ambulatory *in vitro* fertilization program. *Fertil Steril* 1988 **49:** 468–478.

25 Tummon IS, Colwell KA, Mackinnon CJ, Nisker JA, Yuzpe AA. Abbreviated endometriosis-associated infertility correlates with *in vitro* fertilization success. *J In Vitro Fert Embryo Transfer* 1991 **8:** 149–153.

26 Chillik CF, Acosta AA, Garcia JE *et al.* The role of *in vitro* fertilization in infertile patients with endometriosis. *Fertil Steril* 1985 **44:** 56–61.

27 Mills MS, Eddowes HA, Cahill DJ *et al.* A prospective controlled study of *in-vitro* fertilization, gamete intra-fallopian transfer and intrauterine insemination combined with superovulation. *Hum Reprod* 1992 **7:** 490–494.

28 Oehninger S, Acosta AA, Kreiner D *et al.* *In vitro* fertilization and embryo transfer (IVF/ET): an established and successful therapy for endometriosis. *J In Vitro Fert Embryo Transfer* 1988 **5:** 249–256.

29 Simon C, Gutierrez A, Vidal A *et al.* Outcome of patients endometriosis in assisted reproduction: results from *in-vitro* fertilization and oocyte donation. *Hum Reprod* 1994 **9:** 725–729.
30 Medical Research International, Society for Assisted Reproductive Technology, American Fertility Society. *In vitro* fertilization–embryo transfer in the United States: 1988 results from the IVF-ET registry. *Fertil Steril* 1990 **53:** 13–20.
31 Medical Research International, Society for Assisted Reproductive Technology, American Fertility Society. *In vitro* fertilization–embryo transfer (IVF-ET) in the United States: 1989 results from the IVF-ET registry. *Fertil Steril* 1991 **55:** 14–23.
32 Tan SL, Royston P, Campbell S *et al.* Cumulative conception and livebirth rates after *in-vitro* fertilisation. *Lancet* 1992 **339:** 1390–1394.
33 Craft I, Brinsden P. Alternatives to IVF: the outcome of 1071 first GIFT procedures. *Hum Reprod* 1989 **4** (Suppl.): 29–36.
34 Yovich JL, Yovich JM, Tuvik AI, Matson PL, Wilcox DL. *In vitro* fertilization for endometriosis. *Lancet* 1985 **ii:** 552.
35 Porter RN, Smith W, Craft IL, Abdulwahid NA, Jacobs HS. Induction of ovulation for *in-vitro* fertilisation using buserelin and gonadotropins. *Lancet* 1984 **ii:** 1284–1285.
36 Medical Research International, Society for Assisted Reproductive Technology, American Fertility Society. *In vito* fertilization–embryo transfer (IVF-ET) in the United States: 1990 results from the IVF-ET registry. *Fertil Steril* 1992 **57:** 15–24.
37 Remorgida V, Anserini P, Croce S *et al.* Comparison of different ovarian stimulation protocols for gamete intrafallopian transfer in patients with minimal and mild endometriosis. *Fertil Steril* 1990 **53:** 1060–1063.
38 Hammitt DG, Syrop CH, Hahn SJ *et al.* Comparison of concurrent pregnancy rates for *in-vitro* fertilization–embryo transfer, pronuclear stage embryo transfer and gamete intra-Fallopian transfer. *Hum Reprod* 1990 **5:** 947–954.
39 Tanbo T, Dale PO, Abyholm T. Assisted fertilization in infertile women with patent fallopian tubes: a comparison of *in-vitro* fertilization, gamete intra-fallopian transfer and tubal embryo stage transfer. *Hum Reprod* 1990 **5:** 266–270.
40 Toth TL, Oehninger S, Toner JP *et al.* Embryo transfer to the uterus or the fallopian tube after *in vitro* fertilization yields similar results. *Fertil Steril* 1992 **57:** 1110–1113.
41 Fluker MR, Zouves CG, Bebbington MW. A prospective randomized comparison of zygote intrafallopian transfer and *in vitro* fertilization–embryo transfer for nontubal factor infertility. *Fertil Steril* 1993 **60:** 515–519.
42 O'Shea RT, Chen C, Weiss T, Jones ER. Endometriosis and *in-vitro* fertilisation. *Lancet* 1985 **ii:** 723.
43 Wardle PG, Foster PA, Mitchell JD *et al.* Endometriosis and IVF: effect of prior therapy. *Lancet* 1986 **i:** 276–277.
44 Dicker D, Goldman GA, Ashkenazi *et al.* The value of pre-treatment with gonadotrophin releasing hormone (GnRH) analogue in IVF-ET therapy of severe endometriosis. *Hum Reprod* 1990 **5:** 418–420.
45 Dicker D, Goldman JA, Feldberg D, Ashkenazi J, Levy T. Transvaginal ultrasonic needle-guided aspiration of endometriotic cysts before ovulation induction for *in vitro* fertilization. *J In Vitro Fert Embryo Transfer* 1991 **8:** 286–289.
46 Rock JA, Moutos DM. Endometriosis: the present and the future – an overview of treatment options. *Br J Obstet Gynaecol* 1992 **99** (Suppl. 7): 1–4.
47 Gleicher N. Endometriosis: a new approach is needed. *Hum Reprod* 1992 **7:** 821–824.
48 McArthur JW, Ulfelder H. The effect of pregnancy upon endometriosis. *Obstet Gynecol Surv* 1965 **20:** 709–733.
49 Lessey BA, Metzger DA, Haney AF, McCarty KS. Immunohistochemical analysis of estrogen and progesterone receptors in endometriosis: comparison with normal endome-

trium during the menstrual cycle and the effect of medical therapy. *Fertil Steril* 1989 **51:** 409–415.

50 Prentice A, Randall BJ, Weddell A *et al.* Ovarian steroid receptor expression in endometriosis and in two potential parent epithelia: peritoneum and peritoneal mesothelium. *Hum Reprod* 1992 **7:** 1318–1325.

51 Bergqvist A, Ferno M. Estrogen and progesterone receptors in endometriotic tissue and endometrium: comparison according to localization and recurrence. *Fertil Steril* 1993 **60:** 63–68.

Index

Italic numerals refer to figures,
bold numerals refer to tables.

ablation/excision techniques 248–62
adhesiolysis 250, 260–1
adhesion re-formation, postoperative 261
associated/radical procedures 256–7
coagulation 251, **261**
complications 257–8, 261
deep infiltrating peritoneal implants 251–2
excision 250–1, **261**
fertility after treatment 257, **258**
male **259**
ovarian endometriosis 253–6
patient preparation 248–9
results 257
superficial peritoneal implants 250–1
vaporization 251, 254, **261**
abortion, spontaneous 155–6
acid phosphatase 54, 77
activin 76
add-back regimes 228–30
adhesiolysis 250, 260–1
adhesion cell molecule 9
adnexectomy 257
aetiology 3–12
Allen–Masters syndrome 122–3
American Fertility Society
classification of mild endometriosis 58
scoring system 188
analgesics 190
androgens 191
angiogenic factors 63
anovulation 152
anovulatory cycles, women with 50
antiendometrial antibodies 85–9, 151
diagnosis of endometriosis 88–9
antiendothelial antibodies 84
antiovarian antibodies 84
appendectomy 257
apolipoprotein-β 225
arachidonic acid 51
artificial insemination by donor (AID) 52
assisted conception 160–1
assisted reproduction methods 282–92
effect on course of endometriosis 289–92
indications 288
miscarriage rate 286–7
treatment outcome 285–6
autoantibodies 83–90
clinial relevance in endometriosis 89–90
cell components 83–4
endometrium 84–8
ovary 84
autologous endometrial antigens, intradermal injection 77
azoospermic men 148

baboons 11, 268
bats 4
B cells (lymphocytes) 60, 75
HLA-DR expression in 78
endometrium 81
peritoneal fluid 77
serum 77
polyclonal activation 82
bone-marrow-derived cells 81–2
buserelin 31–2, 139, 188

CA-125 antigen 88, 271
measurement 272
cadherins 9
E 8, 9, 60
cell adhesion molecules 9, 60
chemotactic factors 76
classification of endometriosis 168–81
American Fertility Society 168, 170–1, *172*, 176–7
pelvic pain assessment 179–81
simplified RAFS classification 176
stage V inclusion? 176–9
description of peritoneal endometriosis 175–6
historical review 168–71
rationale 171–3
expert system 173
language 171–3
staging technique 173–4
collagen type III aminoterminal propeptide 9

collagenese 4
complement 85
congenital menstrual outflow obstruction 6, 59
cytokines 76, 78–9
  macrophage-derived 78

danazol 28–30, 33, 136, **137**, 191–2, 195–8
  clinical effect 197–8
  laparoscopy after treatment 189
  length of treatment 189
  mode of action 195–6
  pretreatment suppression of endometriosis 288
  pregnancy rate after treatment 197–8
  side-effects 196–7
deep endometriosis 264–78
  CA-125 measurement 272
  clinical examination 271
  cystic ovarian endometriosis 269–70
  deeply infiltrating endometriosis 269–70
  definition 264–6
  diagnosis 270–1
    by excision 272
  medical therapy 274–5
    postoperative 275
    preoperative 274–5
  pathology 267–70
  pouch of Douglas involvement 271
  radiology 272
  results of treatment 275–6
    pelvic pain 276–7
    pregnancy rates 275–6
  surgical excision 272–3
    complications 273–4
  types 266–7
defecation, painful 16
1,25-dehydroxy vitamin D 226
diabetes mellitus, insulin-dependent 84
direct intraperitoneal insemination 282
double-antibody immunohistochemistry 86
dydrogesterone 138, 193, 284
dysmenhorrhoea 16, 190
dyspareunia 16

elephant shrew 4
ELISA 86–7, 88, 89
enavid 191–2
endometrial cancer cell line 8
endometriosis
  'activity' 175
  age-related frequency of endometriosis sites **100**
  assisted conception 160–1
  autoimmune response 151
  black lesions 10, 38
  blue-black lesions 148
  cellular immune changes in 76–82
  classification *see* classification of endometriosis
  clear papules 10
  deep *see* deep endometriosis
  fertility effect *see* fertility
  frequency of location in pelvis **122**
  genetics 150–1
  GnRH-A therapy 220–1
  histochemical characterization 26–7
  humoral immune changes in 82–90
  light microscopic appearance 20–5, *26*
  macroscopic aspect 16–18
  medical treatment *see* medical treatment
  natural history 156–7, 187–8
  non-pigmented lesions 17, 38, 123–4, 187–8
  ovarian *see* ovarian endometriosis
  painful 3
  peritoneal 38
  peritoneal fluid in 154–5
  placebo effects 188
  powderburn lesion 148
  progressive disease? 10–11
  proliferation markers 26–7
  red lesions 10, 27, 39, 123–4
  spontaneous resolution 10
  symptoms 16
    frequency **112–13**
  three-dimensional architecture 42–5
    evaluation 43–5
  ultrastructure 20–5
  white lesions 10, 39–40, 123
endometrium
  antigens in 85–6
  attachment to peritoneal lining 8–9
  autoantibodies 84–8
  detachment 4
  ectopic, immune cell population in 81–2
  regurgitated 3, 6–8
epidermal growth factor 8, 63, 64, 79
  monoclonal antibody against 64
erythrophagocytosis 54
excision techniques *see* ablation/excision techniques
expectant management 282–4

fertility, endometriosis influence on 157–60, 287
  no structural damage present 159–60
  structural damage present 158–9
fibrinolysis, intra-abdominal 62–3
fibronectin 8
folliculogenesis 152

gamete intrafallopian transfer (GIFT) 282, 285
or *in vitro* fertilization 288
gestrinone 30–1, 139, 198–9
side-effects 198
gonadotrophin-releasing hormone analogues (GnRH-A) 31–2, 206–31
bone mineral density changes during therapy 225–8
action within bone 226
alkaline phosphatase increase 226
bone chemistry changes 226
calcium absorption 226
1,25-dehydroxy vitamin D reduction 226
measurement 227–8
oestrogen action 226
osteocalcin increase 226
parathyroid action 226
women at risk 228
comparative clinical trials results 215–21
differential responses 220, **221–2**
endometriomas 220–1
impact on endometriotic implants 217–20
symptomatic relief 216–17
comparison of dosage regimens 214–15
endocrine changes following administration 211–12
formulations 212–13
aqueous solutions 212
depots 212–13
differences between 213
intranasal 212
gonadotrophin changes after administration 208–11
initial studies 213–14
lipoprotein changes 225
mode of action 207, *208*
pharmacology 212
pretreatment suppression of endometriosis 288
recurrence rates following therapy 222–3
safety issues 223–5
stimulation protocols 287
structure 207

haemagglutination 86
haematuria 16
heparin-sepharose-binding growth factor 64
histogenesis 18–19
metaplastic theory 19
metastatic theory 18–19
hormone receptors in endometriotic tissue 32–4
hormone replacement therapy (HRT) regimes 229
human leucocyte antigens 76
human macrophage colony-stimulating factor 63
17-hydroxyprogesterone 138
17β-hydroxysteroid dehydrogenase 26–7
hyperprolactinaemia 154
hypo-oestrogenaemia 226
hysterectomy 257

idiopathic thrombocytopenic purpura 196
IGF-1 8
immune system 76–90
decreased cellular immunity 269
immune cell population in ectopic endometrium 81–2
immunodiffusion 86
immunoelectrophoresis 86
immunofluorescence 86
immunoglobulin, endogenous 85
immunological basis of endometriosis 8
implantation theory (Sampson) 59
interferons 76
infertility, endometriosis-related 47, 147–62
autoimmune response to endometriosis 151
endocrine abnormalities 151–2
epidemiology 149
folliculogenesis 152
genetic predisposition 150–1
hyperprolactinaemia 154
laparoscopic confirmation 147
luteal phase deficiency 153–4
luteinized unruptured follicle syndrome 153
male, after laparoscopic treatment **259**
management *260*
mild endometriosis 150
ovulation defects 152–3
peritoneal environment 154–5
severe endometriosis 149–50
subtle lesions 148–9
inflammatory-cell-derived growth factors 8
inhibin 76
innervation of female pelvis 113–16
Fallopian tubes 116
ovary 115
parasympathetic 114–15
sympathetic 113–14
uterus 115
vagina 116
insulin-like growth factor 76
integrins 60
γ-interferon 7
interleukin-1 7, 8, 54–5, 76, 78–9, 155

embryotoxicity 56
recombinant 56
interleukin-1β 63, 78–9
interleukin-2 7
embryotoxicity 56
interleukin-6 63, 78, 79
interleukin-8 63
in vitro fertilization (IVF) 282
or gamete intrafallopian transfer 288
pre-IVF aspiration of endometriomas 289
pre-IVF suppression of endometriosis 288
see also assisted reproduction methods
in vitro fertilization-embryo transfer 257

6-keto-$PGF_{1\alpha}$ 57

laparoscopy 17, 188, 189
treatment assessment by 189
length of treatment 189
leucine aminopeptidase 77
leucocyte common antigen (CD45) 81
leuprolide acetate 188
luteal phase deficiency 153–4
luteinized unruptured follicle syndrome (LUF) 153
luteinizing hormone 50
lymphocytes, large granular 81
lynoestrenol 138

macrophage 7, 8, 49–50, 53–7, 75, 77–8
activity inhibition 155
cyclic activation 54
'disposal system' 77-8
endometrial 81
functions 53
HLA-DR expression in 78
peritoneal 63, 77–8
cytotoxicity 155
phagocytosis of spermatozoa 54
secretory products 55–6
macrophage colony-stimulating factor 76, 78
major histocompatibility complex 75
matrilysin 9
medical treatment 10, 187–201, 284
endocrine modulation 191
morphological changes after 28–32
medroxyprogesterone acetate 33, 138, 193–5, 229
menorrhagia 16
menstruation 3
decidual cell reaction 5
endometrial detachment 4
endometrial entry in abdominal cavity 5–6
metaplasia theory 5
metastasis theory 5
reflex implantation theory (Sampson) 6
metalloproteinases, of stromelysin family 4
methyltestosterone 191
metrorrhagia 16
Meyer–Rokitansky–Küster syndrome 19
micturition, painful 16
mifepristone (RU486) 199–200
miscarriage rate 286
monoclonal antibody against epidermal growth factor 64, 79
monocyte 4
monocyte/macrophage 'disposal system' 77–8
monthly fecundity 52
mushrooms 12
myeloperoxidase 77

naferelin 139–40
natural killer (NK) cells 7, 61, 80, 269
aberrant activity 80
defective activity 8, 80
nerve growth factor 76
neutral protease 54
nociception 116–17
norethisterone 138, 193, 229
norgestrel 138

oestradiol 50
oestrogen(s) 62, 191
receptors 33–4, 62, 226
oestrogen–progestogen combination 191–2
oestrone sulphate 26
oophorectomy 257
opiate receptors 117
oral contraceptives, combined 192
ova, fertilized, transport through Fallopian tube 57
ovarian cystectomy 244, 253
ovarian endometriosis 27, 97–109, 237–46
age-related frequency of sites **100**
classification 107, 237
clinical appearance 100
deep infiltrating 237
diagnosis 101–6
aspiration/examination of content 103
biopsy 102–3
laparoscopy 102
magnetic resonance imaging 101–2
ovarian cystoscopy/guided biopsies 103–6
sonography 101
haemorrhagic cysts (endometriomas) 17, 237, 238

histopathology 106
laparoscopic treatment, conservative 237–46
preoperative evaluation 238–9
laster surgery 239–46
instruments 239–41
ovarian closure 243–4
pregnancy rate after 245
recurrence rate 245–6
results 244–5
techniques 241–3
pathogenesis 98–100
response to hormone therapy 107
superficial lesions 237–8
symptoms 106
torsion 107
treatment 107–9
ovary
autoantibodies to 84
cyclic hormone secretion 62
endometriosis *see* ovarian endometriosis
ovulatory dysfunction 152–3

pain localization, visceral/somatic 117–20
parathyroid hormones 226
passive haemagglutination 86, 89
pathogenesis 3–12
pelvic pain 16, 112–43
chronic 112
endometriosis severity–pain severity correlation 121–4
measurement 124–31
analgesic use 127
Andersch–Milsom score 127, **130**
McGill questionnaire 126–7
numerical rating scales 125, **126**
pelvic pain score 127
medical treatment 135–40
danazol 136
gestrinone 139
GnRH analogues 139–40
oestrogens–progesterones combined 136–8
progestogens 138–9
RAFS assessment 127–31, *132–3*
verbalizing scales 125
visual analogue scales 125–6
mechanisms in endometriosis 120–4
psychological factors 131–5
questionnaires **135**
surgical treatment 140–3
laparoscopic uterosacral nerve ablation 141–2
laser ablation 141
presacral neurectomy 142–3
symptom–site relationship **121**

peritoneal dialysis, blood in dialysate 6
peritoneal fluid 48–65
cellular constituents 49–50
cytokine level after cessation of hormonal treatment 58
development of endometriosis and 59–65
growth factors in 64
inhibiting effect 269
macrophages in 53–7
prostaglandins in 51, 57–9
proteins in 50
steroid hormones in 50–1
sterile inflammation due to 7
subfertility in endometriosis 51–2
volume 7, 48–9, 52, 53
peritoneum, response to menstrual debris 7
phytohaemagglutinin 77
pituitary ovarian function abnormalities 151–2
platelet-derived growth factor 8, 76, 78
pneumoperitoneum 249
polyarteritis, microscopic 84
premenstrual condition 5
premenstrual spotting 16
presacral neurectomy 256
procollagen type II 27
progesterone 50, 62
receptors 33–4, 62–3
progestogens 138–9, 193–5
long-term use 194
side-effects 194
prostaglandin(s) 51, 57–9, 155, 190
F 123
$F_{2\alpha}$ 190
prostaglandin synthetase inhibitors 190
pseudopregnancy regimen 191

rabbit, endometriotic implants in 58
RANTES 63
rectal bleeding 16
regurgitated menstrual blood 62
retrograde menstruation 58, 59, 60, 62, 267
rheumatoid vasculitis 84
Rokitansky syndrome 87
RU486 (mifepristone) 199–200

scoring systems 188–9
sodium etidronate/calcium carbonate 228–9
spermatozoa 55–6
phagocytosis 54, 55
staging technique 173–4
steroid hormones 32–4
stilboestrol 191
stromelysin 4
subfertility 51–2

surgical castration 206
systemic lupus erythematosus 84, 196
systemic sclerosis 84

tamoxifen 200–1
T cells (lymphocytes) 60, 75, 76
  helper 61
  HLA-DR expression in 78
    endometrium 81
    peritoneal fluid 77
    serum 77
thermocolour test 17
thromboxane (TxB_2) 57
tibolone 230
transforming growth factors (TGF) 64, 76
  –α 8
  –β 8, 226
tubal embryo transfer 282, 285
tumour necrosis factor (TNF) 7, 59, 63, 76, 78, 79
  –α 79
  –β 79

ultrasound examination of pelvis 17
uterine cannulation 249
uterine suspension 256
uterosacral ligament section 256
uteropelvic fistula 6
uterotubal junction hypoptonia 6
uterus, fixation of 17

vascularization of endometriotic implants 40–2
visceral innervation, afferent/sensory 119
visceral pain pathways 119–20

zymosan 8